Traditional medicine and health care coverage

A reader for health administrators and practitioners

EDITED BY

Robert H. Bannerman
John Burton
Ch'en Wen-Chieh

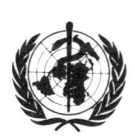

1983

World Health Organization   Geneva

Reprinted 1988

The authors alone are responsible for the views expressed in this publication.

ISBN 92 4 154163 6

© World Health Organization, 1983

Publications of the World Health Organization enjoy copyright protection in accordance with the provisions of Protocol 2 of the Universal Copyright Convention. For rights of reproduction or translation of WHO publications, in part or *in toto*, application should be made to the Office of Publications, World Health Organization, Geneva, Switzerland. The World Health Organization welcomes such applications.

The designations employed and the presentation of the material in this publication do not imply the expression of any opinion whatsoever on the part of the Secretariat of the World Health Organization concerning the legal status of any country, territory, city or area or of its authorities, or concerning the delimitation of its frontiers.

The mention of specific companies or of certain manufacturers' products does not imply that they are endorsed or recommended by the World Health Organization in preference to others of a similar nature that are not mentioned. Errors and omissions excepted, the names of proprietary products are distinguished by initial capital letters.

TYPESET IN INDIA
PRINTED IN ENGLAND
82/5466 – Macmillan/Spottiswoode – 6000
88/7844 – Spottiswoode – 2000 (R)

Contents

	Page
Foreword—*H. Mahler*	7
Introduction	9

PART ONE—*Systems and practices of traditional medicine*

Chapter 1.	An introduction to ethnomedicine—*G. M. Foster* .	17
Chapter 2.	Traditional medicine and psychiatry in Africa . . .	25
	I. *M. Koumaré*	25
	II. *P. Coppo*	33
Chapter 3.	Traditional medicine in Latin America—*C. Goldwater*	37
	I. Humoral theory and therapy	37
	II. Spiritism	46
Chapter 4.	Ayurveda—*P. N. V. Kurup*	50
	I. Ayurvedic medicine	50
	II. Medical astrology	59
Chapter 5.	The Unani system of health and medicare—*H. M. Said*	61
Chapter 6.	Traditional Chinese medicine—*Wang Pei*	68
Chapter 7.	Acupuncture and moxibustion	76
	I. Theory and practice—*Wei Ru-Shu*	76
	II. Research in acupuncture—*R. H. Bannerman*	82
Chapter 8.	Treatment of fracture and soft tissue injury by integrated methods of traditional Chinese and Western medicine—*Shang Tienyu*	86

Chapter 9.	Modern allopathic medicine and public health . . .	90
	I. Allopathic medicine—*J. J. Canary*.	90
	II. Public health—*J. Burton*.	102
Chapter 10.	Homoeopathy—*G. Vithoulkas*	110
Chapter 11.	Naturopathy—*R. J. Bloomfield*	116
Chapter 12.	Divination and exorcism—*P. Coppo*	124
Chapter 13.	Hypnosis—*T. W. Harding*	128
Chapter 14.	Yoga and meditation for mental health—*K. N. Udupa*	134
	I. Yoga	134
	II. Meditation.	138
Chapter 15.	Traditional midwifery and contraception—*S. Cosminsky*.	142
Chapter 16.	Selected individual therapies—*H. A. W. Forbes* . .	163

PART TWO—Herbal medicines and herbal pharmacopoeias

Chapter 17.	Endangered plants used in traditional medicine—*E. S. Ayensu*	175
Chapter 18.	The NAPRALERT data base as an information source for application to traditional medicine—*N. R. Farnsworth*.	184
Chapter 19.	Phytopharmacology and phytotherapy—*M. A. Attisso*	194
	I. Medicinal plants and plant drugs	194
	II. The utilization of local plant resources in primary health care.	198

PART THREE—A profile of traditional practices in the WHO Regions

Chapter 20.	The African Region.	209
Chapter 21.	The Region of the Americas	222
Chapter 22.	The South-East Asia Region	231
Chapter 23.	The European Region	240
Chapter 24.	The Eastern Mediterranean Region.	253
Chapter 25.	The Western Pacific Region	263

PART FOUR—Organizational and legal aspects of traditional medicine

Chapter 26. Organizational aspects—*G. S. Mutalik* 281

Chapter 27. Legal aspects. 290
                I. Patterns of legislation concerning traditional medicine—*J. Stepan*. 290
                II. Policy options in regulating the practice of traditional medicine—*C. Leslie* 314

Chapter 28. The role of traditional medicine in primary health care—*R. H. Bannerman* 318

Index. 331

Foreword

The Member States of WHO are currently engaged in preparing and implementing strategies for the attainment by *all* their people by the year 2000 of a level of health that will permit them to lead a socially and economically productive life—a goal popularly known as "Health for All by the Year 2000". To succeed in attaining this goal, all useful methods will have to be employed and all possible resources mobilized. Among these methods are various kinds of indigenous practices; and among those resources are various types of traditional practitioners and birth attendants.

This approach was endorsed by the International Conference on Primary Health Care, held in Alma-Ata in 1978. The Declaration of Alma-Ata, describing primary health care, referred to the need for a variety of health workers, including traditional practitioners as needed, who are suitably trained socially and technically to work as a health team and to respond to the expressed needs of the community.

For team work to be fruitful, team members must understand one another's functions. Since traditional medicine was incorporated in the World Health Organization's programmes in 1976, the gulf between traditional and modern systems appears to have narrowed to some extent. A genuine interest in the many traditional practices now exists among practitioners of modern medicine; and growing numbers of practitioners of traditional, indigenous or alternative systems are beginning to accept and use some of the modern technology.

In addition, some health administrators in the developing countries have recommended the inclusion of traditional healers in primary health care on the grounds that the healers know the sociocultural background of the people, and that they are highly respected and experienced in their work. Economic considerations, the distances to be covered in some countries, the strength of traditional beliefs, the shortage of health professionals, particularly in the rural areas—all these are factors that have also influenced this recommendation. Suitable training and orientation programmes for healers and traditional midwives have already been developed in several countries.

The purpose of this book is to provide a better understanding of traditional, indigenous and unorthodox systems. This should help to foster team work among all categories of health workers. The book therefore examines the most common patterns of these systems and some of their local or regional variations, and suggests how health practitioners and administrators might best apply this information as they endeavour to improve health care coverage, particularly in the developing countries.

It is hoped that this information will be of use to governments when they consider the most appropriate methods for inclusion in their health strategies. The book is also intended to improve our understanding of why people accept or reject certain practices or why they use or do not use those health resources that are available. Such an understanding should be of help in designing realistic national health plans and related training programmes.

Halfdan Mahler, M.D.
Director-General
World Health Organization

Introduction

Traditional medicine is a rather vague term loosely used to distinguish ancient and culture-bound health care practices which existed before the application of science to health matters in official modern scientific medicine or allopathy. Some frequently used synonyms are indigenous, unorthodox, alternative, folk, ethno, fringe and unofficial medicine and healing. The term is unsatisfactory because it implies broadly that there is some body of principle, knowledge and skills common to all the varieties of traditional medicine; and because it does not distinguish between all-embracing and complex systems of health care such as Ayurveda on the one hand, and simple home remedies on the other.

Traditional medicine has been practised to some degree in all cultures and other terms based on culture include African, Asian or Chinese medicine. Traditional practitioners define life as "the union of body, senses, mind and souls," and describe positive health as "the blending of physical, mental, social, moral and spiritual welfare." The moral and spiritual aspects of life are here stressed, thereby giving greater dimensions to the system of health care by which man maintains his health.

The problems

How countries can make health and medical care available to all their citizens and communities has been one of the major preoccupations of politicians, administrators, the community and health workers in all the Member States which have joined WHO. Since WHO's creation in 1948, debates in the World Health Assembly, in the WHO Regional Committees and in technical meetings bear witness to this concern and reflect the ambitions, the frustrations and the controversial nature of some problems to which such concern gives rise. A new sense of urgency has characterized recent discussions which have culminated in the global resolve to accomplish a total health and medical care coverage for all peoples by the year 2000.

The old debate between advocates of scientific excellence and the champions of minimum effective coverage has been largely resolved by a general consensus that all citizens have a right to health and to medical care of their choice, and that this right should embrace safe maternity, the healthy growth and development of children, maintenance of health in adult life, the protection of individuals and the community from environmental hazards, and the provision of medical care for the sick.

To turn such a principle into practical action is a daunting challenge for most countries. The creation of modern health care services and their dispersal to all classes of the population and to remote agricultural and nomadic communities in the fewer than 20 years which remain in this century would be exceedingly difficult in terms of the provision of personnel, supplies, maintenance and supervision. Apart from the cost, the administrative complications and logistics would require governments to introduce major reforms in planning and mobilizing resources, and in the education and training of staff for many of which problems there is as yet little preparedness. The fact that there are very few places in the world where traditional healers are not practising means that a form of health care coverage that is culturally acceptable to the local population already exists and is dealing more or less satisfactorily with many of the health problems of the local people. It was in view of this fact that the World Health Assembly in May 1976 first discussed seriously the contribution that traditional medicine makes to the health care of the community.

The debate, however, has taken place mainly between doctors and administrators, most of whom think in terms of the technological and organizational assumptions of modern medicine and public health. This background leads many, even of those who are sympathetic to traditional medicine, to think of it as no more than a possibly useful source of manpower to increase the coverage of official health services. Traditional practitioners, many of whom have suffered from official neglect or even persecution, have expressed grave doubts about this relationship. Confident of their own power and skills and unimpressed by the quality and coverage of the official health services, they are confronted by a problem summed up by one eminent practitioner of traditional medicine by asking "who phagocytoses whom?" The question is highly relevant because at the present time there are four main organizational relationships between official and traditional health care services. The first might be termed *monopolistic* because it gives to allopathic practitioners sole legal right to practise medicine; the second might be termed *tolerant* because, while not recognizing traditional medicine, allopathic exclusivity is limited to specific medical and public health activities while traditional and unofficial practitioners are free to work and be paid for services in all other fields provided they do not claim to be registered MDs; the third relationship, which might be described as *parallel*, occurs when practitioners of allopathic and other systems of health care are officially recognized and render services to patients through equal but separate systems; fourthly, there is the *integrated* system in which modern and traditional medicine are merged in medical education and jointly practised within a unique health service.

At the present time about half the world's population resides in countries which have ministries or departments of government responsible for traditional medicine, and in many countries 80% or more of the population living in rural areas are cared for by traditional practitioners and birth attendants. The relationship between official and traditional health care practitioners is therefore one of major importance, although in some countries health administrators will not admit the existence of any such problems.

The background

Until the beginning of the 19th century all medical practice was what we now call traditional. It was then that the great philosophical upheaval of the renaissance began to introduce Cartesian scientific materialism into all human activities and notably into the theory and practice of health care. The new way of looking at things subjected all assumptions to experiment and statistical validation and foresaw the future in terms of research and organization. Of necessity it introduced doubt where previously there had been belief; it emphasized intellect and logic and belittled emotion and intuition.

Its method was to break up complex phenomena into their component parts and deal with each one in isolation. In diagnosis this approach resulted in a search for a single cause; in pharmacology the search was for an active principle that could be isolated; and in the doctor–patient relationship the search for an efficient treatment of the physical cause of symptoms tended to exclude any serious interest in the complexity of the life situation in which the patient was immersed.

The application of scientific method to medicine and public health brought dramatic improvements in all those conditions in which material factors such as infection, poisoning, injury, nutrition or personal and environmental hygiene play a major part in the etiology. In degenerative conditions, however, the results have been less striking, and in conditions where behavioural, emotional or spiritual factors play a major role it would be difficult to argue that the scientific method has produced noticeable improvements; some would contend that deterioration is evident. Since psychosomatic disturbance is today one of the commonest of human afflictions, the philosophy and functioning of modern health and medical services is being questioned in many quarters. Add to this the fact that only in the richest countries has the modern allopathic health service been able to achieve a significant coverage of the population—at what is becoming an intolerable cost—and the search for alternatives seems highly topical.

The official backing which crowned the application of science to individual and social well-being blinded most people to its limitations. Today, it is precisely in societies which have a long experience of scientific medicine that a serious reawakening of interest in the emotional, spiritual and irrational aspects of health is expressing itself by the rediscovery of local traditional systems of health care and the importation of traditional practices from abroad.

In countries into which the scientific approach was imported by nationals who had studied abroad, it often remained isolated in the higher centres of learning and administration. Even today in many such countries research of international significance has greater prestige than that devoted to local problems. It is striking that the amount of research devoted to the indigenous health and medical care system, even in countries where it caters for the majority of the population, is meagre. However, in countries where the scientific approach was imported by a colonial administration, independence has brought about a reactive revival of interest in indigenous health beliefs and practices. This is explained partly as an assertion of cultural identity, partly as a possible means of escaping the spiralling cost of modern health services, and partly as a serious reassessment of the efficacy of many traditional practices in the local setting.

This revival of interest in traditional and unorthodox systems of health care is by no means confined to the so-called developing countries. In urban societies in all parts of the world, health care is being provided by official and unofficial practitioners and in some wealthy countries self-care has become of major public interest.

Some department stores and certain major airports have installed self-operated sphygmomanometers for measuring one's blood pressure; where the reading is not within normal limits, the client is advised to consult a physician.

Even in well served towns with a free general practitioner service, hospitals and clinics, large numbers of people choose to pay for the services of unofficial practitioners. The reasons are many. Apart from the inconveniences of crowds in waiting-rooms, hospital routines etc., the shortcomings of the seemingly cursory or impersonal interviews with the doctor, the difficulty of communication and the sometimes complicated ineffective treatment, many patients feel that there is more to their illness than the system deals with.

In their wisdom the founding fathers of WHO proposed a definition of health as "physical, mental and social well-being". This definition fits the outlook of many of the great systems of traditional medicine as well as, if not better than, it does the current practice of allopathic medicine. The more leisurely and personal interest taken by many healers, the attention paid to the total life-style, diet, rest, exercise, human relations, sexuality and even moral and spiritual factors, does much to satisfy the patient's desire to be understood. The belief that the healer can call on vital and even cosmic forces to reinforce his own skills and release the patient's own will to recover may add greatly to the confidence which all medical practitioners recognize as important in the healing process.

Whatever the health administrators' point of view may be, the fact is that, wherever he is working, traditional and unofficial health care and medicine exist and enjoy the confidence of large sections of the population.

The epidemiology of traditional beliefs

How can this confidence and the accumulated wisdom of many thousands of years be used to improve the health of the population for which health administrators are responsible? The first step, as in all health work, is to know one's area and its people; the second is to use this understanding to plan for improvements and total health care coverage.

To complement the standard epidemiological information, the health authorities that wish to incorporate the practitioners of traditional medicine among the resources available for extending health care coverage to the entire population should determine the numbers and location of these practitioners, the diagnostic and therapeutic methods they employ, their role and functions in their respective communities, what training and orientation they have had, if any, which of them would be suitable for collaboration or integration, and what types of training and orientation they would require to improve their services. An analysis of such data could indicate the impact of the services given by these traditional healers and unorthodox practitioners on the general health of the community and country. Certain Member States have already embarked on this formidable exercise.

This book is intended to assist the health workers and administrators responsible for extending the coverage of health services to develop a fruitful relationship with the practitioners of traditional medicine who are already living and working among, and enjoying the confidence of, the local population. This book is the first of its kind, and no doubt many shortcomings will become evident in the course of time. However, the editors hope that readers will participate in the achievement of its purpose by communicating with WHO in order to correct errors, make good any omissions, supply examples, discuss theories and review administrative arrangements, report on results of experiments and suggest improvements.

ROBERT H. BANNERMAN
Formerly, Manager, Traditional Medicine Programme, World Health Organization, Geneva

JOHN BURTON
Formerly, Chief, Fellowships Programme, World Health Organization, Geneva

CH'EN WEN-CHIEH
Formerly, Assistant Director-General, World Health Organization, Geneva

Acknowledgements

In addition to the named authors of the various contributions in this book, the World Health Organization would like to thank the many other people who contributed to the preparation of this work, including Mr K. Grinling, Mrs M. Brown, Dr J. Haworth, Mrs C. Brelet and Mrs S. Murray.

Part One

Systems and practices of traditional medicine

CHAPTER 1
An introduction to ethnomedicine

George M. Foster[1]

Medical systems

As our primate ancestors evolved into human form, the diseases they brought with them, and those they acquired along the evolutionary way, became social and cultural facts as well as pathological states. For human beings disease threatens not only the well-being of sufferers and their fellows, but also the integrity of the community. Illness and death are disruptive events that impose high economic, social, and psychological costs wherever they occur. Quite apart from humanitarian reasons, therefore, it is of primary importance to the members of every group to try to maintain their health, and to restore to health those who fall ill.

Every human community has responded to this challenge by developing a "medical system", i.e., "*the pattern of social institutions and cultural traditions that evolves from deliberate behavior to enhance health*" (*1*). Written sources tell us about the history of some medical systems; in addition to contemporary scientific medicine we know much about the origin and development of traditional Chinese medicine, of Indian Ayurveda, of Moslem Unani, and of ancient Greek medicine and its modern descendant, the humoral pathology of Latin America and the Philippines. Other medical systems—those of peoples who until recently have lacked a literature—reveal little of their antecedents but, through the studies of anthropologists and others such as missionary doctors, they have been well described in their present forms.

The published accounts of the world's medical systems have made possible the new discipline of "ethnomedicine", i.e., "those beliefs and practices relating to disease which are the products of indigenous cultural development and are not explicitly derived from the conceptual framework of modern medicine" (*2*). Although this is the most commonly accepted

---
[1] Professor Emeritus of Anthropology, University of California, Berkeley, California, USA.

definition of the term, increasing numbers of writers expand it to include contemporary allopathic medicine as a part of ethnomedicine. Most of the topics discussed in this chapter are included in Hughes' (2) definition; the expanded definition covers *all* topics.

A reader who for the first time approaches the literature of a subject new to him is overwhelmed by the apparently infinite variety of data; structure and order are not immediately apparent. The same is true of ethnomedicine; one's initial impression is that the ordering and systematization of the data found in accounts of traditional medical systems is an impossible task. The very need to label so many different types of systems, of illnesses recognized, of therapists, and of forms of treatment adds to the impression of limitless variation.

Fortunately, familiarity with some of this vast body of literature leads to the realization that the data of ethnomedicine lend themselves to orderly classification and reduction to relatively few general principles. Many of the similarities found are due to the principle of limited possibilities: there are only so many causes to which illness can be attributed, so many ways in which a doctor can acquire knowledge and skill, so many ways in which a patient can be treated. Similarities in the medical systems of Africa, native America, and Oceania, for example, are probably due to this fact. Other similarities are at least in part due to historical contact; although we know very little about the earliest periods, the congruences in the traditional medicine of China, India (Ayurveda), and Moslem Asia (Unani), in classical Greek medicine and modern humoral pathology certainly reflect ancient cultural exchanges.

It is to provide a unifying framework for the reader of the accounts of medical systems in the following chapters, to bring order into what at first glance is bewildering variety, that this introduction has been written. The three categories discussed to illustrate this order—causality concepts, therapists, and therapy—vastly oversimplify the picture, but space limitations make this inevitable. Also, with a topic as extensive as traditional medical systems, it must be remembered that every generalization must be qualified by such adverbs and phrases as "usually", "commonly", or "in the majority of cases".

Causality concepts

Representative "causes" of illness listed in ethnomedical accounts include such things as:

(1) Angry deities who punish wrongdoers, for example those who violate taboos.
(2) Ancestors and other ghosts who feel they have been too soon forgotten or otherwise not recognized.
(3) Sorcerers and witches, working for hire or for personal reasons.

(4) Loss of the soul, following a bad fright that jars it loose from the body or as the consequence of the work of a sorcerer or supernatural spirit.
(5) Spirit possession or the intrusion of an object into the body.
(6) Loss of the basic body equilibrium, usually because of the entry of excessive heat or cold into the body.
(7) The evil eye.

In ethnomedical accounts causes such as these are commonly described as "magical" or "supernatural", in contrast to "natural". Illnesses caused by angry deities, ghosts, ancestors and witches fall into the first category, while those due to an upset in body humours and consequent loss of bodily equilibrium, fall into the second. Yet this common classification system is not entirely satisfactory, since witches and sorcerers are hardly "supernatural", while the work of deities and ghosts is not really "magical". In reading the accounts that follow we are better served if we think of one major category of cause as characterized by the purposeful intervention of sensate agents (deities, evil spirits, sorcerers) who, whatever their reasons, seek out a victim who falls ill. We can call this category *personalistic* in that aggression or punishment is directed against a single person as a consequence of the will and power of a human or supernatural agent or being.

This category stands in contrast to that of natural causes—we can call it *naturalistic*—where illness is explained in impersonal, systemic terms. The intrusion of heat or cold into or their loss from the body upsets its basic equilibrium; the balance of humours, of the *dosha* of Ayurveda, of the *yin* and *yang* of Chinese medicine must be restored if the patient is to recover (*3*).

Personalistic explanations appear to predominate (although not to the exclusion of naturalistic explanations) in the traditional systems of such vast areas as Africa, preconquest America, Oceania and indigenous Siberia. They also underlie the more complex systems of contemporary China, South Asia, and Latin America. In contrast, naturalistic explanations (also not to the exclusion of personalistic causation) predominate in humoral pathology, Ayurveda, Unani, and traditional Chinese medicine. Homoeopathy and naturopathy are also marked by naturalistic causality concepts.

It is important to remember that classification systems are imposed on data by classifiers; they are not (as Sydenham, Linnaeus and others believed three centuries ago) inherent in the data themselves, in the laws of nature. Taxonomic models are no better than the contributions they make to bring order out of apparent chaos, and opinions on any topic differ as to relative contributions of different taxonomies. With respect to the classification of disease causality, it must be remembered that both personalistic and naturalistic causes are invoked to explain some illnesses in every society, including those most addicted to allopathic medicine. For example, traditional Chinese medicine, Ayurveda, Unani and humoral pathology are essentially naturalistic systems in so far as causation theory is concerned. Yet in the countries where these systems exist one also finds other "layers" of belief and practice that are purely personalistic: witchcraft, spirit possession, and the like. If, for example, we restrict our discussion of traditional medicine in India to Ayurveda and Unani, we overlook a major underlying substratum of "folk" medicine that largely invokes natural and supernatural agents as the cause of illness.

Traditional medical systems are often marked by "levels" of causality; we find both efficient and proximate causes. In personalistic systems, deities, ghosts, witches and sorcerers are efficient causes, the prime movers. But they require operational techniques such as ability to steal a victim's soul, possess him, poison him, or cause a snake to bite him. This distinction, as we will see, is important in understanding the procedures and roles of many traditional curers.

The nature and role of therapists

As in industrialized societies, in traditional societies a variety of types of therapists, each with a specialty or specialties, is usually found. The most common types are shamans and priests, with supernatural attributes, other curers possessed of great magical power (such as the African witch-finder), herbal therapists, bonesetters and midwives. The last three are probably to be found in all societies; the others, while widespread, are not universal. They are particularly associated with the treatment of illnesses we have called personalistic, marked by dual causality levels. The distinguishing mark of the shaman is power acquired supernaturally. Usually the shaman-to-be is possessed by a tutelary spirit who causes a grave illness, from which the person slowly recovers. The power inherent in the spirit, and transmitted through illness to the novice, may be augmented by formal study under older shamans, but it is the shaman's ability to go into trance and communicate with the tutelary spirit that permits him to aid the sick. In contrast, African witch-finders usually acquire their magical powers through lengthy training and the purchase of magical spells and incantations from their tutors. Whatever the source of power, *the primary role of shaman, priest, or witch-finder is to identify the deity, ghost, or other agent that has caused the illness*, and then to determine how to placate or overcome him. Until the causal agent has been discovered, therapy is believed to have little effect. We see in this belief the reason why so often traditional peoples happily accept the ministrations of physicians but also insist simultaneously on traditional rituals and ceremonies. The physician alleviates the symptoms, but until the ultimate cause is uncovered and dealt with, improvement will be temporary.

In contrast to supernaturally and magically endowed curers, herbal and other therapists, such as the *curanderos* of Latin American humoral pathology, usually acquire their knowledge of herbs and their skills in treatment procedures from older practising curers; supernatural or magical elements are absent in their repertoires. This is significant with respect to the expectations patients have of their therapists. In communities where the equilibrium model of health predominates, patients commonly believe they know what has happened to them: how cold entered their body, how fever struck them. Self-diagnosis is the rule; from the therapist they want treatment, the appropriate combination of herbal remedies, teas, massages and the like. Thus, two major classes of curers emerge from the data of traditional medicine: those with supernatural or magical powers who diagnose (i.e., identify the efficient cause) and who also may administer therapy, and those who accept the patient's self-diagnosis and administer the appropriate remedies.

Forms of therapy

The therapies found in every society stem largely from prevailing causality beliefs, which form the rationale for treatment. Object intrusion? The California Indian shaman went into a trance, identified the offending spirit, attempted to placate it, and sucked out the intruded quartz crystal. Soul loss? The curer identifies the responsible human or supernatural being and through placation or a battle of wits returns the wandering soul to its body. A child afflicted by the evil eye? The carrier of the "eye" must be persuaded to slap or spit on the child; by showing symbolic disdain evidence is given that the accused does not envy the mother nor seek to destroy what is dear to her.

Illnesses believed to have natural causes are handled in non-magical, non-religious fashions. Excessive cold may be extracted from the body by warm baths, teas of "warm" herbs, or by "hot" poultices. Excessive heat may be removed by treatment with "cold" herbs: "cold" leaves applied to the temples for "hot" headaches, cold sponge-baths for fever, and bleeding (in equilibrium medical systems blood is usually considered to be heating; reducing the quantity is, quite logically, thought to reduce body heat). In studying the medical systems summarized in the following pages the reader will note that with a good understanding of causality beliefs the nature and role of curers and the logic of their therapies becomes readily apparent.

Preventive medicine

No society lacks beliefs and practices having to do with the avoidance of illness. The positive acts and the avoidances that constitute preventive medicine in traditional society are often quite different from those of scientific medicine, but they are equally rational (if not always as effective) in that they are functions of what is believed about what causes sickness. In contemporary societies we believe that much illness is caused by germs;

the appropriate preventive acts are to eliminate or reduce the frequency of germs through sanitation, to render the body immune to them by vaccination, and to avoid places where they are believed to exist in dangerous quantities (e.g., crowded theatres during epidemics of colds or influenza). Among peoples subscribing to the tenets of traditional Chinese medicine, Ayurveda, Unani and humoral pathology, health-maintaining behaviour is seen in the great care paid to the "heating" and "cooling" qualities of food. Excessively "hot" or "cold" foods that can cause illness are eaten only when these qualities are counterbalanced by foods of the opposite quality.

In Latin America, where much illness is attributed to cold air, the cautious person keeps the head and face well covered with rebozo or serape, especially at night, and does not emerge from a warm room after sleeping until the excess heat from deep sleep is dissipated by a few minutes of wakefulness. Where the glance of a barren woman is believed to cause a child to fall ill, the careful mother places the appropriate charm around the infant's wrist or neck to deflect the envious stare. In societies where lengthy mourning rites and annual remembrances are expected by the dead, the living reduce the likelihood of illness by meticulous observation of traditional rites. Where witchcraft is feared, people are careful to avoid giving offence to neighbours who might resort to professional sorcerers or magical charms to strike back. All of these examples are just as much preventive medicine as are immunization and environmental sanitation. Moreover, it is well to remember that in many traditional societies houses and yards are meticulously cleaned and refuse is burned or removed from the immediate vicinity of the house. Defecation often occurs in fields or the surrounding bush and (except for very small children) not in the village. Sweat baths (often taken for ritual purposes) and frequent bathing, especially in hot countries, also contribute positively to the prevention of illness.

Stereotypes

In weighing the evidence in favour of the utilization of traditional medicine in contemporary health programmes, and particularly in primary health care, it is important to note that several stereotypes contrasting traditional and scientific medicine have been popularized in recent years. If uncritically accepted as a basis for health planning, these stereotypes may in fact be counterproductive.

(1) *Traditional medicine is holistic; modern medicine sees only the disease.* A basic argument advanced in favour of enlisting traditional curers in primary health care programmes is that they know the family background of their patients and hence can weigh psychosocial as well as clinical factors in diagnosis and therapy. In relatively isolated tribal and peasant villages this is certainly true. But contemporary villages are

modernizing rapidly: transport is more readily available than in former times, and both traditional and allopathic care are often sought well beyond village borders. Charismatic healers, such as El Niño Fidencio in Mexico, draw patients from hundreds, and even thousands, of miles away (4). Spiritual healers, who tend to practise in urban areas, increasingly replace more traditional types. In impersonal settings such as these, improvement in the patient's condition can hardly be attributed to the therapist's knowledge of the family background.

Even in stable villages the cures for such illnesses as *empacho*, *susto*, *bilis* and *mal de ojo* (to cite Latin American examples) are remarkably standardized. Sufferers are treated in much the same way, regardless of how different family situations may be. The *curandero's* knowledge about family conditions and sociopsychological factors that may have contributed to the illness plays a minimal role in therapy. The evidence suggests that the family-oriented holistic argument for the incorporation of traditional curers into primary health care programmes may be considerably weaker than is often assumed.

(2) *Traditional healers are relatively old, highly respected people, and because of their status they should be valuable allies in primary health care.* It is certainly true that elderly herbalists with a profound knowledge of traditional remedies, or famous shamans and priest curers, may inspire confidence in patients and their families. But to assume that because they fulfil their roles well in traditional settings they will do so equally well as formal participants in modern health services is to generalize carelessly. For example, officials of the Mexican National Indian Institute working in the state of Chiapas initially assumed it made good sense to work with and through local shamans in introducing improved health services to the Indians. But it was found that, in this instance at least, old and prestigious specialists were *not* the best intermediaries to promote sociocultural change. Health training for young literate people proved to be a more practical approach to providing primary health care (5). This is not to argue that mature traditional curers who enjoy high community respect should never be considered for new health roles. But the evidence suggests that a particular stereotype should not be accepted automatically as justification for health policy and planning. It is also well to remember that in many traditional societies shamans and other therapists are amoral: they cure, but they may also cause illness through sorcery; they take no Hippocratic oath. Ambivalent feelings often mark the relationships between patients and therapists in such societies.

(3) *Traditional peoples dichotomize illnesses into two categories: the first, illnesses that physicians can quickly cure; the second, "folk" illnesses the very existence of which physicians deny.* This "adversary" model has been widely accepted as a predicator of the choices traditional peoples will exercise in seeking medical help. While it does appear to have some validity in the first years following the introduction of modern medicine to

traditional peoples, after a relatively short time it loses its predictive value. Recent research shows that the health care decision-making process is marked by a great many factors: economic and social costs, prestige factors, distance, convenience, time, traditional beliefs, the personality or fame of specific curers and the like. No single model can predict care-seeking behaviour in times of a health crisis. In the final analysis people chose therapists, not medical systems.

(4) *Physicians practising in traditional settings are frequently ignorant of traditional medicine; they fail to understand its vocabulary and rationale, and hence have difficulties in communicating with patients.* Like the adversary model this is also an early stereotype developed by anthropologists. Yet increasingly it fails to describe reality because it is based on the image of Western missionary doctors in developing countries and upper class physicians in these countries treating their lower class fellow countrymen. Recent evidence indicates that medical doctors in growing numbers *do* understand the etiologies to which their patients subscribe and that they communicate with them effectively. In Latin America, for example, few physicians are puzzled when a patient explains a headcold by saying "I was struck by *aire* [air]". It is probable that the physician's mother used the same expression. Moreover, in many Third World countries medical education is no longer the monopoly of upper-class youth. Increasing numbers of young people from traditional communities are now entering medical school and graduating as physicians. They are not faced with a doctor–patient communication problem.

The foregoing stereotypes have been discussed, not with the intention of discouraging the incorporation of traditional curers into primary health care programmes, but rather as a caution against the uncritical acceptance of untested or untrue assumptions which will hinder rather than promote sound health policy and planning.

REFERENCES

(*1*) DUNN, F. L. Traditional Asian medicine and cosmopolitan medicine as adaptive systems. In: Leslie, C., ed. *Asian medical systems.* Berkeley, University of California Press, 1976, p. 135.
(*2*) HUGHES, C. C. Ethnomedicine. In: *International encyclopaedia of the social sciences.* New York, Free Press/Macmillan, 1968, vol. 10, p. 99.
(*3*) FOSTER, G. M. & ANDERSON, B. G. *Medical anthropology.* New York, Wiley, 1978, pp. 53–56.
(*4*) MACKLIN, J. Folk saints, healers and spiritist cults in northern Mexico. *Revista Review Interamericana,* 3:351–376 (1974).
(*5*) AGUIRRE BELTRÁN, G. Training programs in intercultural medicine. In: Velimirovic, B., ed. *Modern medicine and medical anthropology in the United States–Mexico border population.* Washington, DC, Pan American Health Organization, 1978 (PAHO Scientific Publication No. 359), pp. 10–13.

CHAPTER 2
Traditional medicine and psychiatry in Africa

Section I	Mamadou Koumaré[1]

Traditional medicine caters for most of the health needs of at least 80 % of the African population. Health is envisaged in all its physical, psychological and social dimensions and the following review will therefore be general in scope and illustrated by examples from psychiatry, which may be considered as the most comprehensive of the disciplines.

The all-embracing outlook of traditional medicine cannot, as will be seen later, be dissociated from religious concepts and the knowledge possessed by traditional healers of the causes, classification, diagnosis and treatment of disease and of the anatomy and physiology of the human body.

Thus African traditional medicine may be described as the total body of knowledge, techniques for the preparation and use of substances, measures and practices in use, whether explicable or not, that are based on the sociocultural and religious bedrock of African communities, are founded on personal experience and observations handed down from generation to generation, either verbally or in writing, and are used for the diagnosis, prevention or elimination of imbalances in physical, mental or social well-being.

African traditional medicine is thus a distillation of African culture, but the spirit that moves it is that shared by all forms of medicine, since the fear of disease and death and the need for food and health have led men in every age and clime to seek assistance from all that nature can offer them.

Undoubtedly, therefore, it is environment and social evolution that are responsible for the differences between the various health care systems now in existence.

The fundamental concepts regarding health and sickness are based on the idea of balances and imbalances (organic disorders, physiological disorders or social conflicts) between the component parts of the organism,

---

[1] Director General of the National Institute for Research in Traditional Medicine and Pharmacology, Bamako, Mali.

and between those components and elements of nature such as earth, water, air, fire and metals, and heavenly bodies such as sun, moon and stars. Each element is capable of exerting a specific influence on certain organs. Thus from birth the newborn infant is subject to the control of elements of nature, and survival depends on the capacity to establish equilibrium in an environment containing both favourable and unfavourable elements. A knowledge of these elements can give the power to preserve or disturb the equilibrium that represents health, even at a distance.

The Bambara of Mali, for example, consider an equilibrium of the same kind to exist within the body, where *kalia* is said to dwell in symbiosis. They have no instruments, however, such as the microscope or devices for recording electromagnetic force, to give concrete and visual expression to the idea of *kalia*, which is much more than just a symbol. It must be pointed out that the traditional African system includes not only the visible, sometimes tangible, elements of nature, but invisible and intangible elements too; this highlights the concept of "natural" and "supernatural" causes of illness and leads the traditional healer to seek such causes in invisible as well as visible elements, sometimes as a routine measure but more often at the request of the patient himself, who may be the first to be alarmed by the circumstances under which his illness developed or by the abnormal course it has taken. It should be noted that, as far as healer and patient are concerned, a "non-natural" disease may well take the form of a "natural" disease when, for instance, it is inflicted as an act of vengeance. This dual outlook on disease often gives rise to much confusion and to mistakes in interpretation when it is referred to the nosology and nosography of modern medicine.

The power that attaches to words, which some refer to derisively as "incantations", forms no small part of African traditional medicine and may even be said to be its characteristic feature.

Might not "incantations", which are mere words, inducing sound waves, have some effect likely to induce endogenous secretions and influence the biosynthesis of substances produced by plants?

Under these conditions, could it be possible that only those "in the know" are given the "power" of inducing activity with the result that some plants do not acquire their therapeutic properties unless collected and prepared by such persons?

Some traditional healers would agree with this, whereas the scientist might consider it to be nothing but trickery and superstition. Nevertheless, the experiments described in Tompkin & Bird's book *The secret life of plants* (1) prompts us to a more detailed consideration of the problem.

Dualism is another basic concept, which goes hand in hand with the concept of equilibrium, and exists at several different levels. "Hot" and "cold" are an example. The concept of dualism leads readily to the idea that for every disease there is a substance that will prevent or cure it. Hence, sometimes by application of the theory of "signature", in which a resemblance between the disease and the therapeutic substance suggests its use, folk medicine, which may take the form of self-medication, has been developed.

It is apparent that traditional medicine concerns itself mainly with curative practices, but it also includes preventive measures involving immunization, the wearing of conservation objects to stave off illnesses, sacrifices and offerings, and the observance of prohibitions, taboos and a number of rituals including bodily hygiene.

Admittedly, some of these preventive measures are difficult for scientists to accept, but here again the underlying concept of "intangible forces" deserves some consideration. These "intangible forces", which may be termed "protective and restorative forces", are as difficult to generate as the "force" of hypnosis. The latter and other similar forces have been called "direct forces" and the rest have been classified as "indirect forces" as they need to be sustained by the "inductive power" of the traditional healer.

Who then are these traditional healers? They are persons recognized by the community in which they live as competent to practise medicine. At present, there is one traditional healer to every 500 inhabitants whereas there is only one doctor for every 40 000 inhabitants. There is thus a social consensus conferring a special status (given different names depending on the language concerned) on such healers and according them the power to heal or even to prevent illness or any other misfortune, or to promote the happiness (social advancement, increasing wealth, marital harmony, etc.) of those consulting them.

Traditional healers therefore engage in medical and non-medical activities, which are sometimes connected only by the divination rites such healers use in the various fields in which people seek their services.

The all-embracing nature of African traditional medicine is a reason for the wide variety of practices encountered and these may be used as a basis for classification. Three categories are proposed:

(1) *Practices using medicinal substances.* Here it should be pointed out that it is not strictly accurate to talk of phytotherapy or even "new-style phytotherapy" since plants are often used in association with animal or mineral products or both. Practitioners in this field may be considered as dealing with somatic aspects and they are not very different from the experts in popular medicine or self-medication mentioned earlier.

(2) *Practices concerned with "intangible forces" and rites.* The methods employed may in some cases be influenced by religious trends. This group is very complex and diversified and is the category principally concerned with the psychological and social aspects.

(3) *Practices combining in various degrees those of the two previous groups.* This category appears to be the largest.

In each of these three categories it should be noted that there are general practitioners and specialists, who may or may not have recourse to divination. However, the term "specialist" should not be understood in the narrow sense applied to modern medicine. In African traditional medicine the term "specialist" refers to a person dealing with a limited number of pathological conditions and not just with one organ or system of the human body, although it is possible to find traditional healers who confine themselves to fractures, cataract or mental disorders. A consultation with either a specialist or a general practitioner in traditional medicine is often a fairly lengthy procedure. Based on anatomical and physiological concepts acquired as "dynamic knowledge", diagnosis in traditional medicine also involves the concepts of natural and supernatural causes. Traditional healers, despite their lack of sophisticated technology, are helped by meticulous observation of clinical signs. A number of elements such as body temperature and the blood are most frequently used. It should be noted, however, that the meanings attached to the terms "heat" and "blood" may sometimes overlap.

Thus, "driving out heat" from the body should not always be taken literally and translated as "febrifuge", as sometimes it means "hypotensive", the term "heat" being also used to describe an increase in the blood pressure. This illustrates the difficulty of communication in any collaborative effort when inexperienced intermediaries are used as translators. It must also be realized that some substances are administered merely to guide the traditional healer in his diagnosis, otherwise it may be mistakenly thought that he is giving treatment on a hit or miss basis. Early in the course of treatment he may use certain substances that he knows will aggravate the clinical signs of a given disease in order to be certain of his diagnosis.

Another very important factor is the use of divination techniques, which may in some cases help to determine prognosis and thus play the part of additional paraclinical analyses. Mention should also be made of the considerable help the patient himself may give and which may be used to establish a diagnosis in certain cases of diseases attributed to supernatural causes. In such cases, a ritual act places the patient in a state in which he can give the required assistance.

Treatment itself is most often directed both to the body and to the mental state taken in the context of social environment, ancestral spirits, family, community, etc. It is thus as all-embracing as the diagnosis. Three categories of action are always found corresponding to "natural" causes, "supernatural" causes and the different degrees of association between these factors.

The overwhelming emphasis is on symptomatic treatment, but this does not mean that etiological treatment does not exist. Here again, the care taken to find a treatment suited to the case, and hence related to the evolution of the disorder, may also give the impression of a hit or miss approach but is, in actual fact, a basic principle aimed at avoiding impersonal treatment.

The use of aromatic plants and fumigation in dwellings to "drive out evil spirits" in general is likewise linked to the disinfection of premises, even if the traditional healer is unable to express these actions in such terms. Detailed analysis shows clearly that acts and attitudes are controlled by the therapeutic objective which in turn determines the mode of administration of drugs, etc. to the patient.

The therapeutic objective is, of course, dominated by the pharmacopoeia and the remedies it contains. Traditional remedies are prepared from vegetable, animal or mineral substances. Plants undoubtedly play a major part in the pharmacopoeia, but this does not justify restricting the scope of the traditional remedies or referring to those who prescribe them as essentially "herbalists".

Experience has shown that the methods used to determine the dosage of traditional remedies are reasonably accurate, bearing in mind that dosage is adjusted to the case under treatment. This, at any rate, has been the conclusion of the author's field studies.

Posological equipment is still rudimentary and is very similar to kitchen utensils. When studying the posology of traditional remedies, an attempt has been made to find a parallel between the screens of known calibre used in Western pharmaceutical practice and the different sorts of kitchen sieve used.

Although African traditional medicine covers 80% or more of our populations, its practice is barely tolerated by most health authorities. In many countries, local administrative authorities have given some traditional healers the right to practise even though there is no national legislation on the subject. For lack of a coherent policy, healers therefore continue to be severely penalized for their failures, but are rarely commended for their successes. Similarly, the methods of their remuneration still vary widely. They may be paid in kind according to local custom, or in cash.

As a result of current enthusiasm some traditional healers have become full-time or part-time salaried employees. It is usual for remuneration to be symbolic in rural areas. There is, however, a current tendency to charge high fees, particularly in urban areas.

Traditional medical practitioners often feel that they form a "corporate body" in society. Sometimes this stems from the fact that they belong to an identifiable group like that of hunters, for example. The realization of their position as a result of current enthusiasm has led to a desire for the establishment of official associations, but mistrust among the healers is still prevalent and one can hardly speak of national associations comprising a substantial body of practitioners. There is likewise considerable suspicion between the health professions and the healers. The public therefore needs to be given statutory protection against malpractice, and for this purpose the provision of legislation under the control of a state institution and under the authority of the minister of public health is mandatory.

Few countries have taken such action and, depending on the country concerned, traditional medicine may come under the ministry of arts and culture, the ministry of research, or some other ministry. Clearly, such departments have relatively little to do with the health care of the population. It is thus apparent that if research is to be conducted effectively, it must primarily be directed to a public health goal. Admittedly, such research has not yet been properly organized in most African countries. In the first place there is no consistent policy on the subject and, secondly, the all-embracing nature of traditional medicine calls for multidisciplinary research. Although national research institutions have been established in some countries, their operation is subject to difficulties despite the efforts made to assist them by agencies such as the Organization of African Unity (OAU), the World Health Organization (WHO), the Agency for Cultural and Technical Cooperation (ACCT), and the African and Malagasy Council on Higher Education (CAMES). The non-availability of information on the work done by these institutions is one reason for the duplication in their activities. However, the problem of dissemination of results is being solved by means of the bulletins of a number of institutions and of the OAU, and by means of the records of CAMES meetings.

None of these praiseworthy efforts is likely to prove at all useful unless people are on their guard against becoming overexcited by the "picturesque" aspects of traditional practices, a trend which could alter and completely destroy them. Their impact no longer requires to be proved, but they need to be linked up in some way to the official system based on Western medicine in order to obtain a more equitable and wider health care coverage.

If frank and sincere collaboration on this basis is to succeed, the following guiding principles should be applied:

a) exclusion of any tendency to eliminate traditional medicine by an attempt simply to take over remedies and techniques that are effective;

b) provision of the traditional healer with a place in the health team that corresponds to his skills and abilities; this would apply at all levels;

c) adoption of the concept of a health care network based on both systems and to the benefit of the community; and

d) creation of awareness through educational activities rather than a publicity campaign.

There have already been some instances of collaboration and some aspects of those relating to psychiatry will be mentioned here.

Mental disease is unmistakably connected with individual and community behaviour, and the special qualities of African psychiatry are derived from the specific nature of the culture that has produced it. We are, therefore, in full agreement with Collomb when he says "As the individual is dependent on the group he never experiences anything as an isolated person. The depersonalization from which the group benefits produces a need for equality, a sense of justice, solidarity, a lack of competitiveness and of dependence. When on his own and far from the group to which he belongs, his status as an individual is undermined and becomes prone to distress, he may fall victim to drug dependence or even a psychotic state" (2).

African cultures often require total acceptance of a highly structured universe of magical forces that permeate everyday life and often go far beyond their purpose as social regulators to produce an effect of overwhelming persecution and exert a harmful influence on the body and soul of a person whom chance rather than disease has placed in an unaccustomed or dangerous situation. To this must be added that "physical integrity does not survive dissolution of the social personality". This sort of approach to mental disease makes understandable the tolerance accorded an "insane" person in the community provided he is not too aggressive. It also explains the traditional psychiatrist's approach to treatment by means of medication, ritual, sacrifice, etc.

It is in this context that the practitioner–patient relationship develops. The psychiatrist's "power" is a direct expression of his personality, and the "energies" he transmits are its fundamental element. For this reason, some forms of collaboration undoubtedly could pose a serious threat to traditional psychiatry, particularly in urban areas in cases where traditional psychiatrists are likely to have suffered "alienation" if not a complete change of cultural background. Nevertheless, a harmonious working relationship is attainable judging from what has been achieved at the Fann Psychiatric Hospital in Dakar and the Aro Hospital in Abeokuta, Nigeria. If collaboration with the traditional psychiatrist is to be effective and comprehensible it must be based on the whole body of his psychosocial, anthropological and pharmaceutical knowledge. The modern psychiatrist does not necessarily need to know the incantations and remedies used by the traditional psychiatrist before collaboration can begin.

The surrender of the traditional psychiatrist's "secrets" should on no account be a condition for collaboration. On the contrary, a process of mutual exchange should be envisaged with a reasonable understanding of both concepts of madness and cultural systems. What must be avoided is any attempt to compare or contrast the two techniques, in so far as the traditional psychiatrist treats the "insane" mainly within his own family and community and not in a padded cell, while the modern psychiatrist is beginning to accept this mode of therapy.

This review has endeavoured to demonstrate the diversity of traditional medical practice, which is inseparable from religion and forms a coherent system. In point of fact, whether the emphasis is on amulets, self-discipline, the *kwalwa* (period of retreat in which a marabout, a Moslem leader, invokes spirits to communicate with), holy water, or a fetish, religion is the predominant factor. The inherent and inevitable multivalence of traditional practices must also be emphasized. Since by means of magic, sorcery, fetishes, etc., it is possible, through the intervention of forces in opposition to those we have termed "restorative" or "protective", to provoke "imbalance", i.e. disease, the traditional healer must, according to his nature, act as a sorcerer, magician, fetishist, etc., in order to obtain a better understanding of the patient's illness and of the appropriate way to treat him.

As mentioned earlier, the traditional healer draws on his knowledge not only of magic and religion but also of physical disorders and major syndromes and thus proceeds to assemble what amounts to a case history that will culminate in his diagnosis.

His task does not end there for he still has to dispense his own prescription, whether for remedies or therapeutic rites.

This illustrates the indivisibility and unity of the knowledge, techniques and acquired or innate "power" combined in traditional medicine.

The healing art and the pharmaceutical art, the two main components of any health system, are here intermingled. Although the knowledge and techniques involved are relatively easy to impart, the "power" of the traditional healer is, by its very nature, a different matter. It is not given to everyone to be a traditional healer, especially a traditional healer with every attribute, as family tradition is not always enough.

It would therefore not be a good idea to restrict traditional medicine solely to its pharmaceutical aspects, particularly when account is taken of the fact that it deals with disease on a psychosomatic basis and thus ties in with the new trends in psychiatry.

It is to be hoped that the new direction being taken by the Western medical disciplines will lead to harmonization of the two systems each respecting the other's essential nature while gaining from it.

REFERENCES

(1) TOMPKIN, P. & BIRD, C. *The secret life of plants*. London, A. Lane, 1974.
(2) COLLOMB, H. Aspects particuliers de la psychiatrie africaine, *Cliniques africaines*: 419 (1966).

FURTHER READING

KOUMARÉ, M. Le remède traditionel africain et son évaluation. *Santé pour tous*, 3: 28 (1978).
SOW, I. *Les structures anthropologiques de la folie en Afrique noir*. Paris, Payot, 1978.

Section II

Piero Coppo[1]

It is much more difficult to separate the physical from the mental in African traditional medicine than it is in modern medicine. In African culture the distinction and contrast between mind and body is less profound and significant and this may go some way to explaining why all traditional treatment is directed to both the mind and the body. This is not surprising in view of ancestral beliefs, generally animist in nature, which encompass systems in which all things are animate and there are spirits everywhere and in every substance, no matter how inert.

Every African therapeutic act may thus be said to be psychiatric in the etymological sense of "seeking to cure disease of the life force", even though it may be directed to a patient with what "scientific" medicine would define as a "physical" ailment. The incantations accompanying the preparation and administration of a medicament, the part played by the healer as mediator between spirits and humans, and his occult powers are components of every therapeutic act.

However, to return, for greater convenience, to the outlook of "scientific" medicine and the culture that produced it, we shall restrict our discussion of traditional psychiatry to the traditional art of treating insanity.

About ten years ago European investigators (H. Collomb among others) became aware of the fact that Africans had always considered the treatment of insanity and other psychiatric ailments well within the competence of indigenous healers and that patients attending colonial hospitals for treatment had often already received some form of treatment from traditional healers. It was this situation, which still persists, that led modern physicians, both European and African, to appreciate the importance of traditional psychiatry and the particular features of the

---

[1] Medical practitioner and psychiatric specialist, Usigliano, Italy; Visiting Consultant, National Institute for Research in Traditional Medicine and Pharmacology, Bamako, Mali.

psychological and psychopathological states for which it gives treatment. It therefore became clear that it was inadvisable to superimpose an imported psychiatry on communities steeped in a different culture and tradition. Since then there has been an increasing trend among investigators to take an interest in psychology, and in psychopathological conditions and their treatment in traditional, modernizing or modern African societies.

The traditional psychiatrist's main function is the treatment of insanity, but he may treat other diseases, and in his capacity as mediator between his community and the gods, he may be called upon in any crisis such as flooding or famine.

Traditional African societies are rather rigidly organized with well defined systems and roles, the degree of rigidity being directly related to the difficulties the community faces in its environment. Nevertheless, the characteristic features of African societies and the many group systems that exist for controlling any irrational individual or community action lend a certain flexibility to this ordered structure. If the action is contrary to the cultural or traditional pattern and is important, and if the disorder is excessive, then insanity will be declared and treatment by a "specialist" immediately initiated.

The traditional psychiatrist is never solely a medical practitioner. He may be a farmer, hunter or fisherman, occasionally a herdsman, and usually supports himself by these other activities. The healing art is acquired through family tradition, or through having a vocation for it, or by having survived a severe illness oneself. In addition to the above attributes, the traditional psychiatrist has to go through a long period of apprenticeship during which he has to learn not only the therapeutic properties of plants but also the mysteries of nature such as the world of night and darkness and sacred objects, a world barred to the other members of the community who fear such mysticism.

Relations with the sacred include interaction with natural and supernatural beings and with ancestral spirits. The healer is thus a teacher and a leader, who can take the patient by the hand and lead him through the labyrinth of insanity. Moreover, because of the cultural affinity existing between patient and physician and the fact that both usually belong to the same community, each therapeutic act is culturally meaningful and psychologically effective. The long period of initiation allows the healer to free himself of any narcissistic, sadomasochistic or aggressive tendencies to the point where his relationship with the patient becomes a model of what the doctor–patient relationship should be. Briefly, the healer assumes complete authority over the patient, who in turn obtains all the security he so much needs.

There are many therapeutic techniques and these may differ from one subculture to another or within the same culture. Divination, for example, serves to determine the time the disease started, to supplement the medical case history and to specify the most useful remedies to apply. The medicaments, some with specific pharmacological properties, are prepared and administered in accordance with ritual practices that are said to increase potency. Massage, incantation and ablution may precede or accompany their administration. There is liberal use of musicotherapy, often associated with tribal dances and with ritually induced "trances" or hypnotism.

The traditional psychiatrist may treat his patients on an "outpatient" basis or keep them in his own home for several months or shorter periods. In such cases, a member of the patient's family will stay with the patient throughout the time required for treatment and will assist with nursing care. This reduces the risk of the patient being "dumped" by his family or of too sudden a severance from the surroundings of treatment when he returns home, as someone who has witnessed the curative process will continue to attend him at home.

As regards payment for services, the patient or his family generally makes a token presentation of a small sum of money, or small quantities of cola nuts, tea, etc. at the first interview with the healer. Once treatment has been completed, payment is proportional to its duration and complexity, and depends also on its success.

In psychiatric practice, collaboration between the modern physician and the traditional psychiatrist is highly desirable with a view to combining the two systems for more effective care through due regard for original beliefs and traditional therapeutic practices. It is precisely in the psychiatric field that the contrast is most striking between the great storehouse of traditional practices with their tremendous originality and the limits placed on them by rapid social transformation which severs people from their original cultures and roots and alienates them, through rapid exposure to Western culture in the wake of national development and industrialization. This severance from the ancestral world, even if deep down there remains a strong ambivalent tie to the original system of beliefs, is also likely to impoverish the African mentality (making it more vulnerable to psychopathological phenomena) and to remove all their effectiveness from traditional psychotherapeutic practices, leaving intact only that part of the psychotherapeutic heritage whose validity has been "scientifically" confirmed.

This is one reason why traditional psychiatry in its present form is a valuable therapeutic tool, particularly in a society, such as that in rural areas, which is still organized along traditional lines. Here traditional psychiatry can develop its therapeutic potential to its maximum, and the modern physician could also gain considerable understanding. To send an illiterate country-dweller in an acute psychotic state to a psychiatric hospital in a distant town some hundreds of kilometres away where his mother tongue is not understood, for treatment with neuroleptics, when there is available in his neighbourhood a traditional healer capable of treating his condition successfully, is a negation of good sense and is dangerous for the patient. Similarly, it would be unwise to use traditional treatments on a city-dweller who has been subjected to acculturation and severed from his ancestral world, since that would force him, in a defenceless and acute psychotic state, into an abrupt confrontation with the sociocultural pattern he has repudiated. In such circumstances, a doctor wearing a white coat and sitting in a modern consulting room would give him a much greater sense of security.

There is a third possibility, however, which seeks to integrate both therapeutic techniques into one system, applying whichever aspects are most useful in the given circumstances.

The author has found it very useful to exchange information with the traditional psychiatrist on the appropriate use of modern and traditional psychotropic drugs. There are indications that integration of the two pharmacological approaches is now being made in an intelligent manner— for instance, industrial drugs are administered in the acute agitated phase and traditional medicaments, generally slower but more balanced in action, are used to effect a cure. Some modern medical concepts, such as the distinction between secondary psychopathological manifestations of physical disease, which require hospital treatment, and manifestations of "essential" disease, also seem useful to the traditional psychiatrist. We have, in turn, learnt from the traditional psychiatrist to consider the "safe" distance between physician and patient as less important, where possible not to interpose a third party between them, to have the patient accompanied by a member of his family and, perhaps, to use some indigenous medicaments.

Both systems of treatment and both concepts of insanity may thus in the long run be of benefit to one another. Otherwise, if integration is attempted in one direction only, there is a danger either of a psychological weakening of the effectiveness of the traditional healer, which is much more vulnerable than traditional medical structures, or of his repudiation of an ancestral art in favour of too hasty identification with an approach which appears to have the force of history behind it, namely the modern Western approach and its most important by-product, scientific technology.

FURTHER READING

COLLOMB, H. Les niveaux d'intervention du guérisseur. In: *Actes du colloque du CAMES sur la médecine traditionelle et la pharmacopée africaine.* Niamey, Conseil africain et malgache pour l'Enseignement supérieur, 1976.
HARDING, T. W. Traditional healing methods for mental disorders. *WHO Chronicle,* 31:436–440 (1977).
LAMBO, T. A. Services for the mentally handicapped in Africa. *Royal Society of Health journal,* 93 (1): 20–23 (1973).

CHAPTER 3

Traditional medicine in Latin America

Carmel Goldwater[1,2]

I. Humoral theory and therapy

The term "humoral theory" refers to the "hot-cold" classification of living and inanimate matter known throughout Latin America[3] and applied by Indian and other peoples[4] in the maintenance of health and treatment of disease. Hot and cold do not refer to measurable physical characteristics such as temperature, but rather to the effect attributed to qualities or properties inherent in the substances themselves.

The origin of this classification and the suggestion that it represents a truncated form of the Hippocratic humoral theory and the Galenic system of medicine (see *Appendix*) has been subject to debate (*1*). This concept could well have been in use by the indigenous population prior to the conquest, and there is evidence supporting this suggestion (*2*). The acceptance of this concept may also help to establish whether or not there is a valid distinctive Latin American humoral theory and therapy comparable to the "large" systems described in subsequent sections of this chapter.

Before going into further details, some thought should be given to the sheer size and complexity of Latin America. The extremes of climate and habitat, the diversity of life-styles and occupation, and the increasing population and urbanization all make for considerable variety. The unity of understanding and cultural identification provided by a common language, Spanish or Portuguese, is not shared by the entire Indian population (*3*). Whatever their common background before migration to

---

[1] Specialist in Public Health and Social Anthropology, London, England.
[2] In collaboration with V. Lenart Lunny.
[3] Latin America refers to the 20 Republics.
[4] The knowledge regarding hot–cold exists in all sections of the community, Mestizo and white, but its extent is uncertain. In the context of this chapter "traditional" is taken to refer to the Indian indigenous population.

the region, there is currently a multiplicity of separate ethnic groups ranging in size from as few as 50 to as many as 1 million.[5] In spite of this diversity, certain common denominators are found, besides the hot-cold categories. Concepts regarding the various types and causes of disease, healers and their specialties, ideas and beliefs regarding the non-material world, are often distinguished only by their names at local level. Just as nomenclature may vary, so will the possible range of conceptual expression in each language, reflecting the particular experience and world view of the population concerned.

Basic concepts

Hot and cold represent two opposite states. The ideal is a balance between the two. A state of balance is conducive to maintaining good health, while imbalance leads to disease. An individual goes out of balance through changes resulting from excess of hot or cold affecting the body, and restoring balance by means of the opposite or similar, as relevant, also involves change. Hot and cold are therefore processes whose action presupposes change. Balance is a state of dynamic equilibrium, and is relative because to attain it involves change in the process; balancing as a static phenomenon is a contradiction in terms of life processes.

There are two main ways in which an individual is exposed to hot and cold. One is internal, through daily consumption of food and beverages; the other is external, a result of physical activities including exposure to the elements.

In the case of food and beverages, the two categories would be taken into account both in preparation and consumption, if relevant knowledge and interest exists and food availability allows for the necessary choices. The classification of foods can extend to extremes of very hot or very cold, or more modified and indeterminate (temperate) degrees including substances which do not have any real or known intrinsic hot-cold effect. An excess of hot food (not hot in the sense of temperature or taste, though this can be an added factor) will result in fever, while too much cold food leads to general debility. These states would be regarded as having a direct relationship to diet and corrective measures would include withdrawing certain foods and including some of the opposite kind.

In the second case, heating and cooling are the result of physical factors, the element of the temperature being relevant. Exposure to heat at work or to the sun may overheat the body, and working in the cold or in water, or

---

[5] The descriptions given here are most relevant to Central America and the Andean region, where the concentration of Indians is greatest (54% Bolivia, 16% Mexico). The language complexity can be illustrated by the fact that in Bolivia alone there are 24 linguistic families and 123 dialects, even though 1 million speak Quechua and 660 000 Aymara. The various groups may be found in more than one country.

exposure to cold air and wind when hot, will result in a chill or cold. In both cases there may be clear-cut symptoms indicating whether the condition is hot or cold, but there may be symptoms common to both. Therapy aims to restore the balance by using foods and remedies of opposite or similar type as indicated. Such measures may require the use of more specific remedies, mainly herbal. Treatment for hot-cold beyond the home treatment or self-care level becomes the responsibility of the indigenous herbalist.[6]

The picture may not always be so clear-cut. Though illness may still be categorized as hot or cold, its origin may be supernatural and will then require the services of a diviner to elucidate, and special rituals for treatment. Hot and cold are part of a spectrum embracing the overall belief system regarding causation of disease, the non-material forces at play in daily life, ranging from individual emotions and actions to the evil eye and the work of malefic spirits, and man's interrelationship with nature and universe.

Hot and cold as a health regulator

This is one of the most important functions of the hot-cold categorization, which can provide a simple and effective method of self-care and preventive medicine. It is applied by proscribing, mainly in the regulation of health; and prescribing, mainly in the context of treating illness.

One must first know how to classify all the foods, plants, mineral and other substances into the appropriate category, hot, cold, (very hot or very cold) or temperate. This is learnt as fact and reinforced by direct experience. Classification has been found to vary in different areas, and inclusion of recently manufactured items does not appear to follow a consistent pattern. It has hitherto been difficult, therefore, to establish how substances are allocated to one or other category, other than on an empirical basis.

To illustrate these points, examples of foods in daily use in five different ecological environments[7] and their categories are given here. The most consistent classification was that of water, always cold whatever its state, becoming hot when a substance is added to it, such as honey or cane sugar. Tea, beer, lemon, potato, rice, barley, tomato, eggs, were

---

[6] In view of the differences in non-Spanish names applied to the indigenous practitioners in the region, and to specification of illnesses, it has been decided to give only general descriptions which can then be identified locally. The extensive range of possible diagnoses has been shortened to include only those related to the topic and others providing the necessary perspective.

[7] Chiloe, South Chile; North Patagonia, Argentina; near Calca, Peru; Cania, Ecuador; and near Cartagena, Colombia.

consistently cold. Coca leaf, coffee, cocoa, chocolate, quinine, coriander, mint, salt, consistently hot. Disagreement occurred on such common items as beef (mainly hot), chicken (both), beans, frijole (mainly cold), onions, pork (mainly cold), maize depending on colour (yellow, hot; white, cold). Hot and cold can be modified by mixing with proportions of the opposite, and by cooking. As individuals are themselves continually subject to and undergoing change in the hot-cold context, classification may be relative at any given moment.

Within this framework, proscribing aims at avoiding extremes. For example coffee, being hot, should be taken in the morning, a cool time, but not in the middle of the day. In the evening it would be preferred initially to a cold drink, which should be avoided until the body has cooled down naturally after heating during the day. Food combinations such as pork and tea would be too cold, and lemon being cold is best avoided in the cool of the day unless balanced. In special circumstances such as pregnancy, dietary restrictions are tailored to the hot-cold relating to the particular trimester and the postnatal period. Avoidance of eggs and milk appears to be related to the infant's development, which will also be affected by the mother's breast-milk.

Prescribing of foods is limited to some extent by availability. More frequently it involves choosing food considered suitable for the task at hand, for example, maize and potato for manual labour and beer in moderation to provide strength.

Hot and cold in therapy

Put in the simplest way, excesses of diet cause fever and debility, which can be alleviated by prescribing suitable foods of an opposite nature, cooling or heating, respectively. More obvious illness is precipitated when external factors come into play. Overheating at work through exertion, or exposure to the sun, can cause skin eruptions, kidney and liver diseases, and sore eyes. Too rapid cooling or exposure to damp, wind and severe weather produce bone and joint pain, rheumatism, lung complaints and colic.

Treatment consists of using both food and medicinal plants to obtain a cure, choosing those with known opposite qualities to the causes of the illness diagnosed (though there are exceptions, as when hot treatment is advocated first in hot conditions, as noted). If the remedies prove ineffective, they will be replaced by their opposite, the assumption being that diagnosis was incorrect as regards hot-cold. This applies particularly to the inexperienced healer and in certain conditions such as cough or dysentery, which might be classified as either hot or cold ailments. However, it must be stressed that remedies are chosen for their specific action (e.g., expectorant, costive, etc.) from a wide variety of medicinal plants.

The category of cold diseases includes illnesses resulting from air. Air (cold) can be "caught". It can act suddenly as a fulminating agent causing spasms, convulsions or vertigo. A lightning-like air causes respiratory complications, alters the atmosphere and contaminates man and animal. The circulatory system can be affected directly or indirectly by air, resulting in blood and urine infections. Internal toxins and bad air may combine, leading to paralysis of the limbs and rheumatism. Another type of air can cause cutaneous eruptions. Emanations from spirits of the dead, in earth and air, can combine to affect the living, inflicting scrofulous and other abnormal states. Like air, wind can be a harbinger of disease causing facial palsy, migraine, mental illness and other ills. At this stage it is difficult to say whether the illness was caused by cold as such.

General treatment for these conditions consists of the use of herbs, fumes (inhalation of tobacco and incense), sweating and massage with various types of oils. Hot poultices may also be used to draw out the cold.[8]

Heat may surface as the result of toxins generated in the body by decomposed ingested food, causing skin complaints. Treatment is by hot baths, mud packs, and herbal enemas. Just as cold, in its external aspect, has a wider connotation, so heat in its internal aspect can be viewed in another context, such as anger and suppressed rage. In both cases the therapeutic and balancing measures required extend beyond the hot-cold concept defined at the beginning of this paper.

Beyond hot and cold

The interface between individual reaction and external forces is further illustrated by a well known condition caused by fright. Fright (*mal de susto*) affects the central nervous system and manifests diversely as shivering, anguish, nervousness, restlessness at night, lack of strength, palpitations and gastrointestinal symptoms. The fright experienced results in a dissociation of the spirit (or a portion of the soul) which abandons the body. The severe psychic shock alters the body's metabolism and the functioning of the central nervous system in particular. A ceremony is performed to call back the spirit (or soul), and to complete the cure a form of massage and ceremonial bathing is administered by the practitioner.

Illness may also be caused by spirits, as mentioned in connexion with emanations carried by the air. Those of the dead can enter the body, for example when a person walks near graves. Similarly, such spirits can contaminate clothes left out at night and affect the wearer. A breast-fed baby is endangered when its mother sees a dead body.

---

[8] Hot steam baths are in use more in Central America. The treatment here refers to that used in Bolivia. Tobacco and hallucinogenic plants are not used there as part of divining or ceremony. The term "drawing out" is literal; it does not refer to the practices used in Amazon, to suck out illness thought to be an intrusion.

A more active source of induced illness is the evil eye (*mal de ojo*). This may be applied deliberately or inadvertently by someone who has a tendency to do so. Children are particularly susceptible. As envy is a prime factor in the situation, care must be taken to avoid praise, criticism being less likely to attract attention from persons of ill will. Treatment is carried out by specialists through prayer and blessing, and in severe cases the person carrying out the cure may develop the symptoms himself.

Aberrant behaviour, such as neglecting to pay homage to the spirits of home, mountains or fields, may result in the member of the family being "caught" by the earth. Pain and swelling develop and can only be alleviated by making some form of payment to the earth mother. This ceremony is performed by the indigenous practitioner at night, burning a specific type of offering and burying the ashes. Illness may also be a more direct punishment by the higher divinities for behavioural transgressions, including alcoholism, and is cured by prayers and offerings.

Situations of this kind call for more specialized skills than the use of simple medicinal plants. These include divining the general somatic and psychic state of the individual and more specific matters relating to future events, guarding against evil, and undoing its consequences by ceremony and prayer and by protective amulets and talismans.

Such persistent age-old beliefs and practices are no mere anachronisms. They are an inescapable part of the overall view of man in relation to the universe and the immediate environment, enforced by experience and the interpretation of religious precepts.

A view of the universe

The oldest known distinctive group of indigenous practitioners in South America, the Bolivian *médicos* or *Callawaya*, are agriculturists who come mainly from two cantons in the northern area of La Paz. They have practised their art for centuries and during Inca times were reputed to use various moulds of fermented green bananas, moss of corn and other products, and special hot poultices of black mud. Gentian, ipecac, quinine and Peru balsam, among other substances, were introduced by them to the Spaniards (*4*).

Today training is still passed on orally, to the men only, by the older men of knowledge, who teach the collection and preparation of plants used in their pharmacopoeia. These are gathered from all the ecological zones, from high altitude to tropical. Animal and mineral as well as excretion products are also used. The professional teaching, ultimately subject to examination by a family council, is supplemented by learning in the home environment, acquiring skill in making amulets and in divining. Other skills include the preparation of special offerings used in prayers and intercessions. Treatment of animals is an important part of their work and is carried out in the home or other appropriate place. Traditionally the

Callaway travel throughout the continent, for periods of two or three years, providing herbal and other treatments, the wife being meanwhile responsible for the agricultural work and family.

Methods of diagnosis depend on the origin of the illness, and physical signs including pulse and urine. Urine is used in divining the site where a person may have received the fright (or *susto*). In other divining methods coca leaves and different coloured maize grains are used.

Both colour and music are important adjuncts to therapy, colour for its significance and symbolism, and music as a background for healing and divination ceremonies. Music is thought to frighten away evil spirits and also to act as a form of prophylaxis.

Behind all this lies a specific and universal belief system. There is a trinity of divinities: He who is the energy maintaining the universe and giving life to all beings, whose will decides human destiny; Supreme day or light, father of the third member of the trinity, the divine Mother of the Indian, a saint sent by God who preached love and advised banning envy and grudge from the human heart, with severe penalties for those not heeding.[9]

Man, too, is a triune being. The soul, the spirit of divine breath conveying the power of thought, sensitivity and movement; a fluid-like small soul or astral body which can leave the body (when it leaves the body, as in sleep or fright an altered state or illness supervenes); and the material body. The soul is eternal and may return to nature.

The heart of the plant

Within the universe, cosmic reality manifests the union of that which exists and that which does not. The entire world is said to be full of forces of energy through which matter is animated—sun and heat often producing good crops, and cold and hail resulting in bad crops. These opposites are in an endless continuous cycle conceived in the mind (of man) as the development of life's events proceeding in a rightward clockwise movement. This direction reverses in the case of misfortune or illness. Man tries to deflect the inevitability of the coming bad times by actions such as rites and prayers for the fertility of soil and animals, and keeping pure in heart, at the start of the year's agricultural cycle. Illness is also conceived as a state which can be "given away" by reversing the leftward movement, inverting and turning over the unfavourable to the right order. There are a number of methods to do this, including the use of thread carded in a left-

---

[9] Tutujanawin, the supreme being, beginning and end of all things. The *Callaway* say we cannot understand such divine existence because our intelligence is too limited. Pachaquanan, father of Pachamama, the mother earth who brings life and happiness, protects crops, flowers, fruit and animals and fights with inclement elements. Similar concepts appear elsewhere in the region.

hand way, wound round an injured or sick limb leftwards, and symbolically cut.

Similarly, the way in which terminology is used in the context of the body can indicate concepts of life. The word for heart (in Quechua, for example) can be used to denote and express any state of mind, personality, behaviour, good or bad intention, a whole range of meanings without clear-cut boundaries. In the plant terminology, the expressions to stone, to core, to pare green beans, the marrow of wood, the pip of a fruit, all point to the interior, the heart of objects and reflect the idea that everything is alive or vital (5). This vitality extends to a concept of quality inherent in medicinal plants, as used by the indigenous practitioner.

Indigenous peoples have to develop their own system of classifying plants and establish the authenticity of naming. The above simple example indicates that the method and classifications may be both extensive and detailed. Observations include habitat, size, shape, length and width, thickness, moisture content, colour, smell, taste, edibility, maturity and potency, and these will have many subdescriptions and relate to different parts of the vegetation.

However, according to a study of plant classification in Mexico, the terms hot and cold are not applied (6). The nearest indicator might be potency or strength, as hot and cold categories may be likened by their appearance, in the plant's growth and nature, to male and female. Medicinally their actions would differ, the former having more intrinsic energy and speedier and stronger action, the latter being more benign, acting slowly and gently. In spite of the indigenous custom of envisaging all plants as hot or cold, the thousands of medicinal plants recorded by the Spanish on their arrival in the New World were described by their medicinal action, but seldom as hot or cold. The same situation applies to the oldest herbals in use in Europe, and to the extensive records of medicinal plants in other Latin American countries.

Nature and nurture

The fact that hot-cold is not recorded regularly in the plant classifications, herbals and lists of plants collected from indigenous practitioners, may be due to a number of factors. The quality may not be considered relevant and therefore not recorded, or the information is not obtained.

It is the indigenous herbalist's life task to train and acquire the in-depth knowledge of the plants used in treatment. The symptoms of illness which he may encounter far exceed those which can be attributed to hot-cold. Yet without this classification, an extensive range of medicinal plants are used successfully, on the basis of their specific actions. This action will be learnt by practice, as will the ability to identify the plant and know exactly when to pick it according to time of day, moon, month, and also the knowledge of its properties including colour, flavour, and smell, all of which determine its therapeutic value.

The nature of an illness, the variety of organs involved and the degree of the disequilibrium produced will determine the hot-cold category of the illness. The actual hot-cold phenomenon cannot exist other than in relationship to a process in the body or the composition of a plant, food or mineral. It echoes an understanding of the flows of energy inherent in all biological rhythms, and signifies the tendency of action or reaction to the particular substance, whether food or medicine. The information obtained, and the practitioner's ability to classify, are based on an understanding of the various factors involved. This knowledge is unlikely to be imparted, and hence is not recorded, because it is part of a skill or trade secret whose practice presupposes a certain approach, ethic, reverence, acknowledgement of the remedies and their virtues as belonging essentially to God.

The same applies to food. Hot-cold at its simplest represents the fruits of experience in daily life, and diet as such is a minor consideration in conditions where food is eaten in season and fresh, or where availability is limited. This will function best when the awareness of food as it affects the body is more easily recognized. The modern concept that the link between diet and subjective feeling (behaviour) is at best circumstantial is belied in the context of the practitioners of hot-cold as discussed here. The practices would not be continued unless their observance produced some tangible benefit, or were based on ingrained belief of proven value. Where they conflict with current dietary theory, it must be remembered that foods and medicinal plants act by virtue of the nature of their totality, which does not equal the sum total of the analysed parts; and that the whole depends on, and varies with, conditions of soil, climate, time of year, all of which will affect the nutrient and medicinal properties of plants. In some areas plants are being adversely affected by agricultural practices and medicinal plants are losing their efficacy, or even dying out, virtually unnoticed.

Collaboration and conclusion

The majority of research carried out in this field has been done either by social scientists (anthropologists or ethnographers), nutritionists, or other personnel introducing health projects. This research is important in the context of attempts to improve the nutritional status of the people of Latin America. On the whole, the food habits and therapies related to hot-cold have had little in the way of a "good press". Certain aspects have been considered negative, others tolerable. The evaluation does not perhaps do justice to the wisdom behind these practices, because they are not seen in the overall context. "Hot" and "cold" do not in themselves constitute a "humoral theory", or any theory for that matter. They are simply aspects of a set of characteristics, or a reflection of processes within the body which can be learnt and understood, using the criteria relevant to the viewpoint of the system itself. Once learnt, as by the indigenous practitioner, hot-cold is not separate from the inherent properties of a medicinal plant, or food used as medicine, but rather a reflection of these. For the untrained the methods employed are based on their own experience, and are no different from the application of home remedies elsewhere. The fact that a detailed elaboration of the hot-cold classification of food would require paying attention to the underlying qualities and properties of the food (flavour, colour, taste, etc.), and its origin, climatic factors and so on, need not invalidate its use by those who have learnt the classification by rote in their own locality as a means of achieving a balance, a dynamic equilibrium.

However, these factors do not lend themselves to quantitative analysis, an inherent difficulty for a medical administrator. A solution to this situation was initiated by the *Callawaya* themselves, by setting up a National Institute of Natural Medicine, Aymara and Inca Culture. The purpose, which is already being fulfilled, is to teach knowledge of medicinal plants and other remedies to the medical profession, health workers and others at a basic level, as well as diet, i.e., a positive approach to nutrition, based on the Hippocratic doctrine that "there are no illnesses, only sick people" and "food is [the sole] medicine, and medicine, food", without reference to hot-cold, but using locally available foods and incorporating modern knowledge of food values. The absolute thrust of this move is to improve the overall health of the rural and urban population by recognizing and applying the understanding that the system, of which hot-cold is but a part, is fundamentally one of "man inseparable from nature", and that the potential for health and balance lies within the dynamics of nutrition and the ability of man to benefit from, and live with, the climatic and other conditions of the environment. Given the involvement of the medical profession at all levels, there is every prospect that this could become a model for future developments in the region. By providing basic insight, it could also assist in evaluating those aspects of hot-cold which are beneficial though out of favour in the light of present medical theory.

The advent of medicinal plants to Europe from Latin America in the Middle Ages revolutionized European medicine which had been stagnant for 14 centuries. Perhaps history is about to repeat itself in a different form.

II. Spiritism

Spiritism has its origins outside Latin America, in two main streams, both of which found a place in Brazil. The first had its antecedents in the 16th century when African peoples were transported across the Atlantic in a trade which continued for over three centuries. The Yoruba deities as spirit possessors and African language, music and chants provide the focus for both the older *candomble* and the more recent *umbanda* movements. Each involves, in its own way, large sections of the community, many of whom will be seeking help, guidance or healing. Each also incorporates rituals based on old knowledge, the nature and power of plants and symbols, links with medievalism and indigenous Indian, the latter being very tenuous. These deserve mention but will not be considered in detail here.

The other stream, which is more relevant in the sphere of medical practice and healing, and in relation to modern scientific discoveries, originated in France. Kardec (Léon Hippolyte Denizard Rivail, b. 1804) became interested in spirit manifestations popular in France in the early 19th century (following Mesmer and Swedenborg). His studies convinced him that there was "something beyond the control of mere man" and culminated in the *Book of the Spirits* (1857). This dealt with primary causes (universe, human diversity, life, and death), the spirit world (origin and progression of different kinds of spirits, their mission in the mortal world, why past lives are not recalled, and clairvoyance), moral laws and rewards on earth and hereafter.

Kardec's book was brought to Brazil in 1858 and taken up by a group of physicians who were engaged in the practice of homoeopathy (through correspondence with Hahnemann in France), laying on of hands and free treatment for the poor. Spiritism has continued since and provides daily sessions for thousands of people, as well as hospitals, orphanages etc., all free, the key being to work for charity without gain.

Man is seen as a physical body and surrounding fluid-like body (perispirit or aura), a counterpart of the physical, reflecting illnesses in the body, and leaving it at death. Outside of this is a second aura whose colours indicate the state of thought, emotion and desires. These can affect the surrounding current of electrical particles running clockwise. A black space separates these from an outer envelope of similar particles running in a counterclockwise direction, which can be affected by the cosmic forces to which humans are constantly subjected. Thus everything is mental (mind) or cosmic, registered on these auras and visible to a trained medium.

Training requires first of all wanting to cure, being able to receive an advanced curing spirit from the astral plane (an ability depending on one's place on the path), learning about anatomy and positive and negative (electrical) areas on the body, selflessness towards others, purity in heart and body, and great faith in God and His powers. Treatment consists in healing passes, magnetic fluids discharged from the medium's finger tips which realign the disturbed currents, hot and cold breaths (for example, for inflammations and nervous disorders respectively), prescriptions if indicated (usually homoeopathic), and other counselling. The key to cure lies in an absolute faith in the healing power, and in retaining this faith, applying it in daily life along with the practice of charity and service, and recognizing that man reaps as he sows and that the quality of life and progress on the spiritual path lies in his hands now.

Appendix

The Galenic system of medicine

The Galenic system conceives of things as composed of the four elements of fire, air, earth and water, formed by the union of matter, and the four qualities of hot, cold, dry, and moist. The food and drink which humans consume consist of these elements, and in the process of digestion turn into the humours, or bodily juices: blood, phlegm, yellow bile and black bile. They are the nourishment of the tissues, which are formed by them. The elements as such do not exist in the body, but are represented by yellow bile (fire), black bile (earth) and phlegm (water), air being directly supplied by respiration. There are, however, nine possible types of qualitative mixtures, or temperaments—the ideal, in which all qualities are well balanced, four in which one of the qualities, hot, cold, dry or moist, predominates, and four others where the qualities appear in pairs of hot and moist, hot and dry, cold and dry, or cold and moist. The classification extends to other aspects, including age. Youth is hot and moist, manhood hot and dry, and senility cold and moist. Colours, red, white, yellow and black, are due to balance or excess of humours, and to direct external temperature of hot and cold. Faculties, such as imagination, cogitation and memory, are located in the fore, mid and hind brain respectively, and also voluntary motion and sensation. Three spirits (spiritual forces) are recognized: natural (liver, nourishes the body), vital (heart, wrath and desires) and psychic (brain, thinking and passion).

The art of diagnosing and prescribing lies in being able to detect the imbalance, and correct it by choosing a corresponding opposite. The palm of the hand is suggested as a reference point, but pulse is also used.

Knowledge of materia medica was acquired by observation of action, testing (by the physician himself) and study of properties such as taste, colour and odour, and of the primary qualities producing the action (therapeutic). For example, bitter would be hot and dry, sour cold and styptic in action. The need for mixtures arose because more than one organ might be affected in the body. A hot remedy required for a stomach chill might be bad for a sclerotic liver (hot would weaken it), so a strengthener must be added. The method of mixing remedies in proportions or degrees developed into the realms of mathematics. However, it was considered that the ingredients in the compound acted on each other and the mutual interaction produced the result perceived by the body. (Note that food when ingested produces the humours by virtue of the elements contained. Medicines, and food used as such, are not incorporated in the body but act by their form as perceived by the body.)

Difficulties arose increasingly because of the ensuing complexity of procedures designed to provide experimental methods whereby physicians could avoid personally the need to test and trust the results which seemed obvious to their senses. This desire for standardization effectively fossilized medicine for 14 centuries.

REFERENCES

(*1*) AUSTIN, A. L. *Medicina Na'huatl*. Instituto de Investigaciones Históricas, Universidad Autónoma de México, 1975, pp. 16–30.

(*2*) AUSTIN, A. L. & ROYS, R. L. *Ethnobotany of the Maya*. New Orleans, Tulane University, 1931 (Middle America Research Series No. 2).

(3) ACUÑA, H. R. Cross cultural communication, its contribution to health in the Americas. *Bulletin of the Pan American Health Organization*, **13**:111–116 (1979).
(4) DELGAR, M. *Terapéutica indígena de 1493–1588*. Sucre, 1911.
(5) DEDENBACH, S. *The lexical unit sonqo*. St. Andrews University, Department of Spanish and Latin American Linguistics (unpublished document).
(6) BERLIN, B., BREEDLOVE, D. E. & RAVEN, P. *Principles of Tzeltal plant classification*. New York, Academic Press, 1974.

FURTHER READING

Reference *1* above and the following give a comprehensive picture of indigenous medicine, including hot-cold, with ample bibliographies covering both historical and modern studies, also of work undertaken by researchers from outside Latin America. Several of the works are written by doctors, whose interests lie in the educational, social and psychological aspects of indigenous practices and their implications for medicine. Publications and journals suggested include recent articles on the topic.

BALDIZAN, H. & MALDONADO, A. *Historia de la medicina popular Peruana*. Lima, 1944.
BASTO, L. *Salud y enfermedad en el campesino Peruano del siglo XVII*. Lima, Instituto de Etnología y Arqueología, 1957.
CAVERO, G. V. *Supersticiones y medicinas Quechuas*. Lima, 1965.
ESTRELLA, E. *Medicina aborigen*. Quito, 1977.
FRISANCHO, P. D. *Medicina indígena y popular*. Lima, 1971.
FRIZ, F. A. *Antropología, cultura y medicina indígena en América*. Buenos Aires, 1977.
HOMERO, P. N. *Estudio antropológico de la medicina popular de la Puna Argentina*. Buenos Aires, Ediciones Cabargon, 1973.
LABRADOR, J. S. *S. J. la medicina "el Paraguay natural" 1771–76* (ed.) Hannibal Ruiz Moreno. Universidad Nacional Tucumán. 1948.
OBLITAS, P. E. *Magia hechicería y medicina popular en Bolivia*. La Paz, 1971. (incl. reference to two previous books on the subject of *Callawaya*).
PARDAL, R. Medicina aborigen americana. *Boletín de Americanista Moderna* (1937).
PINEDA, D. *Medicina indígena popular*. Lima, Librería Editorial Juan Mejía Bac., 1973.

Publications by Instituto Indígena Interamericana in Mexico, Instituto Indigenista Nacional in Guatemala, Andean Institute in Cusco, Peru, and others by National Universities series. Books on medicinal plants available in print for most countries. Journals: *América Indígena, Ethnomedizin, Medical Anthropology*.

ACKNOWLEDGEMENTS

Thanks are due to Professor D. Gifford and the staff of the Department of Spanish and Latin American Linguistics, St. Andrews University, Scotland, for valuable information and discussion. Some of the material included in this chapter was obtained as a result of a research travel grant made by the Bau Foundation to V. Lennart Lunny.

CHAPTER 4
Ayurveda

P. N. V. Kurup[1]

I. Ayurvedic medicine

Ayurveda means the science of life. This is one of the oldest formulated systems of medicine, which has spread to East and West and also contributed to the development of contemporary medical science. It is considered divine in origin and is widely practised in southeastern Asia, especially in Bangladesh, India, Nepal, Pakistan, and Sri Lanka. There are scattered references to health as well as to diseases in the Vedas (the book of wisdom) especially in the Rig Veda and Atharvaveda. Atharvaveda has as many as 114 hymns which describe the treatment of diseases. Ayurveda originated from this Veda, which is the most ancient text and gives more information than any other extant literature.

According to Hindu philosophy the universe and all the laws of the universe have been decreed by Lord Brahma. He is believed to have taught Ayurveda to Daksha Prajapati who taught it to the Ashwinkumar twins. They in turn taught Lord Indra, who is considered to be the common teacher of all the branches of medicine.

Doctrines of Ayurveda

Ayurveda is based on certain fundamental doctrines known as the *Darshanas* which encompass all sciences—physical, chemical, biological and spiritual. Ayurveda, born out of intuition and revelation, developed in due course into eight well defined specialized branches as indicated below and

---

[1] Formerly, Director, Central Council for Research in Ayurveda and Siddha, and Adviser on Indigenous Systems of Medicine to the Indian Ministry of Health and Family Welfare, New Delhi, India.

two major schools, the School of Physicians (*Atreya sampradaya*) and the School of Surgeons (*Dhanvantri sampradaya*).

The specialties comprise the following:

1. Internal medicine (*kayachikitsa*).
2. Paediatrics (*balachikitsa/kaumarabritya*).
3. Psychological medicine (*grahachikitsa*).
4. Otorhinolaryngology and ophthalmology (*urdwangechikitsa/shalakyatantra*).
5. Surgery (both general and special) (*shalyatantra*).
6. Toxicology (*damshtrachikitsa/agadatantra*).
7. Geriatrics (*jarachikitsa/rasayanatantra*).
8. Science of eugenics and aphrodisiacs (*vrishyachikitsa/vajikaranatantra*).

The basic theories of Ayurveda arise from the concepts of *Panchamahabhutas* and *Tridosha*, which embrace the process of creation and evolution of the universe and all laws of life therein. According to Ayurveda the human body and all matter in the universe are composed of *Panchamahabhutas*. So far as the function of the body is concerned this system considers the body, mind and soul as complementary to one another.

All the physical and physiological processes in the human body and the pathogenesis of various diseases and their symptoms are explained by the theory of the *Tridosha*: three basic constituent complexes in the physiological system—motion (*vata*), energy (*pitta*) and inertia (*kapha*); and the seven *dhatus*: body fluids (*rasa*), blood (*rakta*), muscular tissue (*mamsa*), adipose tissue (*meda*), bone tissue (*asthi*), nerve tissue and bone marrow (*majja*), and generative tissue including sperm and ovum (*shukra*). There are also the waste products (*malas*).

Vata, pitta and *kapha*, the three basic biological elements derived from the five basic physical elements, constitute the bodies of all the living creatures from microbes to man. *Vata* particles control the utilization of energy by various cells and organs for their anabolic as well as katabolic activities. *Vata* also controls the movements of *pitta* and *kapha* and thus controls all the functions and activities of the body. Energy exists in the body in the form of *pitta* particles. *Pitta* particles are responsible for all the biochemical reactions and metabolic processes and supply heat and energy to the body. *Kapha* particles constitute the cellular as well as intracellular structure of the body and maintain the internal environment of the body. They impart strength and stability to the body. The balanced state of *vata, pitta* and *kapha* is health. The imbalanced state of these three *doshas* gives rise to disease. A detailed study of the *Tridosha* principles may reveal that these are nothing but motion, energy and inertia.

There are seven *dhatus* or tissues in the body as already stated. These tissues constitute the supporting or structural units of the body. Each tissue has its own specific metabolic capability which helps it to digest the specific food and to manufacture its associated higher tissues. During such metabolic activity, each tissue forms its specific waste products or *malas*. There are many *malas* or waste products in the body—stool, urine, sweat, nails, hair, etc. Health depends on the balanced state of all the *dhatus*, *doshas* and *malas* both quantitative and qualitative. Ayurveda defines a healthy person as one in whom there is equilibrium of the humours (*tridosha*) and the body tissues with normal digestive as well as excretory functions associated with the gratification of the senses, mind and soul. In the light of these principles Ayurveda considers human beings in their totality and in their subtle relationship with the universe. Its approach is that since disease or proneness to disease occurs due to imbalance in the equilibrium of the three *doshas*, restoration of the equilibrium eliminates the disease. The treatment aims at not only curing the disease but also enhancing the body vitality to combat the disease and minimize the chances of relapse. Ayurveda epitomizes the philosophy of total health care, and naturally the patient as a whole is given considerable importance. The aim of care is therefore to improve his vitality to resist the disease and to strengthen his immune mechanism so that disease automatically is prevented or cured.

For the promotion, prolongation and maintenance of positive health and prevention of disease, Ayurveda prescribes the observation of certain principles: daily routine (*dinacharya*), nightly routine (*ratricharya*), seasonal routine (*ritucharya*) and ethical routine (*sadvrata*), and also emphasizes that one must follow a regulated diet (*ahara*), sleep (*nidra*) and regulated gratification of sex (*brahmacharya*). Thus Ayurveda is not merely medical science but is in fact a way of life.

Diagnosis and treatment

Before starting the treatment the physician examines the patient as a whole and takes a careful note of his internal physiological characteristics and mental disposition. He also studies such other factors as the affected bodily tissues and humours (*dushya* and *dosha*); the individual bodily state (*desha*) and the site in which the disease is located; the strength, resistance and vitality of the patient and the severity of disease in terms of vitiated humours and bodily tissues (*bala*); the time or season of onset of disease or the gravity of the clinical condition (*kala*); the strength of digestion and metabolism (*anala*); individual constitution (*prakriti*); the age of the patient as well as the relation of age with the principal vitiated humour (*vaya*); psychic power (*satva*); the habits of the patient in relation to the vitiated humour (*sathmya*); and dietary habits (*ahara*).

The classics of Ayurveda prescribe two types of examinations—examination of the patient (*rogi pariksha*) and examination of the disease (*roga pariksha*).

In the examination of the patient one or more of the following methods are employed:

1. Pulse examination (*nadi pariksha*). This is undertaken to determine the state of disturbed *doshas* (*vata, pitta* and *kapha*), vital phenomena indicative of particular disease (*roga*), and prognosis with reference to a particular sick person (*rogi*).
2. Urine examination (*mutra pariksha*)
3. Examination of the faeces (*pureesha pariksha*)
4. Examination of the tongue (*jihwa pariksha*)
5. Examination of the eye (*netra pariksha*)
6. Examination through auscultation (*sabda pariksha*)
7. Examination of tactile stimulation (*sparsha pariksha*)
8. Examination of body structures (*akriti pariksha*)

Roga pariksha

Ayurveda advocates *roga pariksha* for the examination of the disease and for the determination of the pathological condition. The line of treatment is based on the presence of a number of etiological factors (*nidana*), such as the degree to which metabolic activity in *dhatus, doshas* etc. is affected and their mode of premonitory signs (*poorva rupa*), onset and the severity of symptoms (*rupa*), on an assessment of the response to possible causative factors (*upashaya*), and on the stage of pathogenesis of the disease or the symptoms.

The following are the mechanisms which determine the manifestation of the disease state and the pathological signs and symptoms in the body.

Due to the etiological factors responsible for the vitiation of humours (*doshas*), a qualitative and quantitative increase of humours takes place (*sanchaya*). These vitiated *doshas* will create imbalance in various body tissues and also liberate waste products (*malas*) that could spread or circulate all over the body (*prasara*) through channels (*srotas*) which may be large (macroscopic) or small (microscopic) in calibre (*khavaigvaya*) and eventually create blockage in the channels (*sthanasamsharva*), or settle in particular body tissues to cause pathological changes. The expression (*vyakti*) of the pathological changes occurs in the form of signs and symptoms, thus permitting a differential diagnosis (*bheda*) to be made.

Treatment of disease consists in avoiding the causative factors, in advising medicines, suitable diet, activity and regimen which will restore the balanced state of the body, or in surgical procedures. It requires the combined effort of the physician, nurse, patient and medicine. The treatment of disease can be mainly classified as *shamana* therapy and *shodana* therapy.

Shamana *therapy*

Elimination of vitiated *doshas* or humours. The process by which the vitiated *dosha* subsides or returns to normal without creating imbalance or other *doshas* is known as *shamana*. The administration of carminatives (*pachana*), digestives (*deepana*), the creation of hunger (*kshudha*) or thirst (*trishna*), exercise (*vyayama*), the sun's rays (*atapa*) and exposure to sun (*marutha*), etc. come under *shamana* therapy.

Shodhana *therapy*

Emesis (*vamana*), purgation (*virechana*), enemas (*basti*), and blood-letting (*nasya* and *rakta mokshana*) are classified under the *shodhana* type of treatment. They are also called *panchakarma* treatment. Ceremonial washing of the patient (*snahna*) and diaphoresis (*swedana*) are two important techniques of treatment in the above categories.

Surgical treatment

Ayurvedic classics also advocate surgical treatment for those diseases which are not curable by medical treatment or in cases where surgical treatment may provide immediate relief. Details of preoperative, operative and postoperative methods are also discussed in the ayurvedic classics.

Diet

Ayurveda lays great emphasis on regulation of diet and other regimens as part of the treatment (*pathya-apathya*).

All therapeutic measures can be classified under *vipareeta chikitsa* and *vipareetathakari*. In *vipareeta chikitsa*, the therapeutic measures, i.e., medicine, diet and activity, antagonize the disease. They include *hetu-vipareeta*, i.e., treatment counteracting the etiological factors; *vyadhi-vipareeta*, i.e., treatment counteracting the various manifestations of disease; and *hetu-vyadhi-vipareeta*, i.e., treatment counteracting the etiological factors as well as various symptomatic manifestations. In *vipareeta-thakari chikitsa*, the therapeutic measures, i.e., medicine, diet and activity, appear to exert effects similar to the etiological factors of the disease process.

Drug sources

The practitioners of Ayurveda normally prepare the medicines needed for their patients in their own clinics. For simple decoctions, powders etc., the physician often advises patients to prepare them in their own homes from locally available herbal resources. However, in urban areas the practitioners give prescriptions to the patient for dispensing by chemists. They also prescribe patent drugs. The large-scale production of ayurvedic drugs is now undertaken by modern technology. These include patent and proprietary drugs and classical preparations. There are as many as 4500 pharmacies which produce these drugs in southeastern Asia. Statutory controls over the manufacture of ayurvedic drugs are also enforced in some countries.

Pharmacopoeia

Ayurvedic scholars have compiled all the available information about the drugs and their therapeutic uses. There are some 70 such books containing about 8000 recipes. Besides these publications there are large numbers of recipes which have not been published but which are in use in everyday practice. Ayurvedic medicines are prepared in the form of distillates (*arka*), fermented preparations (*asava* and *arista*), linctus (*avaleha*), incinerated matter, minerals, shells etc. (*bhasma*), powder (*churna*), ghee (*ghrita*), tablets, pills (*vati gutika*), decoction (*kwatha*), and so on.

Drug action

In Ayurveda the drugs have been classified according to the predominance of one or other of five *bhutas* and in view of this the drug action can be correlated with the particular property of the *bhuta* which is predominant. In addition to pharmacodynamics, the drugs exert their effect through one or more of these properties, though ultimately an action entirely different from the ascribed properties might appear, which is known as *prabhava*.

The various tastes (*rasas*) of the drugs are also the results of permutation and combination of the five *bhutas*. Ayurveda attributes the action of the drug to its various therapeutic qualities. They are indicated as taste (*rasa*), property (*guna*), potency (*veerya*), metabolic changes of taste (*vipaka*), and special action (*prabhava*). The knowledge of the above qualities of a particular drug will assist the physician to select the suitable drug for medication.

Patient-physician relationship

The ayurvedic practitioners are closely related to the society in which they live and practise, and their advice as elders in the village is much sought after in all village activities, whether cultural, social, economic or political. They are accorded great respect by the villagers; the village physician is not merely regarded as a physician but considered as a friend, philosopher and guide by the community. Even today in rural areas these physicians remain the first contact of the villagers in times of illness and difficulties. The village physicians do not normally charge any fees, but the village people generously compensate their services by giving them small gifts. However, in cities and semiurban areas the physicians charge fees like modern practitioners. But in general the charges for treatment by this system are lower than those of modern medicine.

Duration of diagnosis

Even though the physicians in Ayurveda have to carry out detailed examinations of the patient and the disease from various angles, applying a methodology, including intuitive knowledge, as briefly listed above, the time taken to make a diagnosis may be similar to that taken by an allopathic physician.

The preparation of physicians for practice

Ayurvedic practitioners fall broadly into the following groups:

1. Traditionally trained practitioners.
2. Institutionally trained practitioners.
3. Institutionally trained practitioners who have undergone training concurrently in traditional systems of medicine and, to some extent, in modern medicine.

The traditionally trained practitioners, who may be generalists or specialists, possess thorough knowledge, having been directly under the guidance of an expert either as an apprentice or as an understudy over a number of years. The second category comprises practitioners who are trained systematically for 3–5 years in institutes imparting training only in the traditional system of medicine. Even in the olden days renowned schools of ayurvedic medicine existed in southeastern Asia. At present about 150 well established colleges are giving training both at undergraduate and postgraduate levels in various countries. In India a uniform syllabus has been formulated and adopted throughout the country. The duration of undergraduate courses is $5\frac{1}{2}$ years after secondary schooling and the doctorate course is a further 3 years after graduation.

There are a number of professional associations of Ayurveda in the region which are engaged in various activities, including ayurvedic education. The practice in this system is being regulated through registration of both institutionally qualified and traditionally trained practitioners in the registers that are maintained by the Governments concerned. Their sincerity and devotion to service remain exemplary, and malpractice is said to be minimal. This may not be altogether true of some of the considerable number of practitioners who, while not registered with any competent authority, practise nevertheless, especially in the villages.

Research

Research is essential in every department of human endeavour and preeminently in Ayurveda, which has been the mainstay of the people of southeastern Asia for several centuries and continues to contribute largely in medical relief programmes. Research, while rehabilitating and popularizing Ayurveda, will be able to provide a meaningful interpretation of the fundamental principles, medicines and modes of treatment. The methods of research employed in Ayurveda should be such as do not deviate from the basic principles of the system. In considering the different areas of research, the common man should remain the focal point, and the entire gamut of ayurvedic knowledge should be fully utilized for his benefit and welfare. At the moment, research in Ayurveda is being conducted in the following fields:

1. Clinical research oriented not only to determine successful drug therapy but to establish the pathogenesis of disease.
2. Research on the drugs used in Indian medicine and folk practice at multidisciplinary level.
3. A medicobotanical survey of the entire region to assess the availability of medicinal resources.
4. Collection of folk information and recipes not described in classical works.
5. Development of quality control for drugs and pharmaceutical preparations used in Ayurveda.
6. Research into fundamental doctrines on which the medical system is based.
7. Medicohistorical research concerned with Ayurveda and its influence on contemporary systems and society.
8. Research into medical literature interpretation, and the publication of critical editions.

Clinical research is one of the fruitful lines of approach to clarify the principles and methods of diagnosis and treatment of diseases mentioned in classical works. It covers research into the mechanism of causation of a disease, its prevention and cure. As already stated, such investigations should give due regard to the concepts and doctrines enunciated in Ayurveda. Scientists should be well qualified investigators belonging to both ayurvedic and modern systems of medicine. Several advantages could be realized by utilizing the following scheme: (1) diagnosis and treatment strictly according to Ayurvedic principles, (2) diagnosis under ayurvedic and modern principles and treatment in accordance with ayurvedic medicine, (3) diagnosis under modern medical principles and treatment in accordance with doctrines of Ayurveda, and (4) diagnosis and treatment according to modern medical methods.

However fruitful and potent the clinical research might be, it cannot be forgotten that drugs play a key role in the success or otherwise of the treatment. This naturally highlights the subject of drug research, which includes a number of components such as medicobotanical survey, plant cultivation, and pharmacognostic, chemical and pharmacological studies.

The pharmacognostic studies have to be planned so that there can be scientific and uniform methods of checking for authenticity of drugs and plants. There is a need for standardization not only of the raw drugs but also of the methods of manufacture and finished products so that genuine medicinal preparations with proven efficacy can be available for clinical application. The results of research should be evaluated on the basis of possible utilization by the profession and by industry. Such results could be disseminated through workshops, seminars, conferences, and the publication of monographs.

The countries of southeastern Asia permit parallel functioning of their traditional, indigenous systems with the modern health care system. Although integration of the various systems is considered the ultimate goal, certain prerequisites are mandatory, such as the introduction of basic elements of Ayurveda into the curriculum of modern medical education in order to bring about a closer relationship between the two systems.

Every system of medicine has its own merits and demerits. No medical system in isolation can fully meet all the challenges and complexities of health problems in modern times. The various systems must therefore collaborate and pool the available knowledge to their mutual advantage and for the good of the community they endeavour to serve. A realistic approach which appears to have a better chance of achieving the ultimate goal of providing adequate health care coverage for all peoples is to adopt whatever is best in the various health care systems.

The Siddha system of medicine

The Siddha system of medicine owes its origin to the Dravidian culture which is of the prevedic period. An examination of the ancient literature would reveal that the vedic Aryas owed allegiance to the cult of Shiva and the worship of the phallus (*linga*) which was later on absorbed by and incorporated into the vedic culture. The Shiv cult is associated with its medical counterpart, the Siddha system of medicine which is mainly therapeutic. Mercury, sulfur, iron, copper and gold, bitumen, white, yellow and red arsenic, and other minerals as well as vegetable poisons are extensively used in the pharmacopoeia of the Siddha tradition. The Siddha system of medicine is prevalent in the southern states of India, and in Sri Lanka, Malaysia and Singapore where the Dravidian civilization was dominant. The principles and doctrines of this system, both fundamental and applied, have a close similarity to Ayurveda, with specialization in iatrochemistry.

II. Medical astrology

Ayurveda postulates the theory that the human being is a replica of the universe in miniature and has therefore close mutual relationships with it. Permutations and combinations of the influences shed by 12 zodiacs, 27 stars and 9 planets is the basis of astrology. This is yet another area of knowledge based on scientific astronomical facts; it deals with the close relationship between the various celestial bodies and human beings. Astrology therefore supports and runs parallel to the doctrines postulated by Ayurveda. It is for this reason that since ancient times the study of astrology, without which the study of medicine is considered incomplete, has been given great importance in the course of ayurvedic studies.

It is believed that various celestial bodies exert varying degrees of influence on individuals depending upon the position of the planet at the time of their birth and its subsequent placement at different periods of their life. Every human being is radiating energy which is not visible to the naked eye, and the health and general well-being of the individual depend on the harmonious relationship or interaction between the amount of radiation or energy received from the universe and the amount radiated by his own body. A detailed astrological study of the individual horoscope provides the information required for the prediction of an individual's proneness to illness and even the severity and duration of the illness that he is likely to endure. For both Ayurveda and astrology the planetary influences categorize individuals into three groups according to their mental constitution; the *sathvic*[1] characteristic is influenced by the sun, moon and Jupiter, the *rajasic*[2] is influenced by Venus and Mercury, and the *Thamasic*[3] by Saturn, Mars, *Rahu*[4] and *Kethu*[5]. The planets likewise have direct influence on the three humoral factors and together with the sun and Mars cause disturbances of energy (*pitta*), while Venus, the moon and Jupiter cause disturbances of inertia (*kapha*), and Saturn, *Kethu* and *Rahu* cause disturbances of motion (*vata*)[6]. Mercury causes disturbances of all the three *dhatus*.[7] The planets also influence the functioning of the various organs of the body, in the same way as they influence animate and inanimate objects. Therefore astrological studies give the ayurvedic physician the knowledge to select the requisite herbal medicines (which are ruled by the planet having opposing influence to the planets that rule the *doshas*[8]) for correcting the imbalance of *doshas* to cure the disease. Thus

---

[1] Existence, entity, goodness. [2] Royal, kingly. [3] Ignorance, vile, vicious. [4] A demon said to be the cause of eclipses. [5] The last of the 9 planets, flag. [6] Air, wind, rheumatism, gout. [7] Metal, any constituent of the body. [8] Pathological conditions.

the study of astrology enables the ayurvedic physicians not only to diagnose patients accurately but also to make a correct assessment of the root cause of the disease and prescribe the appropriate remedy.

Medical astrology has made an elaborate classification of diseases and the particular planetary combinations that could be influencing them. As an example, the moon rules the mind, the sun controls the soul and Mercury influences the nervous system. Afflictions by the moon and Mercury, and Mars or Saturn generally indicate mental disorders. The influence of the sun, Jupiter, Mars centred on Mercury, or the moon induces schizophrenia. Melancholia is produced by the conjunction of the moon and Saturn. Planetary positions also have an important effect on the periodicity of epidemics of malaria, influenza, etc.

The astrologer's main function is, however, to make a realistic assessment of the personality of man, his physical and mental characteristics, his strengths and weaknesses, and the influences exerted over him by various planets at any given time. Thus it is possible to make predictions about the disease before its occurrence, through astrological study as opposed to the diagnosis made by an ayurvedic physician after the onset of the disease.

Much of the mystery of the human body and its intricate working, and of the life force which controls it, still remain inexplicable despite scientific advances. A study of medical astrology could prove to be of great use to the physician by supplementing his own knowledge. Another contribution that astrology offers to medical science is to provide a working knowledge about diseases that might strike an individual during a certain period of his life and to suggest methods by which he can strive to lessen the adverse effects if not altogether ward off the illness. Here astrology recommends the use of *mantras*. Astrological literature from ancient times is replete with references to this important aspect of *mantra sastra*. The afflictions (*arishtayogas*) merely indicate the deficiency of the requisite or normal energy-quantum and this can be compensated by *mantras* which are nothing but packets or bundles of adjusted forms of sound vibrations.

CHAPTER 5

The Unani system of health and medicare

Hakim Mohammed Said [1]

Unani Tibb or Graeco-Arab medicine may be traced to that system of Greek medicine which was developed during the Arab civilization. The Moslems still call it Unani (Ionian) medicine out of adherence to its true historical derivation, whereas European historians would call it Arab medicine. It is now practised in the Indo-Pakistan subcontinent.

Basic concepts of health and disease

The basic framework consists of the four-humour theory of Hippocrates, which presupposes the presence in the body of four humours: blood, phlegm, yellow bile, and black bile.

The body is regarded as comprising the following:

(1) *Arkan* (elements) comprising the different states of matter and materials entering into and forming a part of everything in the universe.
(2) *Mizaj*—the bodily temperament.
(3) *Akhlat*—the structural components.
(4) *A'da*—the fully developed and mature organs.
(5) *Ruh*—the vital force or life-force.
(6) *Quwa'*—the bodily power.
(7) *Af'al*—the corporeal functions.

It will be seen that these seven working principles are comprehensive in that the *arkan* include the elementary constituents of the body; the *mizaj*, the physicochemical aspects of the body; the *akhlat*, the bodily humours; *a'da*, the anatomy of the body; *ruh*, the life-force or vital force; *quwa'*,

---

[1] Adviser on Tibb to the President of Pakistan, and President of the Hamdard Foundation, Karachi, Pakistan.

energy; and *af'al* the physiology of the body including the biochemical processes.

Temperament (*mizaj*) occupies a very important place in Unani Tibb and forms the basis of pathology, diagnosis and treatment. The temperament of the person to be treated is expressed by the Galenic concept of its being sanguine, phlegmatic, choleric or melancholic, according to the respective preponderance of the humours. In other words the temperament of the individual is equal to the uniqueness of the individual or, in modern terminology, the psycho-neuro-endocrinal system with its orientation tempered differently in each individual. Any change in the temperament brings about a change in the person's state of health. Thus disease is an expression of the imbalance of the humours or the disturbance to their harmony, and of the failure of one or more parts of the body to eliminate pathogenic waste.

The humours are assigned temperaments, i.e., blood is hot and moist, phlegm is cold and moist, yellow bile is hot and dry, and black bile is cold and dry (in their physical temperaments).

Drugs are also assigned temperaments and there are degrees of these temperaments. The temperament of a given drug is assessed by its action on the temperament of the body itself. Thus a drug said to be hot means that, when it enters the body and interacts with the vital faculties, it produces a temperament which is hot. Hence drugs are principally used to correct the abnormal pathological temperament of the body itself or of any particular system or organ.

Concept of preventive medicine and self-care

The basic philosophy of Tibb is that the body, composed of matter and spirit, is taken as a whole because harmonious life is possible only when there is a proper balance between the bodily (physical) and spiritual functions. Unani Tibb seeks the restoration of the body as a whole to its original state.

There is formulated also a power of self-preservation or adjustment (*vis medicatrix naturae*) which strives to restore any disturbance within the limits prescribed by the constitution or state of the individual. This corresponds to the defence mechanism which is called into action in case of injury to the body. In the Unani system of treatment, great reliance is placed on this power, the aim of the physician being to help and develop its action. The consequence is that by the use of Unani medicines not only is the system enabled to overcome the present disturbance through its intrinsic power, but it emerges after recovery with a greater power of resistance to future disturbances. Only in case of immediate and imminent danger to life is it considered necessary to resort to drastic methods of treatment.

In time of epidemics, every precaution in maintaining a balance in diet and general health habits is recommended. Unani practitioners recommend inoculation and immunization against diseases. In the classical literature of Tibb, there are certain prescriptions and prophylactic measures along with general preventive measures against the spread of infectious and contagious diseases.

The healer–patient relationship

The Unani practitioner holds a respectable place in society, particularly in rural communities. In urban areas, *tabibs* are often consulted for treatment of diseases and in matters relating to the protection of health. The *tabibs* adhere to the traditional moral and social values while treating their patients. This ensures an excellent healer–patient relationship which can be favourably compared to the old-style relationship between general practitioner and patient.

Consultation, diagnosis, treatment and management of disease

In large clinics and practices, individual case reports are made on the patients and submitted to the chief physician for study and prescribing. Lady physicians (*tabibas*) examine women, who usually observe purdah, and prescribe or give a report of their ailment to the physician who, after a study of the report, examines the pulse and accompanying pathological reports and then prescribes the medicine.

Diagnosis is carried out in the following manner:

(1) Body heat is measured by pulse, palpation and thermometer.
(2) Urine gives many indications of disorders in kidney and liver and in the organs of digestion, and plays an important part in the Unani system.
(3) Examination of stools helps in the diagnosis of certain diseases. (Laboratory examinations of urine and stools are made.)
(4) Observation, palpation and percussion are used to diagnose diseases of internal organs. Every disease is fully described in Unani literature with its symptoms, points of differential diagnosis, and all its complications. A detailed examination of a patient entails studying the person as a whole. The tongue gives an indication of the condition of the blood and functions of the digestion. The eyes, lips, teeth, throat and tonsils have all indicative signs together with other physical conditions and secretions. Sleep, fear or grief, anger or happiness also provide indicative signs.

The prescriptions are begun with the legend *Howash Shafi* (God is the Healer), generally in the Persian language. The prescriptions contain detailed instructions about the dosage and the preparations of medicine. The medicine is prescribed initially for three days, the treatment being continued or changed according to the response of the patient. A strict diet is also prescribed.

General features of the pharmacopoeia

The pharmacopoeia consists of an extremely rich armamentarium of natural drugs, mainly herbal but also including animal, mineral and marine drugs. The drugs can be used singly or as polypharmaceuticals, in the form of decoctions, infusions, tablets, powders, confections, syrups and aquas.

It is true that the Unani pharmacopoeia is lacking in detailed experimental, physicochemical and biomathematical data, but it is nearly always safe. One keynote of Unani medicine is that the drug should not serve as a quick curative and in the end generate serious side-effects such as those sometimes observed with synthetic drugs. Another aspect of its approach is that the physical faculties (temperament) should be allowed to function according to their own nature and at their own speed under the operation of the natural laws, and that their functioning should be given help in every possible way.

Professional services and remuneration

Most of the *tabibs* either conduct an individual practice or operate in hereditary clinics or larger clinics with a chief physician and junior physicians under him. Generally no consultation fee is charged but, on account of rising costs, some *tabibs* have started charging nominal fees. In the case of house calls, a *tabib* does not take fees from patients living in his own locality or home town.

Generally, dispensaries are attached to the clinics, and the *tabibs* derive their income from the sale of the medicines dispensed.

Medical education

There are two categories of Unani practitioners:

(1) Academically qualified from recognized institutes.

(2) Academically unqualified, but having long practical experience in the family tradition.

There are Unani medical colleges for the education and training of practitioners. The course of study is four years, but recommendations have been made to make it five years to bring it in line with the allopathic course of studies. The syllabus and curricula include anatomy, the Canon of Avicenna, physiology, pharmacology, psychology, hygiene, pharmacy, medicine, fevers, medical jurisprudence, surgery, clinical diagnosis, obstetrics, pathology, gynaecology, paediatrics, and infectious and tropical diseases.

A special feature of Unani medical education is that modern medical knowledge is juxtaposed with Unani medical knowledge in such a way that a *tabib*, while specializing in his own system and techniques, also acquires knowledge of contemporary medicine.

Organization of practitioners, discipline, and recognition

There are national and provincial Tibbi associations responsible for the professional and collective problems of *tabibs*. Since the official recognition of Unani medicine by the Governments of Pakistan and India, regulating bodies have been set up in the ministries of health. In Pakistan, the National Council for Tibb has come into being; its Chairman is the Adviser on Tibb to the President of Pakistan. This Council represents the whole country, and its members are nominated by the Government. The Council prescribes the syllabus, holds examinations, awards certificates, and is responsible for registration. In India, a separate Directorate of Unani medicine has been set up under the Ministry of Health and Family Welfare to perform similar functions.

Special laws promulgated by the Government regulate the practice of medicine and protect people from malpractices. A Drug Control Bill is in preparation, with special emphasis on the manufacture of medicines, their standardization and use.

Research

Since time immemorial man has made use of natural medicines in the treatment of disease. Although purely synthetic compounds are being employed in increasing measure in modern clinical practice, interest in the examination of plants as potential sources of new drugs has never waned. No medicinal plant traditionally employed in the treatment of disease can be dismissed as an "old wives tale". Many active antibiotics occur in plants and this is still an unexploited field. In fact we are on the threshold of plant analysis and research. When it is said that *Saraca indica* is useful in menorrhagia, or *Cephalandra indica* (= *Coccinea cordifolia*) in diabetes, or *Boerhaavia diffusa* in dropsy, the scientific mind is not satisfied with mere statements, no matter from what source they originate, unless they are corroborated by clinical and experimental evidence. The active principles responsible for the therapeutic action have to be isolated and analysed; the way in which the effect is brought about and the manner in which the important organs are affected have to be studied. For example, *Podophyllum* and its resin have long been known to cause irritation of mucous membranes and even skin. It is probably knowledge of this which initiated the use of *Podophyllum* resin to destroy soft warts or condylomatas. The excellent work done by Dr Salimuzzaman Siddiqui, Sir Ram Nath Chopra and others has demonstrated the vast scope for research in medicinal plants. In Pakistan, investigations of *Tamarix dioica* and *Peganum harmala* have disclosed astounding results. The efficacy of *Tamarix dioica* in jaundice and *Rauvolfia serpentina* in hypertension are beyond doubt, and the abundance of *Artemisia, Ephedra,* and other medicinal botanicals warrant pharmacological studies on their therapeutic value. With the growth of pharmaceutical institutions and chemical laboratories in universities both in Pakistan and India, a good deal of progress in research has been done. Plant drugs like *Adhatoda vasica, Psoralea corylifolia, Swertia chirata* (= *Agathotes chirayta*), *Plantago ovata, Nardostachys jatamansi, Lavandula stoechas* and others have come under investigation. Still another 2000 plants remain to be investigated and there is a likelihood that some of these may be effective in the treatment of disease and in medical care.

Research studies are being carried out in the Councils for Scientific and Industrial Research and the results published in their respective journals. In Pakistan, recently, an official programme for research has been instituted with the setting up, under a Presidential ordinance, of a National Council for Tibb which has activated the National Council for Tibbi Research with hakims, doctors and scientists constituting its members. As a result, three high-level committees have commenced work: the Pharmacopoeia Committee, the Herbs Committee and the Tibbi Drugs Act Committee. A five-year plan for research in medicinal plants costing about Rs. 1.5 crore[1] has also been prepared.

Interest in medicinal plants is being manifested in the Middle Eastern countries. The Government of Kuwait has already started a programme for a large and modern research centre for medicinal plants. It is expected that other governments will follow suit.

Coordination or integration

The future of medicine lies in a tripartite alliance of the *tabib*, the doctor and the scientist. Traditional practitioners, modern doctors and scientists must make joint efforts for new developments in the field of research. The following is a classic example of such efforts.

Acupuncture, a traditional form of therapeutics in China in unbroken practice over four millennia, used to be dismissed by modern medicine as a lot of old-fangled nonsense. In recent years, however, the alliance of the traditional physician, doctor, scientist and politician has reestablished it not only as a curative measure but also as a form of anaesthesia in surgical

---

[1] Rs. 1.5 crore = US $1.8 million.

operations with astonishing results. Instances like this can be multiplied and exploited for human health and welfare.

In developing countries such collaboration depends to a great extent on official or governmental attitudes. There can be no individual approach to the problem of coordination. The starting point should be the hospital, where a separate wing for coordinated therapeutics should be established and the patient given the choice of treatment, i.e., Unani only, or a combined form of treatment after mutual consultation between the Unani practitioner and the modern doctor. But this can be done only when the modern medical curriculum includes the Unani system of medicine as a subject for short-term study. This too requires a basic change of attitude on the part of modern medicine and a swing to innovative or universal medicine—a combination of traditional and modern medicine—which will rightly be the medicine of the future.

FURTHER READING

BAQUAI, F. U. *Traditional medicine in Pakistan.* Karachi, Hamdard Foundation, 1977.
CAMPBELL, D. *Arabian medicine and its influence on the Middle Ages.* New York, AMS Press (reproduction of the 1926 edition).
CHOPRA, R. N. *Indigenous drugs of India.* Calcutta, U. N. Dhur & Sons, 1958.
GRUNER, O. C. *Commentary on the Canon of Avicenna.* Karachi, Hamdard Foundation, 1967.
HAMEED, H. A. *Attemperament in medicine.* Karachi, Hamdard Foundation, 1979.
NADKARNI, A. K. *Indian materia medica.* Bombay, Popular Book Depot, vols. 1 & 2, 1954.
SAID, H. M., ed. *Hamdard pharmacopoeia of eastern medicine.* Karachi, Institute of Health and Tibbi Research, 1969.
SAID, II. M. *Traditional Greco-Arab and modern Western medicine: conflict or symbiosis.* Karachi, Hamdard Foundation, 1979.
SHAH, M. H. *Canon of Avicenna* (English translation). Karachi, Interservices Press, 1966.
Theories and philosophies of medicine, 2nd ed. New Delhi, Institute of History of Medicine and Medical Research, 1973.
The wealth of India: a dictionary of indigenous raw materials and industrial products. New Delhi, Council of Scientific and industrial research, vols. 1-4, 1948-56.

CHAPTER 6
Traditional Chinese medicine

Wang Pei[1]

The splendid culture of the ancient times had a rich store of medicine, some elements of which, with the development of modern medicine, were discarded while others were preserved and handed down to posterity. A few were further developed and spread far and wide among the people. Traditional medicine has made a great contribution to the welfare of all nations in the world.

In the present era of highly developed modern medicine, it is necessary to give due regard to the traditional medicine of all nations, as our experience in the development of traditional Chinese medicine has shown. We firmly believe that the integration of traditional medicine with modern medicine helps to correct the deficiencies of each and will certainly promote the development of medical science in the future.

Traditional Chinese medicine, with its rich clinical experience, its unique theoretical system and its extensive literature has served to combat illness among the Chinese people over many centuries. It represents the crystallization of the Chinese people's wisdom and experience. What has proved effective in clinical practice has been preserved, handed down from generation to generation, and continually improved upon. A few examples only are given below.

The early stage of medical activities dates from the beginning of human society. The historical documents of ancient China contained some legends about it, but the earliest recorded history of traditional medicine was in 1800 B.C., the beginning of the Shang dynasty. Certain oracle-bone writings, the oldest form of Chinese writing carved on scapulae and tortoise shells and used for divination, that were unearthed from the ruins of the Yin dynasty bear inscriptions naming and describing various kinds of illnesses and indicating elementary methods for the classification of diseases. For instance, head disease was called *Ji Shou*; eye disease, *Ji Mu*;

---

[1] Director, Central Laboratory, Academy of Traditional Chinese Medicine, Beijing, China.

ear disease, *Ji Er*; abdominal ailment, *Ji Fu*; diseases of the foot, *Ji Zu* and so forth. The character 蛊 (*gu*), which means a venomous insect, was formerly written like 𮫙, which indicates that there are parasites in the abdomen; and the character 齲 (*qu*), meaning decayed tooth, was written like 𮫚, which indicates that a tooth is being eaten by insects. These are the earliest records on dental caries and parasites.

More remarkable yet are the notions of hygiene and preventive measures appearing between 1400 and 1200 B.C. For instance, the character 浴 (*yu*), meaning "bath", was formerly written like 𮫛 on oracle bones. 𮫜 indicates "person", 𮫝 "water", and 𮫞 "bath tub". Oracle bones also record "sprinkling of water to remove the dust, sweeping, and getting rid of insects". These excavated cultural relics from the ruins of the Yin dynasty show that there were already at that time sties and folds for domestic animals, lavatories and drainage trenches.

The *Book of Rites*, a manual of ceremonies written in the Zhou dynasty (1100 to 800 B.C.), records that there were specialized doctors in four departments, namely: nutrition, internal medicine, surgery, and veterinary medicine. It also stipulates that "Doctors are in charge of medical laws and decrees". "If one gets ill one should be treated. If one dies of a certain disease, the cause of death should be recorded and made known among the doctors." This is probably the earliest medical case-recording system. It also makes it a rule to assess doctors' knowledge and skills annually so as to determine their salary grade. The famous medical book of our country, *Internal Classic* or *Yellow Emperor's Internal Classic*, the oldest and most comprehensive work on medicine still extant, which appeared around 300 B.C., is a combination of medical theory and clinical practice (*1*). This book is in 18 volumes; it emphasizes the basic theory of traditional Chinese medicine and contains substantial information on hygiene, clinical symptoms, prescriptions and drugs, acupuncture and moxibustion, and so forth.

The theory of yin-yang, viscera and bowels, and meridians recorded in the *Internal Classic* has become the foundation for the basic theory of traditional Chinese medicine. Anatomy was already in the embryonic stage and some anatomical data were analysed. For instance, the length of the digestive tract, from pharynx to rectum, was measured by adding up the length of different segments; the recorded length was similar to that found by modern anatomical measurement. Over 300 signs and symptoms were also described. For instance, in dealing with the symptoms of cervical lymphatic tuberculosis, the book also correctly portrays its relation with visceral tuberculosis. Besides medicinal treatment, the *Internal Classic* records many non-medicinal therapies such as acupuncture and moxibustion, massage, *dao ying* (a combination of deep breathing and self-massage) and so forth. Of special significance is the detailed record on the treatment of ascites by abdominal tapping. A thin needle was inserted at *guanyuan* point, 7½ cm below the umbilicus; the abdomen was then punctured with a hollow needle to drain the ascitic fluid, the needle being kept in the abdominal cavity until the fluid had drained to a certain degree. A tight abdominal bandage was then applied to avoid adverse effects resulting from the sudden change in intra-abdominal pressure. Such an operation and postoperative procedure reflect the wisdom and the medical knowledge of ancient doctors. The *Internal Classic* still remains an essential textbook in the colleges and schools of traditional Chinese medicine.

From the Chin and Han dynasties down to the Ming dynasty (A.D. 1700) the empirical medicine of China forged ahead with great success. For instance, the Chinese medical scientists invented the method of variolation or inoculation to prevent smallpox. It was an important invention in the history of human preventive medicine and one that pioneered modern immunology. At the time of Song Zheng-zong (A.D. 998–1022), a Taoist priest in the Mount E-mei had the son of Minister Wang Dan inoculated. Towards the latter part of the 16th century, variolation was widely used in China. In 1688, Russia sent doctors to Peking to learn this method, and it was thereby introduced to Turkey and Europe. It was only after inoculation with cowpox had been invented by Jenner in 1796 that variolation was gradually abandoned.

There are various kinds of treatment in traditional Chinese medicine. Some original non-medicinal treatments such as acupuncture, moxibustion and massage were introduced over 3000 years ago. Some very rich experience has also been gained in using natural herbal medicines to treat diseases. Drug anaesthesia was applied in laparotomy in the 2nd century; harelip operation was performed in the 3rd century; the treatment of scabies, tinea and carbuncles by mercurial ointment was used in the 4th century; couching of cataract with gold needles was adopted in the 5th century; and false teeth with amalgam were introduced in the 7th century. The treatment of vertebral fracture by suspension, reduction, etc. was introduced in the 12th century. These are perhaps some of the earliest methods of treatment recorded in the history of medicine.

China also has a rich store of books on pharmacology. The *Xin Xiu Ben Cao* (Newly Revised Materia Medica) of the Tang dynasty in the 7th century is the earliest pharmacopoeia promulgated by the government. In the 12th century, the Song dynasty published *Tai-Pin Hui-Min He Ji Ju Fang* which is the world's earliest prescription book of pharmacy issued by the government. In the 17th century, during the Ming dynasty, in his *Ben Cao Gang Mu* (Compendium of Materia Medica), Li Shi-zhen, the world-famous pharmacognosist, collected 1892 kinds of herbal drugs and 11 000 prescriptions. Charles Darwin in *The Variation of Animals and Plants under Domestication* referred to the *Ben Cao Gang Mu* as a Chinese encyclopaedia.

To date, traditional Chinese medicine has generated over 10 000 medical books, 5000 kinds of herbal drugs, and a rich experience of clinical therapy. Traditional Chinese medicine and pharmacology have not only contributed much to the development and prosperity of the Chinese people, but have also had an important influence on the development of medical science in general.

It is a matter for regret that, for various historical reasons, traditional Chinese medicine was not able to participate earlier in the experimental sciences. For many decades, modern or Western medicine has forged rapidly ahead whereas the progress of traditional Chinese medicine since the Ming and Qing dynasties has been much slower in comparison. Under such unfavourable conditions, there have been two different attitudes toward traditional Chinese medicine: one tendency was to eliminate the system and replace it by modern medicine, or eliminate the practice but preserve its effective drugs and prescriptions only; and the other was to accept this precious legacy and develop it with modern scientific knowledge and methods into a unified medicine and pharmacology with the characteristic style of China.

In 1929 the central government of Kuomintang passed a bill "to ban the traditional medicine in order to clear the way for developing medical work". But they did not succeed in banning and replacing it. In the first place, people in the vast rural areas and both the common people and the upper class in many cities earnestly believed in traditional medicine. Secondly, the use of traditional Chinese medicine and medicinal herbs did yield rather satisfactory results in the treatment of diseases, including some diseases intractable by modern medicine. Traditional remedies could reduce symptoms and even produce remission. Moreover, Chinese medicinal herbs were readily available at low cost, were convenient and simple to use, and had very few side-effects. They therefore enjoyed much popularity with the vast majority of people. Thirdly, traditional medicine had a unique theoretical system which can neither be replaced nor explained by modern science, including the theory of yin-yang, vital energy and blood, and so forth. Traditional Chinese medicine has thus survived and has never been eliminated in spite of the persecution it suffered before the liberation. However, it was only after the founding of the People's Republic of China that traditional Chinese medicine entered a new period of development.

The liberation

Since the founding of the new China, our Government has attached great importance to traditional Chinese medicine, giving energetic support to it and taking effective measures to speed up its modernization.

"To foster unity between Chinese and Western-trained doctors" is one of the four principal policies for health work laid down by the Government since the inauguration of the People's Republic of China. Later, the policy on traditional Chinese medicine was formulated according to the actual needs of our country. The main points of the policy are as follows:

(1) To strive to inherit, develop, systematize and raise the level of traditional Chinese medicine;

(2) to unite and rely on the traditional Chinese doctors so as to give full effect to their initiative;

(3) to organize ways for Western-trained doctors to learn and study traditional Chinese medicine;

(4) to modernize traditional medicine and pharmacology gradually;

(5) to develop traditional Chinese medicine and conduct research on the integration of traditional Chinese and Western medicine in a planned and rational way;

(6) to protect, utilize and develop the resources of Chinese medicinal herbs.

In order to ensure the implementation of this policy, a parent organization in charge of traditional medicine has been established within the Government. The Ministry of Public Health has set up a bureau of traditional medicine, while departments of traditional medicine have also been placed under the provincial and municipal bureaux of public health.

As a result of the implementation of the traditional medicine policy and a series of effective measures to promote it, traditional Chinese medicine has developed greatly in the last 30 years.

First, the position of traditional doctors and the condition of the traditional hospitals have changed tremendously. Before the liberation, Chinese medicine was regarded as illegal, and was discriminated against and eschewed. It was only after the liberation that Chinese medicine gained its legal status. Since then, 280 000 doctors of traditional medicine have been invited to work in the state and collective medical organizations such as hospitals, medical schools and research institutes. Chinese medicine and Chinese materia medica have become a part of free medical care. In the hospitals of Western medicine, departments of traditional medicine together with its pharmacies and wards have all been accommodated.

In order to enable traditional doctors to master some modern science and technology, many provinces and municipalities have organized various types of training and orientation courses for teachers of traditional medicine and advanced courses for traditional doctors to study and raise their level of modern science. These have brought about fundamental changes in both the social status and the academic position of traditional doctors.

There have also been great developments in the hospitals of traditional Chinese medicine. China now has 552 hospitals of traditional medicine above the county level and almost all the hospitals of Western medicine have set up departments of traditional medicine; the larger hospitals with better facilities have even instituted research laboratories to explore the problems relating to the integration of traditional Chinese medicine with Western medicine. By the end of 1979, 91 county and municipal hospitals had been established in 102 municipalities and counties in Hunan province, not including the provincial hospitals and the general hospitals where traditional Chinese medicine has the chief position. These traditional hospitals have assumed a great many medical functions. For example, in the traditional hospital of Chang De, the number of outpatients has reached 3 700 000, while 20 880 patients have been hospitalized since its establishment.

In addition, the barefoot doctors working in the rural areas have all received appropriate training in both Western and traditional methods of treatment, but most of them mainly apply acupuncture and herbal treatment. These 1 600 000 barefoot doctors have greatly contributed to the medical service in the rural areas, which have an estimated population of 800 million.

The educational and training curriculum for traditional Chinese medicine has been strengthened. At present, there are 24 institutions of higher learning for traditional medicine with 18 000 students, and 18 secondary schools with 10 000 students. Moreover, the students in the Western medical colleges are also obliged to pursue courses in traditional medicine. Faculties of traditional Chinese medicine have been established in 11 Western medical colleges.

The production of Chinese herbal medicines has increased, and has gradually developed into an industrial system in the last 30 years. The staff engaged in purchasing, processing and supplying medicinal herbs now total 220 000. The area under cultivation of medicinal herbs has reached 6 million *mu* (400 000 hectares). The amount of medicinal herbs purchased totals 13 million tonnes. At present there are more than 800 pharmaceutical factories with 80 000 workers in them, which produce some 2000 varieties of medicinal herbs. With increasing modernization in the pharmaceutical factories, the quality of herbal medicine has greatly improved. During the nationwide quality appraisal drive in 1979, herbal medicine won three gold and four silver medals.

Efforts made to integrate traditional Chinese medicine with Western medicine have proved truly worth while. Only through close cooperation between the traditional and Western-trained doctors, each learning from the other, and especially through the study of traditional Chinese medicine with modern scientific knowledge and technology, can the development of traditional Chinese medicine proceed more speedily. For many years, the Central Government, provinces and municipalities have organized many orientation courses for Western-trained doctors to study traditional Chinese medicine; thus many doctors specialized in both Western and traditional medicine have been trained. Now, there are three types of doctor in our country—namely, traditional, Western-trained, and Western-trained with qualifications in traditional medicine. These categories are advancing along the road to an integration of traditional and Western medicine to achieve a unified new medicine and pharmacology. We have obtained encouraging results from scientific research on the combination of Chinese and Western medicine, for example in the fields of acupuncture and moxibustion, acupuncture analgesia, acute abdominal conditions, burns, injury of bones and joints, anal fistulas, lithiasis of the urinary tract, cardiovascular diseases, cataract, and respiratory diseases in infants. The effect of the combined treatment of the above-mentioned conditions is much better than that of either system applied alone. Applying modern scientific knowledge and technology, encouraging research results have been obtained also regarding the hypotheses on which traditional medicine is based. These include the theory of yin-yang, visceral manifestations, vital energy and blood, meridians, the method of promoting the blood circulation and relieving stasis, reinforcing vitality, etc.

* * *

Traditional Chinese medicine certainly deserves attention and high priority. It contains some scientific elements which will surely make a contribution to mankind if we conscientiously explore and systematize it by modern scientific method and technology. A more realistic policy is required to protect and develop the system instead of discriminating against it or trying to eliminate or replace it. Only thus can traditional Chinese medicine develop and progress. The integration of the two systems requires careful study. These two schools of medicine should be mutually supporting and complementary and there should be no strife. Traditional medicine could then contribute more to the welfare of mankind. Much has already been gained from traditional Chinese medicine in the field of public health and in the development of medical science. We would like to share this experience with all interested health workers.

It is encouraging to note that more and more countries have become interested in traditional Chinese medicine. One hundred and fifty scientists and doctors from 34 countries and territories attended the Symposium on Acupuncture and Acupuncture Anaesthesia held in Beijing in 1979 and this kind of international activity will no doubt increase.

What are the future prospects of traditional Chinese medicine? An analysis of our 30 years' experience tells us that traditional Chinese medicine will continue to develop steadily through the judicious application of modern science and technology. The combined treatment of certain intractable conditions such as malignant tumours, cardiovascular and degenerative diseases and senility is likely to be more efficacious. The non-surgical treatment of certain diseases such as acute abdominal conditions will be popularized so that it can alleviate patients' suffering and reduce medical expenditure. At the same time, the mechanism of its therapeutic effect and basic theory will be further elucidated. Consequently, the integration of Chinese medicine and Western medicine has a particularly bright future.

Science and technology are the common wealth of mankind. Traditional Chinese medicine is an old and yet quite a young science, and its development and improvement naturally require the common efforts of scientists all over the world. Traditional Chinese medicine will always have an important role in the cultural exchange between the Chinese people and the people of other countries. Let us carry on the exchange and the cooperation our ancestors initiated!

REFERENCE

(1) VEITH, I., transl., *The Yellow Emperor's classic of internal medicine.* Berkeley, CA, University of California Press, 1967.

CHAPTER 7

Acupuncture and moxibustion

I. Theory and practice Wei Ru-Shu[1]

Acupuncture and moxibustion have been applied as therapeutic medical techniques in China for at least 2000 years since the time when stone knives and other sharp instruments were used. Because of the wide indication of these therapeutic procedures, the simplicity of their application, their minimum side-effects, and their low cost and rapid effect they have permanently remained popular.

Acupuncture is an apparently simple clinical procedure for inducing stimulation in various locations of the body to treat disease and alleviate pain. The term itself is derived from the Latin words *acus* (a needle or pin) and *punctura* (a pricking).

Channels, collaterals and acupuncture points

Acupuncture requires knowledge of the system of anatomy and pathophysiology which is inherent in Chinese traditional medicine. The human body is thought to be pervaded by a system of energy channels or *jing luo*, in which vital energy or force circulates. The majority of the acupuncture loci are in these channels, although systems of loci are also located on the human ear, forming the basis of so-called auriculo-acupuncture.

Some practitioners of acupuncture still adhere strictly to traditional Chinese medical theory, while others use acupuncture empirically, without reference to the Chinese theory, and strictly in accordance with Western-style diagnosis and concepts of pathophysiology. Internationally there is a diversity of opinions regarding the techniques of acupuncture, the prerequisite qualifications of an acupuncturist, the usefulness of the notion

---

[1] Professor of Internal Medicine, Institute of Acupuncture and Moxibustion, Academy of Traditional Chinese Medicine, Beijing, China.

of channels, and the specificity of acupuncture points in acupuncture therapy.

In the network of channels and collaterals, the channels constitute the main trunks which run longitudinally and deeply in the body and relate to each viscus, while the collaterals which represent the branches of the channels run transversely and superficially from the channels.

The system of channels and collaterals includes the 12 regular channels, the 8 extra channels, and the 15 collaterals. A crisscross network of channels and collaterals in which blood and *qi* (vital energy) circulate is spread over the body. Internally they connect with the viscera and externally with the four extremities and the superficial tissues and organs. Their action is to regulate the function of different organs, transport blood and vital energy and connect external with internal organs, thus making the body an organic whole. Dysfunction of the channels and collaterals is an important cause of disease.

An acupuncture point is the site where acupuncture and moxibustion are applied. Points may be either on the regular channels or on the extra channels; the latter are called *ahshi* points. Over 360 points have been identified along the 14 channels. The points which are not on the 14 channels but have specific therapeutic properties are called extraordinary points and number several hundreds. The tender or sensitive spots on which acupuncture and moxibustion are applied are also termed *ahshi* points. Points are not only the pathways for the circulation of nutrient *qi* and defensive *qi*, and the focus of common vital energy, but also represent the points of entry of pathogenic elements, the locus of response to diseases and the site of treatment. Every point has its own therapeutic property.

Three indications are used for selecting points. First, the distal points; according to the principle of minute differentiation of the symptom-complex the points of some channels which are directly connected with the affected viscus or have an interior or exterior relationship to the involved part, named the distal points, are those most frequently used. Secondly, the points which are at the site of the disease or adjacent to it and are termed local points; and thirdly, the empirical points which are specific for certain diseases and sometimes represent *ahshi* points. These three methods of selection are often used in combination. The action at the point is to remove any obstruction of the channels and collaterals, regulate the circulation of vital energy and blood, and adjust the function of visceral organs and the yin-yang balance. By this means bodily resistance to exogeneous pathogens is enhanced and diseases can be combated.

Technique

Thin filiform needles are inserted into various parts of the body for the intended treatment of a variety of disease states and, since 1958, for inducing analgesia for surgical procedures. The needles are usually left *in situ* for 15–30 minutes or longer. They may be manipulated by hand in twirling or push-pull movements and may be electrically activated by pulsatile electrical stimulation. It has been claimed that an acupuncture-like effect can also be obtained by deep finger pressure, so-called acupressure. Other more recent approaches to the stimulation of acupuncture points include the use of ultrasound and lasers.

Moxibustion represents a special form of point stimulation. The procedure involves burning a piece of the Chinese drug plant, *Artemisia vulgaris*, either on the head of the acupuncture needle so as to conduct heat into the body, or in some cases actually on the surface of the skin. The importance of this procedure can be seen from the Chinese term for acupuncture, *zhen diju*, which literally means "needling-moxibustion".

The therapeutic methods of acupuncture and moxibustion

There are many therapeutic methods which make use of acupuncture and moxibustion. Beside the traditional ones which are still widely used today, new methods developed by combining modern scientific techniques with the traditional Chinese acupuncture and moxibustion are constantly being introduced. These include electro-acupuncture therapy, low frequency electric therapy, point injection with minimal doses of drugs, point magnetic therapy, catgut imbedding into the point, and point laser radiation. Some examples of the current practice of acupuncture therapy, finger pressing therapy or acupressure, and moxibustion are briefly given below:

Acupuncture needles. There are filiform needles, three-edged needles, plum-blossom needles and ear needles, all generally made of stainless steel. The filiform needle is the main one used in ordinary clinics and has various lengths (1.0–15 cm) and diameters (0.27–0.46 mm).

The filiform needle is selected according to the depth of the site of the disease, the thickness of the muscle and skin, and the required depth of insertion. Depending on the degree of the sensation of soreness, numbness and distension manifesting itself, either reinforcement is applied to *xu* or the insufficiency syndrome, or reduction applied to *shi* or the syndrome of excess. For those diseases in which neither *xu* nor *shi* is clear, both manipulations may be used.

The three-edged needle is applied for purposes of blood-letting, and often for patients with high fever.

The plum-blossom needle is used for tapping and exploring the skin of the affected area and its adjacent parts.

The ear needle is employed for press acupuncture at the sensitive point of the corresponding region of the ear which is then compressed and the needle fixed with adhesive plaster.

Finger-pressing therapy or acupressure. This method is used to treat disease by pressing the points with the thumb or middle finger or with the free edge of the finger nail. For example, pressing at *renzhong* may relieve an attack of epilepsy, fainting and shock; pressing at *hegu* may stop toothache and check an attack of asthma, pressing at *fengchi* may abolish dizziness and peculiar sensations in the head.

Moxibustion. The main material currently in use is moxa wool or moxa wool mixed with Chinese herbs which can stimulate the energy flow in channels and collaterals, ameliorate syndromes arising from cold or wind, and promote the circulation of blood and vital energy. The moxa wool, shaped into a moxa stick (20 cm long and 1.4 cm in diameter), is made of dry moxa leaves (*Artemisia vulgaris*) ground into a cotton-like substance with any impurities removed.

The methods of application vary and are summarized as follows:

(*a*) Moxibustion with moxa cone: there are two kinds, the direct and the indirect; the smallest cone is like a grain of rice, with the diameter at the base 0.4–0.7 cm and the height 0.3–1.0 cm. Direct moxibustion is performed by placing the cone directly on the point and then igniting it. Two varieties are used; scarring and non-scarring moxibustion. Indirect moxibustion is also called partition moxibustion since some materials such as ginger, garlic, salt, onion, aconite and monkshood are placed between the cone and the point.

(*b*) Moxibustion with moxa-stick: the ignited moxa-stick (2.0 cm long) is placed on the top of the needle handle, or else a piece of moxa wool is so placed, and when the needle has been inserted into the point the moxa is ignited.

The indication for moxibustion is mainly "insufficiency *xu* syndrome" and "cold syndrome". Moxibustion at *zusanli* and *guanyuan* points is said to improve general health.

The basic theory of acupuncture and moxibustion

Acupuncture and moxibustion are not only simple practical skills. They are governed by a comprehensive theoretical system which guides the clinical practice. The theories are based on the concept of yin-yang; the five elements—viscera, channels and collaterals, *qi* (vital energy) and blood. The etiology derives from the theory relating to the viscera: channels and collaterals constitute the core. A good clinician and practitioner of acupuncture and moxibustion applies the above theories. In practice he will ascertain symptoms and signs through a carefully taken case history and appropriate physical examination. A review of the clinical findings enables the practitioner to determine whether the ailment is exterior (muscle or skin, collateral) or interior (yang, yin viscus; *fu*, yang viscus; or channel), in the blood or *qi*; and to differentiate further the nature of the disease such as *xu* or *shi*; cold or heat, yin or yang. By these means minute etiological differentiations can be made and the practitioner can accurately treat the disease and achieve a desirable result.

Indications

Acupuncture is used clinically in several ways, as a primary treatment or in combination with other therapeutic methods, and as an adjunctive treatment.

The textbook, *An Outline of Chinese Acupuncture* (*1*), gives a comprehensive list of indications for the treatment of diseases with acupuncture. These are listed as follows:

(a) Medical diseases. Common cold, influenza, bronchitis, bronchial asthma, heat stroke, pain in the gastric region, spasm of the diaphragm, infectious hepatitis, acute enteritis, dysentery, cardiac diseases, hypertension, shock, strained neck, malaria, arthritis.

(b) Surgical disorders. Lumbar pain, shoulder pain, elbow pain, tendon sheath diseases, sprain of the lower extremities, acute appendicitis, diseases of the biliary tract, mastitis, furuncle, acute lymphangitis, simple goitre and hyperthyroidism, haemorrhoids, prolapse of rectum.

(c) Gynaecological and obstetrical disorders. Irregular menstruation, amenorrhoea, pelvic inflammatory diseases, prolapse of uterus, morning sickness, malposition of fetus, prolonged labour, lactation deficiency.

(d) Paediatric diseases. Whooping-cough, infantile malnutrition, acute infantile convulsion, chronic infantile convulsion, parotitis, poliomyelitis.

(e) Diseases of the sense organs and neighbouring structures. Acute conjunctivitis, photophthalmia, myopia, atrophy of optic nerve, tonsillitis, pharyngitis, chronic rhinitis, chronic sinusitis, toothache, deaf-mutism.

(f) Nervous and mental disorders. Apoplexy, paraplegia, epilepsy, headache, trigeminal neuralgia, facial paralysis, sciatica, multiple neuritis, neurasthenia, hysteria, schizophrenia, intercostal neuralgia.

(g) Urogenital disorders. Enuresis, retention of urine, spermatorrhoea and impotence, infections of the urinary tract.

The inclusion of specific diseases in the list is not meant to indicate the effectiveness of acupuncture therapy, but rather the extent to which it is currently being applied. Furthermore, this list of indications is based on clinical experience and not necessarily on controlled clinical research.

There are certain specific contraindications to the use of acupuncture. These include pregnancy when associated with diseases otherwise amenable to acupuncture, needling of tumour sites, skin infections, presence of a cardiac pacemaker, and coexisting haemorrhagic diathesis such as haemophilia. The risks attendant to any kind of needle insertion into the body are also acknowledged, particularly in areas where puncturing of vital structures could inadvertently occur. Reliable diagnosis according to general standards of medical practice is essential in the clinical application of acupuncture therapy to ensure the appropriate treatment of disease. Further research into the clinical indications and contraindications of acupuncture is considered essential.

Particular note should be taken of the use of acupuncture to effect anaesthesia. The term acupuncture anaesthesia is in fact a misnomer, since the procedure produces an absence of pain sensation, but not other senses, such as temperature, touch, and pressure. Acupuncture anaesthesia should therefore be more correctly termed acupuncture analgesia. Both terms are, however, freely applied.

In the People's Republic of China, 15–20% of all surgical cases are said to be performed under acupuncture analgesia. In other countries, including Austria, the Federal Republic of Germany and the United States of America, acupuncture analgesia has also been used in surgery with success. The limits on acupuncture analgesia in countries other than the People's Republic of China seem to result from lack of suitably trained medical specialists as well as some degree of opposition from the medical establishment. The overall success rate with acupuncture analgesia in diverse surgical procedures is said to be between 70% and 80%, thus leaving a considerable number of patients who require Western-type anaesthesia. Acupuncture analgesia is considered a valuable addition to the therapeutic armamentarium of the qualified anaesthesiologist.

REFERENCE

(*1*) THE ACADEMY OF TRADITIONAL CHINESE MEDICINE. *An outline of Chinese acupuncture.* Peking (Beijing), Foreign Languages Press, 1975.

II. Research in acupuncture

Robert H. Bannerman[1]

During the past decade, knowledge stemming from research in physiology, biochemistry and pharmacology on the one hand and knowledge from research into the mechanisms of acupuncture on the other have tended to converge. It is interesting to note this convergence of modern international science with traditional Chinese medicine.

Important advances have been made in our understanding of the mechanisms of acupuncture, particularly analgesia. In terms of modern medicine, the principal action of acupuncture and moxibustion is to regulate the function of the human body and to increase its resistance by enhancing the immune system and the antiphlogistic, analgesic, antispastic, antishock, and antiparalytic abilities of the body.

In establishing future policy for research in acupuncture, it will be necessary to consider the integration of basic and clinical research. Clinical research requires the foundation provided by the basic sciences, while basic scientific endeavours may be informed by clinical experience. Certainly clinical trials, analogous to the procedures for testing new pharmacological agents, are urgently needed to further the acceptability of acupuncture.

Great progress has also been made in clinical research on acupuncture analgesia, which has been used during surgery on more than 2 million patients in the People's Republic of China. In over 100 different types of operation, its effects have been found to be comparatively stable in 20 to 30 kinds of common operation. Generally, acupuncture analgesia is thought to be more effective in head, neck and chest surgery. It has also been used with satisfactory results in subtotal gastrectomies, splenectomies, total laryngectomies, and open-heart surgery under extra-corporeal circulation. Large numbers of abdominal tubal ligations are done under acupuncture analgesia, and over 80% have been rated as very satisfactory.

---

[1] Formerly, Manager, Traditional Medicine Programme, World Health Organization, Geneva.

Several animal experiments and clinical studies have been performed to elucidate the mechanisms of acupuncture analgesia and advances have been made in studying the role of the nervous system in such mechanisms. In the past two or three years, Chinese scientists have succeeded in developing techniques for the isolation, extraction and determination of endogenous morphine-like substances, as well as for artificially synthesizing the highly active substance encephalin and its derivatives. Experiments in both man and animal have shown that the analgesic effect of acupuncture may be partially antagonized by the morphine antagonist naloxone.

However, many problems concerning the mechanism of acupuncture and acupuncture analgesia have yet to be elucidated. All of the above studies point to the need for further exploration, application and research on acupuncture. These are important not only for the health and welfare of the people but also for the progress of medical science.

Training

Since acupuncture may be considered as part of the practice of medicine, it is necessary to define suitable standards for acupuncture training. Training must be addressed to the different needs of various kinds of trainees, i.e., basic scientists, primary care physicians, health specialists or auxiliary health personnel. It has been estimated that a Western-trained physician may require no more than three months' training to learn acupuncture in theory and practice. Those who follow the three-month Chinese programmes in acupuncture are generally able to study the identification and use of some 300 basic acupuncture loci. The programme also covers the treatment of common ailments both in theory and in practice as well as traditional Chinese medical theory, including yin and yang and the theory of channels and vital energy. Some time is also spent on scalp and ear acupuncture, on the pathogenesis of disease, and on acupuncture mechanisms according to traditional Chinese concepts.

Internationally, acupuncture training is heterogeneous, reflecting different views on what acupuncture is, how it should best be practised, who should be authorized to practise it and under what circumstances. The country reports from Asia and Europe give an impression of the diversity of training policies and programmes. The more standardized pool of trainees at present is composed of those physicians who have trained in the People's Republic of China. It is generally felt that the traditional Chinese techniques and theoretical approach must be combined with established Western approaches to the diagnosis and treatment of disease.

In the People's Republic of China, while medical school graduates are given both theoretical teaching and clinical experience of traditional Chinese medicine, including acupuncture, they are also taught Western-type concepts of the anatomy, pathophysiology, diagnosis and treatment of diseases. It has been estimated, however, that approximately

20% of the students graduating from medical colleges are trained primarily in traditional Chinese medicine. Doctors trained in traditional medicine work throughout the Chinese health care system in hospitals, clinics and specialty areas, and also in primary health care.

The Chinese health workers who have been called "barefoot doctors" in rural areas and "red medics" in urban areas are also taught acupuncture for a limited number of common ailments such as the common cold and influenza, common skin diseases, neuralgias, sciatica, etc. These health workers constitute an extremely important link between the Chinese population and the more specialized or institutionalized levels of the Chinese health care system. It is significant that such health workers practise an integrated form of medical care, including acupuncture.

In a few countries, training is provided for the most part in private institutions, under the supervision of an *ad hoc* professional body involved with acupuncture, or else on an apprentice/teacher basis. Most other countries do not offer any significant form of acupuncture training at present.

Technology transfer and impact on health care

The development of acupuncture as a safe and clinically useful technique depends largely on international transfer and exchange of information and skills. At present, scientific research and communication in this field are still hampered by limited dissemination of information. For example, acupuncture literature is only sporadically represented in standard computerized medical information systems, such as MEDLINE. There is, as yet, no centre where information on acupuncture from international sources is stored and compiled for use by interested investigators. Nomenclature is another important question. In many medical fields, terminology has been standardized on an international basis as far as possible. However, in acupuncture, a variety of systems are used in different countries for the designation of acupuncture loci, and other technical terms also are translated in various ways. This difference in terminology hinders international scientific communication, and steps must be taken to remedy it.

Most research efforts in the field of acupuncture have been made in the People's Republic of China, but access to Chinese literature is limited by its relative unavailability in other languages. No concerted attempt has yet been made to translate the bulk of this material into the major Western languages.

Another serious obstacle to the transfer of knowledge about acupuncture is the antagonistic attitude of many medical colleagues and allied health professionals towards accepting acupuncture therapy as a medical practice. This scepticism is paralleled by an ignorance on the part of the general public which makes patients in search of treatment easy prey for unscrupulous or uninformed practitioners of acupuncture. This difficulty is compounded by problems of manpower development and the lack of high-quality educational programmes which would ensure a consistently high level of research and clinical care.

Clearly, educational programmes for the dissemination of available knowledge and research data are of great importance; and here, NAPRALERT (natural products alert), the computerized system for the surveillance of world literature on the chemistry and pharmacology of natural products that is described by Farnsworth in Chapter 18, could well make a major contribution. Other programmes might be organized to reverse the unfavourable attitudes of medical professionals and to educate the public concerning the safety of the procedure, its indications and its limitations. The elimination of quacks and unscrupulous or uninformed practitioners, thus ensuring a high level of clinical ethics and practice, would do much to make acupuncture respectable. Obviously, a greater degree of international cooperation is required in teaching, education and research on this subject and also in the control of acupuncture practice.

The problem of control concerns mainly the diversity of national regulations dealing with the practice of acupuncture.[1] In some countries, acupuncture is prohibited. In others, regulations for its practice are completely lacking. Some nations stipulate that only physicians may practise acupuncture, while others consider it as suitable only for research at the present time. Some countries license "doctors of traditional medicine" regardless of whether they are physicians or not. Other nations, such as the People's Republic of China, recognize acupuncture as an acceptable medical practice for all types of health care personnel. Clearly, there is a need in many parts of the world for more careful formulation of policies concerning the regulation of acupuncture.

The transferability of acupuncture to countries with differing social, cultural, and medico-legal conditions requires careful consideration. Yet, as described above, acupuncture has already attained a firm foothold in certain countries of Asia, Africa, Europe and the Americas. Established international agencies could play an important consultative role in such efforts.

FURTHER READING

BANNERMAN, R. H. Acupuncture: the WHO view. *World Health*, December 1979, pp. 24–29.
JAYASURIYA, A. & FERNANDO, F. *Principles and practice of scientific acupuncture.* Colombo, Lake House, 1978.
KAO, F. F. & KAO, J. J., ed. *Recent advances in acupuncture research.* New York, Institute for Advanced Research in Asian Science and Medicine, 1979.
Use of acupuncture in modern health care. *WHO Chronicle,* **34**:294–301 (1980).

---

[1] See also Chapter 27, Legal aspects.

CHAPTER 8

Treatment of fracture and soft tissue injury by integrated methods of traditional Chinese and Western medicine

Shang Tienyu[1]

There are two schools of medicine in China, traditional Chinese and Western medicine. These two different medical systems have been formed and developed from distinct historical backgrounds, yet both serve the same object of investigation and treatment and both are effective in the struggle against disease. Each has learnt and borrowed from the other to correct deficiencies in the treatment and prevention of diseases. In this way, a new system of medicine and pharmacology with a unique Chinese style is expected to emerge.

Treatment of fractures

The new method of fracture treatment by the integration of traditional Chinese and Western medicine has great potentialities, and efforts should be made to explore the system and raise it to a higher level. Large numbers of Chinese medical workers have systematically studied the bonesetting experiences of traditional Chinese medicine in the light of modern science, technology and methodology. After extensive clinical practice and constant review of experiences, a new system of fracture treatment has been established, guided by the principle of combination of mobilization and immobilization, and characterized by the use of small wooden splints for external fixation, the surgeon's manipulative reduction and the patient's initiative through functional exercises. The period of clinical union has been shortened by one third (see Table 1) and the whole course of treatment has been halved. The complications of fracture treatment, such as joint stiffness, muscular atrophy, osteoporosis, delayed union or non-union, have been largely eliminated. The rate of satisfactory functional recovery has reached 90%. Nowadays this therapeutic method can be used

---

[1] Director, Institute of Orthopaedics and Traumatology, Beijing, China.

for various fractures, whether fresh or old, closed or open, or infected. It is applied to fractures of the limbs and spinal column as well as to most intra-articular fractures.

Since the 1960s, foreign orthopaedic surgeons have gradually discarded the older principle of extensive immobilization and complete rest. Recently, most Western authors have also adopted the principle of combination of mobilization and immobilization, though opinions differ in regard to its application.

In Europe, some surgeons advocate strong internal fixation with or without a short period of external immobilization and allow the patient to undertake early exercises in order to minimize complications. The process of fracture healing, however, has not been shortened by this method. Besides the possibility of wound infection, the associated bone atrophy due to the strong internal fixation may lead to re-fracture. A new kind of plate more responsive to bone elasticity is therefore being investigated. Other surgeons, especially in the United States, do not agree with either extensive external immobilization or strong internal fixation but advocate local external fixation by functional brace and allow early exercises, with satisfactory results. They claim that their new conservative therapeutic method is similar to the Chinese method integrating traditional and Western medicine.

We, however, stress the fact that limbs are the motor organs of the human body, and their function is motion. Any long period of immobilization therefore constitutes a kind of physiological injury to the

Table 1. Comparison of healing time in days of common fractures in China and elsewhere

Fracture	Authors				
	Campbell	Watson-Jones	Bohler	Shang Tienyu I	II
Lower end of radius	21–49	35	42	42	21
Shaft of humerus	56–84	52	28–56	56	28
Radius and ulna	70–84	70	91	86	42
Shaft of femur	126	84	86	85	54
Tibia and fibula	98–140	86	84	100	52
Ankle	—	70	70	56	28
Supracondylar fracture of humerus	—	21–28	21–28	21–28	14

I = Method of Western medicine
II = Integrated method of traditional Chinese and Western medicine.

limb. The skeleton is a frame which permits leverage in movement and sustains weight and stress. The bone tissues will become atrophied if their biological nature is denied or restricted. The bone itself possesses great regeneration and remoulding ability. Rapid union can be achieved, the fracture complications can be avoided and the functional recovery of limbs can be satisfactory, if reasonable measures are adopted such as relative fixation on the fracture site after manipulative reduction, timely functional exercise, and appropriate compression and stress sustained on the fracture site.

Soft tissue injuries

Based on the study and application of the traditional techniques of Chinese massage and manipulation, a new diagnostic and therapeutic method incorporating modern medical knowledge has been developed for treating soft tissue injuries. This integrated manipulative treatment method is applied in painful conditions of neck, shoulder, waist and leg. In many Chinese provinces and cities special institutes for treatment and research have been established and accept patients with soft tissue injuries for treatment by the traditional or the integrated manipulative method. National academic symposia are often held to exchange experiences in this field and several books on this subject have been published.

A new view on pathogenesis

Soft tissue injuries resulting from fall, blow, sprain, collision, compression or crushing are usually closed wounds. Very often there is a slight local change in the anatomical position of the bone and soft tissues involved, and this becomes the pathological basis leading to acute aseptic inflammation or chronic degenerative changes, adhesion and hyperplasia of the affected tissues. Such injuries mainly affect the spinal column and major joints of the body and their adjacent soft tissues; they are especially common in the neck, shoulder, waist and buttock. The derangement of the anatomical relation is the essential cause of pain and function impairment.

A new method of diagnosis

Besides adequate history taking, this diagnostic method is based on the clinical knowledge of the doctor and the skilful use of his fingers to determine the anatomical and morphological changes of the affected soft tissues and the bone prominence. By palpation, the doctor can usually detect tracks, lumps, masses, etc. For example, in a case of injury of the spinal column, the clinician is able to determine any deviation, elevation or depression of a spinous process and changes in the adjacent interspinous spaces.

A new method of treatment

With precise knowledge of the slight changes in anatomical position gained through careful palpation and following the principles of "derangement of bones" and "soft tissue out of track", the doctor applies the manipulative method with gentle dexterity, aiming specially at restoring the anatomical positions, releasing muscle spasm, harmonizing nerve reflexes and promoting blood circulation so as to relieve pain and restore the functional movements.

The rationale of our methods and experiences is fully outlined in the book *Treatment of Soft Tissue Injury by Integrated Methods of Traditional Chinese and Western Medicine* written by Dr Feng Tienyu.

Extensive clinical practice has proved that this is a satisfactory method with gentle manipulation, little suffering to patients and effective results, and furthermore that it can be easily mastered and popularized. Since 1975, numerous patients have been treated by this method in our Institute and by the doctors trained by us and working in other parts of the country (see Table 2).

Table 2. Results of treatment (in % of cases treated) of some common diseases by the integrated method of traditional Chinese and Western medicine

Disease	Results			
	Excellent	Good	Fair	Poor
Periarthritis of shoulder	60%	35%	5%	—
Cervical syndrome	25%	35%	34%	6%
Tennis elbow	55%	45%	5%	—
Acute lumbar sprain	80%	15%	5%	—
Herniation of lumbar disc	25%	45%	20%	10%
Lesion of superior gluteal cutaneous nerve	36%	54%	10%	—

CHAPTER 9

Modern allopathic medicine and public health

I. Allopathic medicine — John J. Canary[1]

The organized health care system termed allopathic medicine is but one of several systems which have evolved in more technologically advanced nations and societies. The other organized systems which are found more frequently in such societies are the homoeopathic and osteopathic. These latter systems comprise smaller numbers of practitioners and hence are of less significance in terms of the delivery of health care to worldwide population groups.

Allopathy or the allopathic system is defined as that discipline of medical care advocating therapy with remedies that produce effects differing from those of the disease treated. Homoeopathy is the system of treatment employing minute amounts of remedies that in massive doses produce results similar to those of the disease being treated. Osteopathy is a treatment form emphasizing manipulative techniques for correcting somatic abnormalities thought to cause disease and inhibit recovery.

The primary point of separation of allopathy or, as it is frequently termed today, "modern," "Western" or "scientific" medicine, from the traditional or indigenous medical system from which it evolved millennia ago, is unclear but its earliest beginnings would appear to include the detailed descriptions of a number of medical conditions, including diabetes mellitus and urolithiasis, found in the Vedic hymns written centuries before the Common Era by East Indian predecessors of today's ayurvedic practitioners, and the recommendations for the treatment of goitre with burnt sponges (iodine source) by Chinese observers, forefathers of the modern traditional Chinese medical practitioner. Further growth of the modern allopathic system occurred with the keen observations of a few giant figures, including Aretaeus of Cappadocia, Hippocrates of Greece,

---

[1] Professor of Medicine, Georgetown University, Washington, DC, USA.

and Ibn Sina (Avicenna) of Persia, whose descriptive writings on medical conditions were followed by an ever-increasing number of European practitioners and observers. These were aided by the establishment of the great universities at Padua and Paris and their offspring at Cambridge and Oxford. Much later, the universities patterned after these which were established in the colonies and in North America, particularly those in Pennsylvania and Massachusetts, aided the evolutionary process.

Today, the traditional or indigenous medical care system includes a much larger cadre of practitioners on a worldwide basis than the allopathic. Their practices range from individual and often secret procedures to highly developed systems (1).

The two most developed systems of traditional medicine are represented by the traditional Chinese and the Indian ayurvedic practitioners. These two systems are formalized and have been recognized by their respective national governments. Each has developed a large and active pharmacopoeia and materia medica. Specific predoctoral and postdoctoral training facilities have come into existence, and certification and registration of practitioners exist. These two branches of the traditional approach are well established, recognized and accepted.

Growth of the allopathic system

With respect to the allopathic system it should be borne in mind that it is only within the last 100 years that specific qualifications have been required for the practice of medicine, nursing, midwifery, and other health professions, and that the basis for therapeutic recommendations made by the early practitioners were usually without scientific justification (2). It is only within the past half century that, due to the growth and adoption of the scientific method, the allopathic practice of medical care has bloomed. Rapid development and application of methodologies for accurate measurement of clinical findings have characterized this growth phase. Prior to the last quarter century the clinician practitioner had to be content with little more than measurements of body temperature, respiration and blood pressure, X-ray studies with little use of contrast material, and relatively simple chemical determinations of body fluids. The modern development of a wide range of accurate and sensitive analytical chemical measurements, the application of the principles of physiology to life support and measurement systems, the application of radionuclides to both the study and the treatment of body functions and dysfunctions, the ability to provide extensive surgical modifications and to graft and transplant tissues and organs, the rapid and vast increases in knowledge of immunology and chemotherapy, and the development of potent antibiotics have all led to a sharply focused interaction between the attending physician and the patient with disease. The strength of these developments has greatly increased the impact of the allopathic practitioner in these individually focused encounters, and at the same time has often led to expectations from patients and society which cannot be fulfilled.

Concomitantly there has been a vast expansion of the concept of rehabilitation with the development of specific departments and training facilities. Now the allopathic practitioner does not view a patient encounter as an isolated episode in the life of the patient but attempts to place it in the perspective of the entire life process and is as interested in the rehabilitative aspects as in the diagnostic and immediate therapeutic ones.

Much credit for the improved health care status of large segments of the world must be given to the development of formal centres of education, training and research by the allopathic practitioner groups which have organized themselves into national and regional societies, established formal training courses and developed criteria for certification and licensure. Such groups, in collaboration with their universities and teaching centres, have been leaders in the field of continuing specialized postgraduate education and have been among the first in their societies to begin experimentation with recertification for their practitioners to ensure continuation and improvement in their levels of performance.

The same applies to the nursing and midwifery professions which have since their inception set the highest standards for their work. The team concept of medical care has required all members of the health team to improve not only their knowledge and skill but also their interpersonal relations with other members of the team and their patients.

As the allopathic system has grown and developed, it has subdivided into several major disciplines, e.g., surgery, medicine, obstetrics/gynaecology, paediatrics and psychiatry. Within each of these major disciplines, and in others, significant subdisciplines have arisen. This process has led to greater depths of study required for certification of the practitioners of these various forms of the allopathic system and the development of progressively smaller groups of more specialized individuals requiring deeper and more specific training for progressively longer periods of time. Such deep, extended and sophisticated training in educational centres has led to more research activity, the acquisition of more knowledge, and the development of techniques; as a corollary, the increased capacity of technology has led to a burgeoning in the industrial field of medical engineering. This is exemplified by the recently developed computerized axial tomographic technique. This sophisticated research development in one or two centres, which, parenthetically, led to the Nobel Prize for its inventors, was rapidly recognized as a useful tool. Production facilities were established and now the techniques are so widely available that economic and public health issues are being raised and debated concerning overutilization, oversupply, and the cost of the technique and the instrumentation for its application. All this in hardly more than 15 years.

In societies where allopathic medicine is the major health care system, preventive medicine, which until recently has been largely the province of public health, has now become a key element in patient–practitioner interaction. A number of systems fostering this development are in experimental trial status, sponsored by both national and local governmental groups and by private insurance or industrial organizations. There is still no general agreement as to which, if any, of such systems currently under evaluation will prove to be both result-effective and cost-effective.

Self-care must be mentioned since, although it is much more significant in countries and regions where medical care systems are less well developed, it is of growing importance in allopathy as is evidenced by both oral and written statements of many people in technologically advanced societies. A vast array of literature on self-care is available. Some is of excellent quality, some is very poor. Some self-care activities are eminently practical, useful and beneficial; some may be quite hazardous. To take only the experience of my own country, a number of mechanisms for obtaining information on self-care can be found in daily newspapers. Usually there are one or more columns devoted to health matters. Mass distribution media, radio and television, cover items of interest for self-care. A frequently unrecognized source of self-care information is the interaction of an individual with a trained pharmacist. There is also a vast and apparently very loosely regulated supply of medications produced for sale and consumption by the populace for a variety of the more common symptomatic problems of the human condition. For example, skin emollients, soporifics, analgesics and, last but not least, vitamins and tonics.

Doctor–patient interaction

The interactions of the patient and the allopathic healer or practitioner are so varied that it is impractical to describe them in detail. Only the major ones will be outlined. In many communities of city size, the first encounter with the allopathic practitioner is in the form of the paediatrician's care, immediately following delivery. If complications are present, the paediatrician may ask for consultation with individuals specially trained in the discipline of neonatology. The relationship between the paediatrician and the family may continue throughout the course of early life. After the age of 18–20 years the paediatrician is usually replaced by the primary care physician or generalist. Such physicians in the more advanced technical societies today are most frequently certified in the subdiscipline of internal medicine. Such a doctor–patient unit will occasionally require special services from consultants from other subdisciplines of medicine or other major disciplines of the allopathic system, such as surgery and its subdivision obstetrics, or rehabilitative medicine. A growing number of physicians are being trained in geriatrics—the specialized medical field of the dysfunctions and diseases of the elderly.

In less urbanized regions, a slightly different pattern of doctor–patient interaction is found. Other patterns which occur in both urban and more rural settings would involve the family doctor serving as the primary care physician throughout the lifespan of the individual. Most frequently that doctor will perform minor surgery when needed but will refer the patient to specialists for more extensive surgical procedures.

Newer systems of doctor–patient interaction have been developed. Much has been written about these, largely from the economic standpoint. These are mainly group as opposed to individual practices and include the pre-paid health care systems or health maintenance organizations. This pattern of providing health care is by the formation of a small group of healers. Groups usually comprise a number of doctors with experience in various areas of allopathic medical care. Such group practices usually comprise 4 to 10 or 12 doctors. This pattern of medical care delivery in the allopathic system is, on the basis of this writer's experience, perhaps the most cost-effective and result-effective for both patient and healer. Such an arrangement may be found in private, insurance or State-run systems of health care.

The usual doctor–patient interaction involves individual identification usually by name, address, date of birth, and telephone number, information on the patient's sources of economic support, insurance coverage and occupation, and information on the members of the nuclear family. The next step is usually to obtain the history of the patient's problem. This may be done either by a nurse or paraprofessional utilizing a form which can be coded and computerized, or by the doctor directly. Such a history usually comprises past medical problems, details of the patient's present complaint, and the results of a physical-examination including the measurement of vital signs, height, weight, etc. The initial examination may be limited to the system involved in the complaint or may be a more generalized evaluation of all the body systems. Depending upon the evaluation of the complaint by the doctor and the physical findings, recommendations for both symptomatic relief and the performance of measurements designed to exclude or confirm the healer's diagnosis will be made. Depending upon the outcome of these investigations, which may be performed on an outpatient basis or may in some instances require hospitalization, therapy will be instituted which is directed at the basis of the patient's complaint.

The style and duration of such consultative activities vary greatly depending upon the complaint and the setting in which the doctor–patient interaction takes place. Anything from a single visit of short duration to multiple encounters may be required. It is generally recognized that in no more than 60% of initial doctor–patient encounters can the doctor correctly define the basic cause of the complaint. Hence in some 40% of such encounters the correct diagnosis of the cause of the patient's complaint will only be established by periodic follow-up and continued evaluation.

As a general rule, in addition to advice about the specific complaint and recommendations for or institution of treatment, the doctor may inquire into and make recommendations concerning the patient's environmental and social activities, the application of principles of preventive medicine for conditions producing symptoms which are discovered during the course of the evaluation, and advice to other members of the family group, if present, for ongoing and continued care. In general, the doctor attempts to advise therapeutic action which will minimally disrupt the patient's life and will not adversely affect his or her employment preferences. On some occasions, if the doctor's findings indicate that alterations in the patient's situation are indicated, he or she will participate in such decisions as actively as required.

The allopathic pharmacopoeia

There is no generally utilized pharmacopoeia for the allopathic practitioner. The sources of information about available therapies are multiple. In countries where allopathic doctors are the major arm of therapy and systems have been developed for national or regional care, such regional or national systems have developed formularies in which medications are listed for recommended uses, with appropriate dosimetric information. In general, in such countries, a number of other sources for medicaments are available and may be utilized in addition to those listed in the formulary publications. In other areas, where such formal developments are not yet in place, a wider variety of informational systems is utilized. In large hospital facilities, a hospital formulary is usually developed by a pharmacy committee. Here again, the staff of such institutions are by no means limited to preparations in that formulary, but are limited more by availability. However, if unusual or novel forms of therapeutic procedures are to be undertaken such techniques will have to be considered by an expert technical committee and approved before implementation is permitted.

In the United States of America, the US Pharmacopoeia is generally available in medical libraries and hospital pharmacies, and in most retail pharmacies. Organized medical societies, especially the major ones, frequently publish annual evaluations of a variety of newer therapeutic agents in the USA. A private publication, the *Physician's Desk Reference*, gives a very wide coverage of manufacturers and products, publishing in full the insert required to be included with each product by the US Food and Drug Administration (*3*). This is a widely used tool of the practising doctor.

The selection of drugs in the allopathic system of health care delivery depends on the experience of the doctor and the availability of the drug. In the present era, certain combined chemotherapeutic agents of substantial toxicity are utilized, largely in the cancer chemotherapy section of medical care. The majority of practitioners prefer that those agents be handled by specialists in that discipline.

The majority of physician's offices contain simple equipment, including a scale, blood pressure measuring apparatus, stethoscope, tuning forks, equipment and facilities for collecting urine or other excreta, and sterile swabs for cultures (nose, throat, vaginal and rectal material). Depending upon the type of practice there may be disposable minor surgical instruments, sutures and equipment for performing intravaginal examinations or procedures. Some offices contain microscopes and small centrifuges for centrifugation of urine specimens or for the on-site performance of packed cell volume measurements in blood. Not infrequently, an area will be devoted to simple analytical chemistry for blood and urine, including quantitation of glucose, urea, etc. In the main, the allopathic practitioners utilize large commercial analytical laboratory services which, on a contractual arrangement, will pick up specimens, arrange for their central analysis, and use computer systems to print-out results. Depending on the test requested, the results will be returned to the physician's office by special delivery or by mail, usually within hours but on some occasions after a few days and on others within a week or two.

In many physician's offices X-ray machines or fluoroscopes may be found for diagnostic purposes. In general, much larger facilities, community hospitals, professional commercial radiographic facilities, etc. will be required for the performance of more sophisticated diagnostic techniques and for the application of radiation therapy. Nuclear medicine applications, both diagnostic and therapeutic, are also usually centralized in larger medical care facilities.

Medical care

General medical care or, as it is sometimes termed, medical services, usually refers to an organized structure of some sort with a mission for the delivery of medical care, such as the Armed Forces Medical Service or the Public Health Service. It is unfortunate that the term "service" has begun to loom so large in the lexicon of present-day medicine. The term "service" carries with it an industrial production concept of units, and in medical care, if a care function can be discretely defined in terms of its content and/or its time, it can also be assigned a numerical value which in turn can be united with a cost. Hence in that misapplication of the general systems theory of von Bertalanffy (4) medical care activities in this "service" concept can be more specifically audited. In essence, then, the concept of a production unit and the industrial assembly line can be applied to the doctor–patient interaction. This industrial management technique has had no small influence on the widely recognized deterioration and inhumaneness of these encounters in the recent past.

Such services may be rendered in the doctor's office or in a specifically designated medical care facility—a hospital or an outpatient department—or, less frequently, in the patient's home. In industrialized urbanized areas such encounters take place on the job site, in areas specifically designated for health care.

The methods of payment for such care are extremely diverse and may include barter—the exchange of a skill of the patient for that of the doctor, personal monetary payment by the patient to the doctor, or a fee for care on an insurance basis—the patient contributing to an insurance pool with a large number of other patients. Such insurance organizations may have contractual arrangements with participating doctors, with the doctors agreeing to accept set payments for certain specific types of care. In such arrangements, the doctor submits a bill on the form specified by the insurance company, frequently termed the "third-party" in medical care, to the company, and receives payment from the company for the submitted statement. For doctors who choose not to participate in such plans, and some do not, the insurance company pays directly to the patient an amount based upon the doctor's statements to the patient. The patient is then expected to pay the doctor. In several countries, however, medical care is free for the patient at the time of use and the costs are entirely borne by the State. The doctor is either salaried or paid on a per capita basis.

Professional organizations

In the allopathic system, practitioners are, in general, organized into groups largely developed because of common interests and problems. A wide-ranging number of such professional organizations exist. Membership is not required but many find it beneficial to join such organized groups. The organizations generally sponsor journals containing items of interest, accounts of new developments and other worthwhile information for the practitioner. They organize meetings at which new developments are presented and there are opportunities to discuss mutual problems with other practitioners of generally similar type. Usually one or more such organizations are recognized by governments as representing the profession in any negotiations. They also assist practitioners with legal defence.

The organization of these special groups follows the general outline of the overall disciplines; there is a major group and then a multiplicity of subgroups. These professional organizations serve at least two other important functions, namely the enforcement of discipline and the development of recognition for their members. In general, a condition of membership in such organizations is that certain activities should be documented, such as periods and types of training and certification. In many, particularly the subspecialty organizations, evidence of professionally worthwhile activities are a requirement for election to membership.

For higher levels of specialization, national organizations have appointed groups which organize and administer, on a periodic basis, special examinations which are required for qualification and certification as a specialist in any of the subdisciplines. There are similar examinations for surgery, obstetrics etc., and within the broad areas of subspecialization there are specific boards which administer examinations on a periodic basis for such areas as cardiology, rheumatology, orthopaedic surgery or neurosurgery.

In addition to the organizations largely devoted to the practice of doctors, there are organizations concerned with nursing and midwifery. Still other organizations are devoted to research and professional teaching activities. Membership in such organizations is usually by election after nomination by members of the organization and documentation of high levels of performance in the special field. Nomination and election to such organizations on a national or local basis is clearly a recognition of meritorious performance.

One other area of practice that must be considered is the protection of patients against acts of malpractice. In most systems, whether organized nationally or locally, appeal mechanisms are in place to which a patient who feels that he or she has been maltreated may complain. Such groups are capable of obtaining, organizing and evaluating the data and reaching a judgment. Appeals from the decisions of such groups usually mean legal action in the courts of the nation. I am most familiar with the allopathic system within the USA, and while there are variations throughout the nation, most medical societies in the localities have members appointed to a board of grievance, to which patients who feel that they have been mistreated may appeal. Such appeal groups can obtain directly from the physician in question, records, documentation of activities and explanations. Similar activity documents are obtained from the patient and judgments are reached. Here again, depending upon the legal situation in the local area, if the patient is not satisfied with the outcome, he or she is free to obtain legal advice and to bring suit against the physician or hospital. This is true unless, as is the case in some but by no means all regions, there exists a legally established group comprising lay individuals as well as physicians and lawyers which considers the issue and renders a binding judgment.

Medical research

Research is fundamental to the practice and progress of medicine and should characterize the outlook of all teachers and practitioners. It is organized along many lines. In the majority of the training establishments for allopathic practitioners, the tradition of research is inculcated early on. In the very best medical establishments, the student or the doctor is encouraged to consider his activity in regard to each patient also as a research project. Without prejudice to the welfare or peace of mind of the patient, the practitioner attempts to devise a hypothesis regarding the patient's complaint, then develops an experimental protocol to prove or disprove the hypothesis based upon the data developed. The hypothesis may be proven, leading to reasonable therapeutic actions; if the hypothesis is disproved, then another one will have to be formulated. In a more organized fashion, research is conducted at all levels of medical care delivery—ambulatory clinics, hospitals, predoctoral and postdoctoral training facilities, medical schools and universities. Some research is supported formally by federal, state or foundation funds and some by the pharmaceutical industry, while some is carried on as a part of care activity. In general, in the organized areas of research activities, the responsible boards of health care facilities appoint committees to which planned research protocols are submitted. In general, such committees are made up of professionals as well as lay individuals. The proposed research is considered and the risks and benefits are assigned. Consultation with experts in other disciplines is sought if such expertise is not available within the framework of the committee. Before an investigation can be undertaken, a judgment is rendered as to whether the risk–benefit ratio is satisfactory; it may be decided that the information to be developed seems to be so much needed that some risk may be essential. As a general rule, all participation by laymen in such research activities is entirely voluntary. Attempts are made to give sufficient information so that the participant can make a judgment concerning his or her participation in the protocol. The value of such explanations is difficult to judge. In that context a signed agreement to participate, or "consent form" is usually incorporated in the chart or record of the patient or participant. An additional difficulty arises when the patient who is to participate in the research is unable to be informed or is unable to give consent. In that situation, usually more than one family member is involved. Also, a disinterested but highly trained member of the profession is consulted and, after making an independent evaluation of the protocol and the patient, reports to all concerned his or her views of the applicability, feasibility and safety of the planned research.

Usually, the results of research studies are made known in the form of a paper which is submitted to a journal for publication. The data may be presented at a local, regional or national meeting after submission to a programme selection committee. In large part, the validity, soundness and veracity of the information is evaluated by peer groups prior to its presentation and publication.

Integrated health care

There would appear at this time to be ample reason for a closer integration of the major branches of health care—traditional medicine and allopathy. Many present-day medications are derived from traditional discoveries. Equally, there are many very strong and useful techniques, routinely applied by the allopathic discipline, which could greatly enrich the traditional discipline; and there are many traditional concepts, ideas and practices which could serve to enrich the allopathic discipline. The mention of only a few of the contributions of traditional medicine to allopathic medicine will serve to emphasize the need for the development of much closer and more frequent collaboration between their practitioners. The herbal remedy, digitalis, and the alkaloid, reserpine, isolated from *Rauvolfia serpentina* are two major items. Penicillin is another excellent example. The use of fresh citrus fruits, particularly limes, for the treatment of scurvy, which led eventually to the isolation and characterization of ascorbic acid, is still another. The review article by Bannerman (1) which is a very thorough overview of the World Health Organization's programme on traditional medicine, cites many examples of activities among traditional disciplines which should be of great interest to the allopathic system.

A number of areas exist where collaborative activities in research, training and practice could well serve to strengthen both systems of medical care. The most important means of developing closer collaboration and relationships between the two systems would seem to be the initiation of some informational exchanges. International organizations and national organizations devoted to health care could encourage the publication of items of interest by members of the respective systems, or the reservation of small amounts of space for that purpose in journals devoted to traditional medicine in various countries and in those devoted to the allopathic system. An information exchange of that kind should be of great value to both disciplines, as would the publication of a quarterly or semiannual bulletin containing information from both. Such a bulletin should cover organizational, research, training, and care activities and problems. The phenomena of natural curiosity and interest among the practitioners of both disciplines would lead to closer collaborative activities. The availability of such information would also be of great value to the administrators of public health and private health care delivery systems, and would ensure that their colleagues, professional and paraprofessional healers, became aware of the activities of others performing the same type of tasks although utilizing different systems. Such exchanges could stimulate a desire for and even lead to collaborative efforts.

An excellent overview of the allopathic activities of today can be obtained from the further reading list (see below) which covers most aspects of the system.

In summary, I believe that the allopathic medical care system and the traditional discipline have, at this stage of their respective developments, much to learn from and to teach each other. Joint efforts are essential for mutual improvement and to ensure that adequate health services will be available to all peoples of the world.

REFERENCES

(*1*) BANNERMAN, R. H. WHO's programme in traditional medicine. *WHO Chronicle*, **31**:427–428 (1977).
(*2*) GODBER, SIR GEORGE. Measurement in medicine—origin and purpose (Presidential address). *Proceedings of the Royal Society of Medicine*, **58**:664–670 (1965).
(*3*) BAKER, C. E. ed. *Physician's desk reference*, 35th ed. Oradell, NJ, Medical Economics Company, 1981.
(*4*) BERTALANFFY, L. VON. *General systems theory*. New York, G. Braziller, 1968, p. 289.

FURTHER READING

COHEN OF BIRKENHEAD, LORD. Opening address, Inaugural Meeting of the Section of Measurement in Medicine of the Royal Society of Medicine. *Proceedings of the Royal Society of Medicine*, **58**:659–663 (1965).
INSTITUTE OF MEDICINE. *A manpower policy for primary health care*. Washington, DC, National Academy of Sciences, 1978.
SCHEFFLER, R. M. ET AL. A manpower policy for primary health care. *New England Journal of Medicine*, **298**:1058–1062 (1978).
PETERSON, M. L. The Institute of Medicine report "A manpower policy for primary health care". A commentary from the American College of Physicians. *Annals of internal medicine*, **92**: 843–851 (1980).
ABELSON, P. H. A view of health research and care (editorial). *Science*, **200**:845–847 (1978).
HAMBURG, D. A. & BROWN, S. S. The science base and social context of health maintenance: an overview. *Science*, **200**:847–849 (1978).
CHAPMAN, C. B. Doctors and their autonomy: Past events and future prospects. *Science*, **200**: 851–855 (1978).
BALL, R. M. National health insurance: comments on selected issues. *Science*, **200**:864–870 (1978).
LASAGNA, L. The development and regulation of new medications. *Science*, **200**:871–873 (1978).
FRAZIER, H. S. & HIATT, H. H. Evaluation of medical practices. *Science*, **200**:875–878 (1978).
CULLITON, B. J. Health care economics: the high cost of getting well. *Science*, **200**:883–885 (1978).
SAWARD, E. & SORENSON, A. The current emphasis on preventive medicine. *Science*, **200**: 889–894 (1978).
WINIKOFF, B. Nutrition, population and health: some implications for policy. *Science*, **200**: 895–902 (1978).
KANE, R. L. & KANE, R. A. Care of the aged: old problems in need of new solutions. *Science*, **200**:913–919 (1978).
INGELFINGER, F. J. Medicine: meritorious or meretricious. *Science*, **200**:942–946 (1978).

II. Public Health

John Burton[1]

Modern public health and preventive medicine arose as parallel disciplines to clinical medicine during the 19th century. They developed through the application of science and politics to the control of mass sickness and to the widespread social and environmental problems considered to be affecting the health of the public. A major motive force for the development of public health was fear of epidemic diseases such as cholera and smallpox, the nuisance caused to all by environmental squalor, and the social consciousness aroused by mass poverty, all of which were aggravated by crowding in industrial cities. The need to acquire and analyse objective information about the health of the community gave rise to the basic science of public health, namely epidemiology.

Starting with recording deaths and burying the dead, and the sanitation of towns, public health gradually became involved in the control of communicable diseases and quarantine, food hygiene, housing, water supply, drainage, environmental pollution, town planning, laboratories for the monitoring of health hazards and the production of immunizing agents, hospitals, the health of families, particularly of mothers and children, the health of schoolchildren, and occupational and mental health.

From its earliest stages of development, the means it used for ameliorating adverse health factors were:

(1) The creation of public health services backed by legislation, paid for from the public purse and staffed by medical officers, nurses and sanitarians with special qualifications and many other related professional and auxiliary health workers;

(2) The education and involvement of the public in the promotion and protection of its own health;

---

[1] Formerly, Director, Central Council for Health Education, United Kingdom, and subsequently, Chief, Fellowships Programme, World Health Organization, Geneva.

(3) Epidemiological research into all aspects of physical and mental health which affect large numbers of people and are amenable to mass preventive action;

(4) Operational research into measures which promote the health of the community such as nutrition, feeding, school health, occupational health, housing, leisure and geriatrics;

(5) Experiment and political persuasion related to technical and administrative methods for extending the benefits of public health and preventive medicine to the entire population;

(6) The sustained application of its work through flexible legislation and budgeting, monitoring, cooperation with other social agencies, staff education, management and active penetration of the community by services carried out by the public health staff.

The scope of all these activities covers biological, pathological, behavioural, accidental and degenerative factors in health and sickness as they affect the host, the agent and the environment. An important consideration is their cost-effectiveness in terms of economic development and human well-being.

A glance at history

Aesculapius, the Greek god of medicine (most likely synonymous with the Egyptian Imhotep[1]) had two daughters, Hygeia and Panacea. It is said that he preferred Panacea. That he should have preferred the "universal remedy" to the "personification of health" may have ensured his reputation among doctors, but meant that Hygeia had to fight harder for recognition. She has always gone out into the community looking for trouble and has welcomed as her allies all those laymen and women of goodwill who influence human well-being, the mothers in the family, the farmers and fishermen, the educators, employers and traders, public health workers, and finally the law-makers and administrators.

Concern for the environment and a healthy way of life most likely originated in the earliest urban societies some five or six thousand years ago. Excavations in the Indus valley, China, Egypt and Latin America suggest that as the number of people increased and began to share the benefits of civic action and the calamities of civic neglect, food storage, sanitary engineering and town planning developed. More recent examples of the public health consciousness of the ancient world can still be seen by the casual tourist in such monuments as the baths and aqueducts of Greece and Rome.

Many features of some of the most ancient religions, such as Hinduism

---

[1] Imhotep was an Egyptian priest and physician during the reign of the Pharaoh Zoser (*circa* 2680 B.C.) and was later deified as god of medicine.

with its hatha yoga, Taoism with its following of the way, Judaism with its alimentary and sexual rules, and Christianity with its accent on love and altruism, have attempted to guide mankind towards a physically and emotionally healthy way of behaviour. The foundations of present-day public health are to be found in the cultural heritage of all peoples, and most of the environmental and behavioural ideals of mankind took shape long before the emergence of the scientific and technological revolution of the last century. Science and technology, too, have existed since earliest times but were rarely applied to the human condition, which was regarded as outside the scope of its materialistic outlook. Many traditional practitioners of today continue to give greater importance to spiritual and emotional aspects of health than they do to material factors. Much of the public interest in traditional medicine arises from a feeling that medical behaviour is too mechanistic and misses the non-material factors in diagnosis and treatment, as well as in the planning and execution of public health programmes.

Links with tradition

Public health workers are often made aware of the limitations of their education and practice when they find their activities are not appreciated by the community and their scientific explanations are regarded as inadequate. It is particularly in public health and preventive medicine that cultural differences between science and tradition become apparent because the public health worker is dealing with groups and has greater difficulty in adjusting his approach than the clinician dealing with individuals. However, the link between traditional and modern approaches to public health problems is evident in all countries. Health administrators who are aware of the traditional culture in which they work, and who make use of it in their planning and activities, stand the best chance of creating programmes which are accepted by local communities and satisfy the requirements of scientific disciplines.

Combined approaches to the solution of public health problems

The application of science and technology through public health action to the solution of ancient problems is well illustrated by the story of smallpox, one of mankind's most widespread afflictions. Variolation is known to have been used by a variety of traditional practitioners in several parts of the world. At the end of the 18th century, long before any knowledge of viruses existed, Jenner, an observant general practitioner, using only courageous empiricism, converted this haphazard and often dangerous method of acquiring immunity to smallpox into safe and reliable vaccination. He was ridiculed by many colleagues but Napoleon grasped the significance of his discovery and the first mass experiment was the vaccination of his armies. After 200 years of controversy, neglect, voluntary acceptance, compulsion and organized opposition, the world was still spending heavily on the control of a manifestly preventable disease. It was not until the 1960s that the Member States of the World Health Organization decided to embrace Hygeia and rid themselves once and for all of this universal menace.

The difference between smallpox and most other communicable diseases is that it was worldwide, well recognized by people in every cultural group and only transmitted from person to person.

It was surrounded by an immense variety of beliefs and customs in all countries, and large groups in many of them did not accept the scientific explanation. However, the political will and the technical means for its eradication developed. With great managerial skill, the epidemiological knowledge was gathered, and local beliefs and customs were respectfully documented and taken into account when planning the strategy and tactics of smallpox eradication. New techniques for producing vaccine and of vaccination were developed and adapted for use in a vast variety of field conditions. The effectiveness of the new techniques of vaccination was demonstrated to local people, who sooner or later were persuaded that whatever they believed the cause of smallpox might be, the simple act of vaccination did succeed in preventing the disease. As a result, the world has demonstrated to itself that a combination of political will and managerial skill, technical inventiveness and professional enthusiasm, public cooperation and monitoring by laymen and staff can rid humanity of one of its major afflictions in the space of about ten years.

This unique experience illustrates, in its origins and its final adaptation to a multicultural world, the impetus which combining traditional and scientific health concepts can give to one of the most important measures of public health and preventive medicine. The experience provides well founded hope and guidance for all other forms of immunization.

Another example of the necessity of combining modern and traditional approaches in a more complex area of health care can be taken from nutrition. Food habits are deeply embedded in culture and the nutritional health of communities may depend as much on the social customs and beliefs about feeding as it does on the ability to acquire food.

Kwashiorkor[1], as the name implies, was recognized in Ghana as a disease syndrome affecting babies displaced from their mother's breast by the advent of a pregnancy and later by the arrival of a new baby. The discovery that it was due to the lack of protein, consequent on the lack of breast milk and the absence of any suitable substitute, might have taken place sooner if health workers had given heed to the traditional name of

---

[1] Kwashiorkor (local word in the Gha language meaning "displaced child"). A severe state of protein malnutrition affecting children. First described in Ghana by Dr Cicely Williams in the 1930s.

the condition. Dr Cicely Williams, who first described the syndrome, recorded her astonishment and delight when her nurses explained to her what the word kwashiorkor meant.

The immediate causes and the treatment were soon established, but the problems involved in changing customs remained. They included traditional ways of caring for children, gaining acceptance for locally available protein-rich foods suitable for babies, and spacing the birth of children so that the deprivation of breast-feeding would not be deleterious to the child's health.

Whether this nutritional problem of children has been aggravated by the change from polygamy to monogamy, with its consequent short duration of breast-feeding and stripping of the mother's protein reserves by continuous pregnancy, can be debated, but the resulting situation is still relevant to public health programmes aimed at controlling kwashiorkor. The debate should become largely academic because, family planning having been included as a major aspect of most public health programmes, the achievement of birth spacing through the use of modern or traditional contraceptive methods is feasible and is likely to be more acceptable and surer than any attempt to interfere with marital customs. The revival or maintenance of breast-feeding, the simplest preventive measure, has also become subject to cultural pressures. The unfortunate fashion of bottle-feeding, which swept industrial societies and was only mildly discouraged by health authorities, has resulted in a powerful commercial interest in promoting substitute milk products. Providing dried milk in sufficient quantity costs money and using it requires pure water and careful hygiene. When these are in short supply the practice becomes dangerous. However, in spite of this, bottle-feeding is seen by many women and their husbands, in widely different cultures, as synonymous with progress. The far-reaching risks to the health of babies of this custom may therefore be hard to combat, backed up as the custom is by the global cultural manipulator of advertising.

The case illustrates the range of understanding required of public health planners, administrators, and field workers concerned with a health problem where such culturally sensitive matters as food habits and sex life play a major role in the etiology and prevention.

Apart from respect and understanding for the way of thinking of the individuals and groups directly affected by the problem, all health activities can benefit greatly if the public health staff make it a rule to consult the leaders and traditional practitioners whose beliefs and influence sustain existing health habits and can aid or prevent useful change. Margaret Read said that it is difficult to understand any other culture if you do not understand your own (*1*). The culture of most health workers is that of formally educated people from towns and that of much of the world's population is that of tradition and rural life. Both parties think their view of life is the right one. Planners and administrators also come from the former culture. Being the promoters of the health services and being in the key position to decide why, what, when and how a public health programme should be designed and carried out, health administrators have the major responsibility for building the bridge. With the education of health workers in most countries limited to scientific and technical ideas, the importance of the people affected by the programme has had to be learned the hard way, as when expensive public health schemes worked out in great detail fail in the field. Apart from the technical and logistic problems, the check to the malaria eradication programme in many countries may have been partly due to the failure to appreciate the importance of winning the active cooperation of householders. In many cases the connexion between mosquitos and malaria was not understood; malaria itself was not high on the list of problems the local people wanted solved; the effectiveness of spraying was not demonstrated because, in spite of the nuisance of residual spraying, it did not kill the culicines; and people did not like the invasion of their homes by strangers with very different ways of behaving from their own. But perhaps the most important shortcomings were the failure to consult, learn from and enlist the cooperation of people such as traditional and established practitioners in whom the local population had confidence, and the failure to introduce any meaningful activities through which members of the community could feel that they were party to the particular health project and therefore helping themselves.

The scarcity and expense of modern health services is forcing health administrators who desire to increase the coverage of their services to look for new resources. The two major resources which have been largely ignored to date are the considerable body of traditional practitioners who are actually providing health care in both rural and urban areas, and the capacity of the members of the community to organize and carry out health measures in ways that suit their way of life.

The epidemiology of beliefs and customs

The foundation of public health is epidemiology, the science which explores how disease falls upon the community. In so doing, it claims to investigate the host, the agent and the environment. Its explorations have revealed much about the biological and environmental factors in the causation of disease, but as yet it has, as a rule, only considered the host from the point of view of such simple characteristics as age, sex, mortality, etc. It has signally omitted any serious study of the behaviour, beliefs, motives, relationships and capacities of the host, which are frequently major factors in the maintenance of health and the etiology of sickness in every society.

Such studies have been undertaken by some health workers and social anthropologists, but with a few notable exceptions the epidemiology of beliefs and customs has not, as yet, attracted their attention nor have health authorities recognized its potential contribution sufficiently for it to be incorporated automatically in epidemiological work.

In spite of this omission, and whether health authorities like it or not, the traditional culture surrounds and permeates every public health initiative and cannot be ignored. The holistic view of health adopted by most traditional practitioners may differ widely from that of the modern public health officer but, since it embraces spiritual, emotional and social factors which are of importance to members of the community, it can add a dimension to public health planning and action which could very well ensure success in the field. In some enlightened public health programmes the health education branch has gone deeply into the cultural characteristics of the target community, but this is still exceptional. Since the health workers are frequently neither members of nor residents in the community, the action taken is generally too short-lived to gain the confidence of the people and bring about significant change in such a basic and complex matter as a community's way of life. Traditional practitioners are numerous, are generally permanent residents of the locality, and in most cases already have the confidence of important sections of the community. They, like the public health workers, believe that their mission is to benefit their neighbours. A relationship of professional respect, though a challenge to both parties, may be the public health worker's easiest way of gaining an understanding of the motivations and social structure which determine behaviour in the complex network of groups which form a community.

The recent emphasis placed by WHO on extending primary health care to the remotest communities will confront health administrators with problems quite different from anything with which they are familiar. They will not be extending modern health services into virgin territory, as some writers on primary health care seem to believe, but entering often closely knit societies where health care is already catered for by men and women many of whom have strong personalities and an assured position. They will encounter a variety of generally held beliefs and practices with which they will find it difficult to sympathize, particularly the spiritual, social and magical attributes of the kind of calamity which their patients consider sickness to be. There may be little idea of health as a positive good to be striven for and there may be suspicion of any outsider who seems to be upsetting the accepted order or balance of power which characterizes human groups.

Basic health services extending into the remotest rural areas have been a primary concern of WHO since its foundation. They have always been conceived as a combination of clinical medicine and public health measures in one administrative system. Their most recent manifestation as primary health care puts greater stress on involving local inhabitants with some basic training in providing the combined service, and it is hoped that primary health care will be largely operated and financed by the local community. With imaginative management, cheap and effective therapeutic and public health measures could undoubtedly be developed for a limited but important range of problems. Whether primary health care can operate effectively and give as great satisfaction to the local population as the traditional system of health care which already exists remains to be seen. Much will depend on its ability to solve logistic and interprofessional problems such as the supply of medicines, the training and status of its staff, and relationships with the established health professions. A long tradition of independence among traditional practitioners, a distrust of government officials and even a fear of their repressive and sometimes contemptuous behaviour may make cooperation difficult. A worthwhile start has been made in cooperation with traditional midwives, and the lessons learned in this initiative should be useful if health services decide to involve other traditional practitioners in their work.

Gaining acceptance for new health practices is a complex and delicate operation in all cultures, but this has been Hygeia's predicament all along. She has considered the prize worth while and in all her successful activities she has proceeded gently, gathering the relevant information about the host, the agent and the environment, demonstrating the effectiveness of her methods, educating the people within the context of local beliefs and customs and building up a group of assistants capable of initiating, monitoring, adapting and maintaining a service with competence and humanity.

REFERENCE

(1) Read, M. *Culture, health and disease: social and cultural influences on health programmes in developing countries.* London, Tavistock, 1966.

CHAPTER 10

Homoeopathy

George Vithoulkas[1]

Homoeopathy is a medical discipline whose primary emphasis is on therapeutics. It is a low-cost system employing non-toxic drugs exclusively. It can be used to treat both acute and chronic diseases, but its greatest contribution lies in its successful treatment of chronic illnesses that have become difficult to manage by orthodox methods.

Homoeopathy takes a holistic approach towards the sick individual and treats his disturbances on the physical, emotional, and mental levels at once. Its aim is to bring back the lost equilibrium of the sick individual on all three levels by stimulating and strengthening his defence mechanism.[2]

Homoeopathy was introduced into the Western world by the German doctor, Samuel Hahnemann, through his scholarly work *Organan of the art of healing*, published in 1810. The implications of this new science were for the medical profession of his time as revolutionary as quantum mechanics and relativity theory were to Newtonian physics in this century. Controversies lasted for years and are still continuing today.

Homoeopathy emerged as an important therapeutic modality during the latter half of the 19th century in Europe and America. It has undergone periods of expansion and decline during this century. The last decade has witnessed a resurgence of homoeopathy in the West with increasing acceptance from both doctors and patients.

What are the basic homoeopathic assumptions?

Hahnemann presented his system as a complete scientific method of

---

[1] Director, Athenian School of Homoeopathic Medicine, Athens, Greece, and President, International Foundation for the Promotion of Homoeopathy.

[2] Defence mechanism is taken to mean the autoimmune system, the reticuloendothelial system, the hormonal system, the sympathetic–parasympathetic system, and the psychological mechanism which responds to stress.

healing based on demonstrable laws and principles. The basic homoeopathic laws are:

1. The Law of Similars
2. The Law of Direction of Cure
3. The Law of Single Remedy
4. The Law of Minimum Dose

The Law of Similars

The assumptions that led Hahnemann to formulate this law were:

(1) That every symptom complex or syndrome is not the disease *per se*, but the reaction of the defence mechanism mobilized by the body in order to counteract a morbific influence, be it a specific stress such as bacteria or viruses, or a non-specific stress such as climatic changes, environmental pollution, mental and emotional disturbances, etc.

(2) That symptoms are the best possible reaction of the organism under stress[3] and are the means through which the organism tries to regain its lost balance, its homoeostasis.

(3) That in order to help the organism re-establish order, the physician should assist and strengthen these reactions rather than suppress them.

Hahnemann extensively researched the toxicological literature of his day. In addition, he experimented on a group of healthy human volunteers—himself and a group of doctors—taking by mouth medicinal plants, minerals and animal substances. He found that when such medicinally active material was taken by the human body in sufficient quantity it produced a pattern of symptoms which more often than not imitated a natural disease, either acute or chronic. He further noted that each medicinal substance, when so tested on healthy persons (such tests are called provings) produced peculiar symptoms unique to itself, in addition to producing other symptoms which were common to many substances.

These discoveries led Hahnemann to conclude that if he gave a patient a medicine known to imitate that patient's particular symptoms, he could thereby strengthen the reactive powers of the body. He then found that when he administered a medicine whose proving picture closely matched a patient's symptom complex, the patient, after an initial violent intensification of symptoms, would recover fully. To avoid this unwanted aggravation, Hahnemann successively reduced the dose while observing

---

[3] An organized system in equilibrium (such as the healthy human organism) responds to any particular disturbing force in that optimum manner (i.e., with symptoms) which will most effectively reduce the upsetting effect of that disturbing force, thereby permitting the system to resist the force and return to a state of equilibrium. This may be likened to the principle of least action in chemistry and Newton's third law of motion, or most appropriately, to the modern concepts of cybernetics which deal with the adaptive response of highly organized systems to impinging stimuli.

how the patient reacted, until he was using infinitesimally small amounts without impairing their effectiveness. He finally regulated the dose so that the initial aggravation was just barely perceptible.

It has been a puzzling matter even for modern science to understand how these microdosages can elicit such strong reactions. Perhaps immunology has provided us with a clue. It is well known that certain allergic persons can be exquisitely sensitive to certain allergens. In such cases it is almost impossible to comprehend how seemingly insignificant amounts of pollen or other allergens can bring about such a violent reaction.

The correct homoeopathic remedy is chosen on the assumption that the patient is extremely sensitive to that particular remedy, and only to that remedy, which can produce his symptomatology. Hence the well known principle of homoeopathy, "*Similia similibus curentur*" which can be explained as: "Let the same substance which can produce specific symptoms in a healthy individual cure those same symptoms in a sick individual, although the symptoms have arisen from another cause, i.e., bacteria, viruses, etc."

The Law of Direction of Cure

It was Constantine Hering, a disciple of Hahnemann, who formulated into a law what Hahnemann and his students had earlier observed to take place in a homoeopathic cure. What they actually observed was that the restoration of internal order and consequent return to health of the sick individual follow a predictable pattern. In the progressive movement towards cure it is noted that the principal symptomatology moves from the more vital to the least vital functional centres within the organism, in other words, from the vital organs to the skin and, in the larger context of the whole individual, from the mental to the emotional to the physical centres. In the healing process we may also note the brief reappearance of old symptoms as the remnants of previously suppressed disease complexes make their way to the periphery, to be cleared out by the homoeopathically strengthened defence mechanism.

As in all holistic and natural systems of healing, the process of cure may involve a slight initial aggravation of symptoms as the patient becomes more capable of producing a strong symptom complex. This permits the defence mechanism effectively to combat the noxious factors that produced the diseased state originally. In a successful homoeopathic treatment the initial eliminative phase with mildly enhanced symptoms is rapidly followed by the amelioration of all symptoms and a return to health. Cure is considered complete when there is a full restoration of vital functioning and expression, free from limitations of freedom in the mental, emotional or physical spheres.

The Law of Single Remedy

It must have been already understood that the physician who wants to effect a real cure in his patient must find the one and only remedy that has produced in its proving the greatest similitude to the symptom complex existing in the patient. Any other remedy will have no real curative effect as it will not bear the necessary sensitivity towards the peculiar and individualized response of the defence mechanism of the patient, and hence will not resonate with his disorder. On this point lies the greatest weakness of homoeopathy at present, since it requires a great amount of time, energy and single-minded dedication on the part of the physician to master it and to achieve a reasonable success in treatment. Typically it may take a medical doctor three years of intensive postgraduate study before he can have some confidence in his new homoeopathic skill. Today in almost all Western countries there are a few, mostly private, schools that impart this knowledge to the interested physicians. This effort implies that physicians are taught in a few weeks or at best a few months, a science that requires years of application.

The Law of Minimum Dose

Once the physician has found the indicated remedy it is as if he has found the allergen to which an allergic patient is most sensitive. It is therefore understandable why in homoeopathy the physician has to prescribe a very minute dose in order not to bring about an enormous aggravation of the patient's symptomatology. Giving such a patient a dosage of 1 or 2 mg of the raw substance of the indicated remedy could be a dangerously excessive dose. Hence microdosages of frequently imperceptible amounts of material substance are used in homoeopathy.

Once the initial microdose has acted, it will bring about a curative response through a sequence of predictable internal events, as the strengthened defence mechanism re-establishes order. In this the remedy acts as a triggering and catalytic agent and needs not to be repeated too frequently. Therefore the pharmaceutical cost of homoeopathic treatment will be minimal.

The initial aggravation of the patient's symptoms followed by a full amelioration, together with the observation of the Law of Cure (such as, for example, the alleviation of a chronic bronchial asthma after a homoeopathic dosage and the subsequent appearance of a skin eruption) is a confirmation that a lasting restoration of health, i.e., a cure, has taken place.

Individualization

In addition to its different laws, homoeopathy approaches the problem of illness in another unique way: individualization. In homoeopathy every case is treated as peculiarly individual. Although the disease for which different patients are consulting the physician may be the same, the indicated homoeopathic remedy may be different for each one. A highly refined individualizing process is used. The physician uses the homoeopathic interview to solicit from the patient the unique way in which this patient reacts to his illness. The physician has to consider the whole range of mental, emotional, and physical pathology in order to understand the peculiar ways in which the patient's defence mechanism is reacting. In so doing, he seeks the most suitable remedy to further stimulate these reactions. In this approach he will be particularly cautious not to suppress one or two troublesome symptoms to the detriment of the whole organism.

In homoeopathy the physician's interest is not only the alleviation of the patient's present symptoms but also his long-term well-being. Therefore in the interview the physician has to probe deeply into the most subtle and unique response of the patient's defence mechanism to varying stresses. It is obvious then that the physician needs to spend at least one hour with each patient in order to have a really thorough understanding of the totality of the patient's disequilibrium at all levels of both subtle and gross symptomatology.

Homoeopathy in chronic diseases

Homoeopathy has been serving humanity for almost two centuries. Its greatest efficacy is in the treatment of chronic diseases, especially before tissue changes have taken place. Homoeopathy has been of tremendous value in reversing diseases such as diabetes, arthritis, bronchial asthma, epilepsy, skin eruptions, allergic conditions, mental or emotional disorders, especially if applied at the onset of the disease. The long-term benefit of homoeopathy to the patient is that it not only alleviates the presenting symptoms but it re-establishes internal order at the deepest levels and thereby provides a lasting cure.

Homoeopathy can also be used in undiagnosed cases which present a scanty symptomatology, foreshadowing a deep pathology which may not erupt for years. In such cases homoeopathy acts as a real preventive medicine. All diseases have a prodromal stage in which they manifest themselves with functional disturbances. It is particularly at this stage that homoeopathy can reverse the progress of the disease.

The present situation

It appears that, at the present time, several medical doctors and health professionals are showing increasing interest in homoeopathy. In France, for example, there are some 6000 medical doctors employing homoeopathic medicines. However, there are no full-time colleges of homoeopathy in Europe or America.

Unfortunately, the usual way in which physicians interested in learning homoeopathy today can do so is by attending infrequent, brief seminars and courses. Because of the inadequacy of current homoeopathic training, only an estimated 10% to 20% of the potential of homoeopathy is being realized. No doubt when the training of homoeopathic practitioners is given greater priority, the cost of health care, which has been spiralling astronomically in the last decade, could decline markedly. The price of homoeopathic medicines is almost negligible while the benefits to human health are considerable.

Future possibilities

Homoeopathy has been practised for 170 years with current practitioners numbering in the tens of thousands. There are over 100 homoeopathic journals world-wide, and an International Congress meets yearly. India and Mexico are the only countries that maintain homoeopathic colleges and together have about 20 such institutions. Despite these activities, homoeopathy is still very far from realizing its potential in either developing or developed countries. It is true that solid experimental evidence, such as that provided by double-blind clinical studies in reputable medical centres, is needed to demonstrate the effectiveness of homoeopathy before it can be accepted in the West as a major therapeutic modality. Homoeopaths time and again have asked for such an official evaluation. They are confident that the results will support homoeopathy's distinguished record of clinical successes in treating the whole diverse spectrum of acute and chronic illnesses in man.

Once such evaluations are completed and homoeopathy has obtained wide acceptance, governments could help in establishing homoeopathy as a separate and complete medical discipline. Separate homoeopathic medical colleges with their own clinical facilities and hospitals could emerge.

FURTHER READING

HAHNEMANN, S. *Organon of medicine*. New Delhi, B. Jain Publications, 1978.
HAHNEMANN, S. *Chronic diseases*. New Delhi, B. Jain Publications, 1976.
KENT, J. T. *Lectures on homoeopathic philosophy*. Calcutta, Sett Dey & Co., 1978.
KENT, J. T. *Lesser writings*. Calcutta, Sett Dey & Co., 1978.
VITHOULKAS, G. *The science of homeopathy*. New York, Grove Press, 1980.
VITHOULKAS, G. *Homeopathy, medicine of the new man*. New York, Arco Publishing Co., 1979.
COULTER, H. *Homeopathic influences in nineteenth century allopathic therapeutics*. Richmond, CA, American Institute of Homeopathy, 1980.

CHAPTER 11

Naturopathy

Robert J. Bloomfield[1]

The title of Henry Lindlahr's great work *The Philosophy of Natural Therapeutics*, which was reprinted in a revised edition as recently as 1975 (*1*), represents a significant change of terminology from the phrase "nature cure" that he frequently used. The change is symptomatic of a problem of semantics in the international naturopathic scene. In discussing "naturopathy" and "nature cure" there immediately arises the question of what these terms actually involve and which other therapies naturopathy might embrace.

In some countries the word simply singles out those practitioners of traditional medicine who concentrate on very simple formulae involving water treatments, dietetics and fasting, with a background of philosophic and even religious attitudes. Elsewhere, the naturopath operates on a very clinical basis, utilizing all the latest diagnostic and treatment techniques used by latter-day practitioners of natural therapeutics. These might include acupuncture, osteopathy, chiropractic, homoeopathy, herbalism, vitamin therapy, faith healing and so on. So, effectively, naturopathy for some people means *all* the forms of non-allopathic medicine which depend on "natural" remedies and treatments.

For present purposes, however, naturopathy will mainly be treated in its truest and simplest traditional sense, as it is still much practised all over the world, subject to some up-dating to meet the challenge of the times. The editor of the reprint of Lindlahr's book, Jocelyn Proby, makes it clear in a foreword that he is aware that the expression "nature cure" is apt to conjure up a picture of "loosely dressed people dancing in the dew". This certainly pinpoints the kind of public prejudice that still exists toward nature cure and naturopathy.

Lindlahr himself, an American, was well aware at the professional level

---

[1] Free-lance writer, lecturer and consultant, Maidstone, Kent, England; formerly Executive Officer, International Federation of Practitioners of Natural Therapeutics.

of the kind of opposition he might meet from his medical colleagues. He admitted that many of the statements and claims he made would appear "radical and irrational" to the allopathic school of medicine. Later he got down to the central gist of his philosophy when he said, "while allopathy regards acute disease conditions as in themselves harmful and hostile to health and life, as something to be cured (we say 'suppressed') by drug, ice or knife, the Nature Cure school regards these forcible house cleanings as beneficial and necessary—necessary as long as human beings continue to disregard nature's laws."

As another American naturopath, Dr Jesse Mercer Gehman (2), has put it more recently, "Disease is nature's effort to get you well". Naturopathic remedies would not seek in any way to suppress and thereby obstruct natural healing. Of prime importance is the preventive or prophylactic approach, to avoid illness in the first place.

While Louis Pasteur compared the human body to a barrel of beer—completely at the mercy of extraneous and harmful organisms—Antoine Béchamp states that germs do not cause disease but are the result of it. Rudolph Virchow (1821-1902) came up with the theory that germs seek their natural habitat, which is diseased tissue, rather than actually creating the malaise. Mosquitos *seek* stagnant water, he pointed out; they do not cause it to become stagnant. Lindlahr agreed and said, "the primary cause of germ activity is the morbid soil in which bacteria feed, grow and multiply".

Lindlahr's own nature cure hero was Vincenz Priessnitz (1799-1851) an Austrian peasant. Priessnitz, who lived in the mountains, was out herding cows one day when he saw a badly injured stag limping into an eddying pool at the side of a rushing mountain stream. The animal just stood there fairly deep in the water. The following day Priessnitz saw the stag repeat the performance and suddenly realized that it was there for a healing purpose. The animal returned to the pool for many more days until the wound in its shoulder was completely healed. This deeply impressed Priessnitz, and the incident confirmed his belief in hydrotherapy.

Priessnitz clearly had a natural talent. Lindlahr called him the "genial healer" and said, "His pharmacopeia consists not in poisonous pills and potions but in plenty of exercise, fresh mountain air, water treatments in the cool sparkling brooks, and simple, wholesome country fare, consisting largely of black bread, vegetables and fresh milk from cows fed on nutritious mountain grasses". No one would quarrel with the virtues of such an idyllic approach! When Priessnitz died at the rather early age of 52 he had built up a worldwide following and had a large sanatorium near his mountain home.

Even so, such successes have always been regarded with a certain suspicion by the allopathic medical profession. The *Penguin Medical Encyclopaedia* has a somewhat ambivalent entry for naturopathy. This states, "Naturopathy has no need to justify itself—that is amply done by the known results of overeating, smoking, lack of exercise and rest."

According to author Peter Wingate, "The difficulty arises from not knowing what is natural". Wingate also rather unjustly accuses the "purists in this cult" of avoiding *all* drugs and medicines and says they thus "miss the chance of curing some eminently curable diseases", although he does agree that they "also avoid dangers such as poisoning their stomachs with aspirin, their kidneys with phenacetin, or their intestines with purgatives" (5).

Naturopathy would claim that it is the medicine of common sense, where patient and practitioner cooperate fully to take maximum advantage of what has been described by the British Naturopathic and Osteopathic Association as "the self-regulating, self-adjusting and self-healing ability of the human organism". It would also claim to be a holistic system concerned with body, mind and spirit. Lindlahr wrote that naturopathy includes "mental and spiritual remedies such as scientific relaxation, normal suggestion, constructive thought, the prayer of faith".

There is a strong element of religious fervour in what Lindlahr called his "catechism of nature cure", a list of 20 questions with naturopathic answers. The last of these "definitions" sums it all up. It advocates "the return to nature by the regulation of eating, drinking, breathing, bathing, dressing, working, resting, thinking, the moral life, sexual and social activities etc., establishing them on a normal and natural basis." An American naturopath, Dr H. William Baum, has written more recently in his *Creed for the Naturist* that the body is "the residence of the Soul and the Temple of the Holy Spirit".

So naturopathy is for the serious-minded, both in practitioner and patient terms. There can be little doubt that its philosophy, properly carried out, can and does lead to healthier and happier lives for a large number of patients all over the world. No one could quarrel with the "sound mind in a healthy body" motto. The problem is how exactly to achieve this ideal state and how to provide scientific evidence of the efficacy of all the various systems employed.

In certain countries naturopathy is legally recognized and accepted, in others it is generally tolerated. Some countries have well organized schools of naturopathy, but politically it is not a highly organized profession.

Research is limited, and some naturopaths might suggest that it has all been done already by the great pioneers. Others might, with some justice, suggest that orthodox medical research sometimes proves what they have been thinking all along. This still does not alter the fact that many naturopathic systems and therapies have not changed substantially for over a hundred years.

Naturopathic practitioners often use all normal diagnostic techniques including blood and urine tests, palpation, X-rays, observation and so on. There is one exclusively naturopathic diagnostic technique called iridology, or iris diagnosis, by which it is claimed that the skilled practitioner can tell exactly what is wrong with a patient by studying the marks on the irises of the eyes. Ophthalmic surgeons ridicule the notion, accepting only that it is sometimes possible to suspect a brain tumour in this way; but iris diagnosis is used by naturopathic practitioners and others in the Federal Republic of Germany, India and New Zealand, for example. Naturopaths prepare careful case histories, paying particular attention to eating and living habits, environment and so on. It is usually during this case note-taking procedure that a clear course of recommended future action for the patient begins to emerge.

Almost every country has its own versions of nature cure hospitals, health homes, or "drying-out" establishments. These can vary considerably in the therapeutic systems they use, the type of patient they take and the prices they charge. Efficacy is also always open to discussion, particularly when certain establishments specialize in helping people to recover from overindulgence.

The genuine, middle-of-the-road establishments generally take good care of their genuine cases, people of all social groups and ages who are usually suffering from the miseries of chronic illness. Fees for such patients are reasonable, and if need is proven it is not at all uncommon for fees to be considerably lowered or even occasionally waived altogether. After the root causes of disease have been established the patient receives immediate treatment. As it continues the practitioner will offer suggestions on how, through personal and natural hygiene, the patient could alter his way of life, his diet and, perhaps even more important, his attitudes in order to improve his health significantly and to stay healthier generally. The element of preventive medicine is ever present in the naturopath's approach to his patient.

It is becoming more and more common in many countries for patients in nature-cure homes or hospitals to receive the services of an osteopath or a chiropractor to put right any problems with the vertebrae. There may be neuromuscular treatments and various forms of massage and physiotherapy to relax tension and tone up tissue and muscles. There may be infrared and ultraviolet lamp treatments, herbal and homoeopathic remedies; remedial exercises, including the Alexander technique to improve postural habits; breathing education; and advice on how to balance it all out with proper rest and leisure occupations.

Some naturopaths advocate the enema and colonic irrigation; but the majority would not consistently and automatically apply such drastic procedures, regarding them perhaps as emergency measures in the same way as would an allopathic medical practitioner.

Most nature-cure establishments continue to recommend modern hydrotherapy, the kind of water treatments first promulgated by Priessnitz, usually combined with friction in some form. Other initiators of hydrotherapy include Louis Kuhner, Adolph Just and Sebastian Kneipp. Kuhner was a weaver who evolved a shallow cold-water-bath technique which was always followed by a good rubdown, using only the hands. One of his mottoes was, "cool the abdomen", based on the fact that animals tend to keep their stomachs out of the sun!

Kuhner is also credited with the statement "all disease is curable, but not every patient". Adolph Just adapted and developed Kuhner's methods of hydrotherapy, and Sebastian Kneipp, a 19th century Roman Catholic priest, introduced a system (which he adapted from one invented by Johann Hahn) which was called *Wasser Kur* or water cure, involving footbaths or armbaths with various infusions, often sprinkled on as with a watering-can rose.

Mahatma Gandhi is on record as saying, "The writings of Kuhner, Just and Father Kneipp are simple, popular and useful to all". Gandhi was, of course, a firm believer in nature cure and felt strongly that disease came from ignoring the laws of nature. He was convinced that a timely return to those laws could ensure the restoration of health. He also claimed that "nature-cure treatment brings us nearer to God".

Water treatments take many forms, involving steam baths, Sauna techniques, various kinds of compresses, and whole-body and localized mud packs. Balneotherapy is the term used to describe baths to which have been added minerals and salts, herbs and other materials which vary according to the beliefs of the naturopathic practitioner. There are the well-known sitz-baths, where the patient may sit in one bath of hot water while his feet dangle in another bath of cold water, and vice versa. There is the Scotch douche, which involves a pressured hosing down with hot and cold waters, to tone up skin and muscles, and no doubt to stimulate the overall metabolism.

Many nature-cure establishments have grown around the natural sources of mineral or otherwise health giving hot and cold waters. These centres are usually known as spas after the town of Spa in Belgium. Other European examples are Bath and Matlock in the United Kingdom, the innumerable French towns whose names end in *les-Thermes* or *les-Bains*, and almost any German township with a name that starts with *Bad*. Many of these spa resorts date back to Roman times. There is nothing particularly new about nature cure. Some spas have waters that are taken internally and these are often sulfurous and unpleasant both to smell and to taste.

One of the most dramatic locations for a natural spa is an area immediately beside the 80-kilometre long Dead Sea in Israel. The surface of this large lake is 394 metres *below* sea level and it seems that this geological factor has given it some special characteristics. The Dead Sea itself is so full of salt and therefore so buoyant that bathers can without effort float on it. While the Dead Sea water itself has many therapeutic qualities, the area is surrounded by vast chemical concentrations and natural hot springs. This has all been commercialized and there are many hotels, spa treatment centres and health clinics. One of the claims made for the Dead Sea resorts is that a number of skin diseases, including psoriasis, can be helped considerably.

In such a location there are, of course, many other factors at work, not least of them the beneficial effects of fresh air combined with suitable exercise. One of Kneipp's disciples was Benedict Lust (1872-1942), who emigrated to the USA and became what some naturopaths describe as America's "father and founder of naturopathy". Lust was a great advocate of the "air bath", which is meant literally and involves getting as much air to as much of the body as is decently and climatically possible. As a good minimum compromise he suggested a barefoot walk of 5 or 10 minutes in the dew of the early morning, an activity advocated also by Winston Churchill who, during a 1942 visit to President Roosevelt, was observed taking an early morning barefoot stroll on the dew-soaked lawns of the President's estate at Hyde Park, New York.

Looking at the recent history of naturopathy it would seem that perhaps the Federal Republic of Germany and India share the honours for exploiting its advantages to the full. The Federal Republic has some 250 spa resorts and it is estimated that up to 5 million Germans take "the cure" every year, some through social welfare schemes at highly subsidized fees. The Deutsche Heilpraktikerschaft, the Federal German organization of health practitioners, awards an annual prize to the person who is thought to have contributed most to the cause in the preceding twelve months.

All world systems of medicine have a greater or smaller element of naturopathy firmly based within them. The general practitioner advising a patient to give up smoking or alcohol is acting naturopathically. The dentist advising a mother to cut down her child's sweetmeat intake is doing the same. Strict naturopathic diets disallow all processed and refined foodstuffs, including all kinds of white flour, white rice and white sugar. Also taboo in an ideal world are rich and concentrated foods, butter, cream, eggs, fatty cheeses and animal fats. Dietary reform is the keynote.

In a book published in 1939 by the Theosophical Research Centre (*3*), the following comment can be found: "Dietetic treatment has been brought to the point of comedy and disrepute by fanatics and by the fads of single-minded practitioners". This was a specific reference to the so-called monodiets prescribed by some naturopathic practitioners where they feel such drastic action seems appropriate. A monodiet means that only one thing is eaten, to the exclusion of almost everything else.

Monodiet "cures" include lemons, potatoes, raw meats, celery, grapes. Not quite a monodiet is Schroth's cure, which involves doses of dry white wine and dry toast, combined with hydrotherapy. Dr Josiah Oldfield was an exponent of "fruitarianism", which in its extreme interpretation means living on fruit alone.

It would be foolish to underestimate the importance of diet and its effects on health, beneficial and otherwise. Naturopaths, as dietitians, do concentrate heavily on this aspect of every case. A good naturopath would never generalize, knowing that different typologies need different chemical combinations in their nutrition. Too little can be as devastating as too much. Not everyone can manage on a vegetarian diet, let alone a "vegan" one where even animal products like milk and eggs are disallowed.

Even so, there are strong tendencies towards vegetarianism in naturopathy. These have both humanitarian and hygienic motivations, well expressed by Albert Einstein when he said "Besides aesthetic and moral reasons, it is my view that a vegetarian manner of living by its purely physical effect on the human temperament would most beneficially influence the lot of mankind".

The most dramatic and potent, although temporary, food reform of all is the total fast which, carefully supervised, is often applied to suitable patients in most nature-cure establishments. Partial fasting is also advocated to clear the system of toxic buildups. Maybe only water or dilute fruit juices are given for a few days while the body begins to eliminate, but strict supervision is the order of the day, as fasting can have a number of traumatic effects, both physical and emotional.

Rather defeating the object of elimination is what has been called the "medicine of self", so described by Morarji Desai, the ex-Prime Minister of India, who said he employed it personally. Supporters of this unusual natural therapy drink a glass of their own urine every day. It is undoubtedly true that large numbers of people around the world do add their own urine to their diet without ill effects; but there does not seem to be any real evidence that it has detectable therapeutic value.

The ideal naturopath would, it can be supposed, be so successful with his treatment and advice that the re-educated and reformed patient would never need to see him or any other practitioner again, apart from the consequences of external events such as accidents—which are preventable in an ideal world—and other disasters that might be attributable to acts of God. Unfortunately, it is not quite like that. There has to be a real effort of will and proper discipline to follow a naturopathic way of life. To repeat, it is a philosophy rather than just a means of treating illness. To gain his patient's full confidence the naturopath needs to be a combination of priest and guru dogmatist, with medical man coming in a poor third.

So what is the future for naturopathy? Brian Inglis has written of its main advantages: "Apart from being the oldest medical system naturopathy is also the simplest; and it represents, in a sense, the aim of all branches of medicine—or at least what should be the aim; the prevention of unnecessary disease" (4).

Although much is being written about the incidence of iatrogenic illness, there is some neglect of the diseases caused by bad food, bad habits, bad working conditions, bad home environments and other menaces to health that could, in time, be corrected. Much of naturopathy is preventive common sense but to be really effective it must be properly organized. That is how the naturopath sees his job, as a good health organizer.

REFERENCES

(*1*) LINDLAHR, H. *The philosophy of natural therapeutics* (revised version). Maidstone, Kent, Maidstone Osteopathic Clinic, 1975.

(2) BAUM, H. & GEHMAN, J. M. *Living today for tomorrow.* Duncannon, PA, USA, Natural Health Foundation International, 1974.
(3) *Some unrecognized factors in medicine.* London, Theosophical Research Centre, 1939.
(4) INGLIS, B. *Fringe medicine.* London, Faber & Faber, 1964, p. 64.
(5) WINGATE, P., ed. *Penguin medical encyclopaedia.* Harmondsworth, Penguin Books, 1972.

CHAPTER 12

Divination and exorcism

Piero Coppo[1]

Divination is the process of obtaining knowledge of secret or future things by means of oracles, omens or astrology, or from contact with superhuman or divine sources. Examples of these practices are to be found in the earliest periods of the history of mankind and still today in all cultures, whether or not industrialized. Already known and practised by the Babylonians, Assyrians and Greeks, this science was first systematically described in *De Divinatione*. In that work Cicero distinguished two forms, *naturalis* and *artificialis*, the former based on phenomena quite independent of the observer, who interprets them (astrology; weather indications, such as the direction of lightning flashes or the shape of clouds; behaviour and movements of animals; special marks on the hands or other parts of the body; rustling of plants' leaves; features of dreams, and the like); and the latter based on techniques (with playing cards, wooden tablets, bones, small stones, cowries etc.) employed by the diviner, who interprets the results. This means of obtaining information is still operational in various cultures throughout the world, reflecting their particular differences. Although despised as "superstition" by the "science" born of the philosophy of enlightenment, at the beginning of the 20th century divination became the object of scrutiny by specialists in psychical phenomena. Dream analysis (S. Freud in particular) and analysis of "occult" paranormal phenomena (C. G. Jung) revealed the existence of "automatic" non-verbal ways of thinking in analogies, very similar to those used by an "inspired" diviner. Research on trance, ecstatic phenomena and altered states of consciousness, and recent anthropological and ethnological observations, have conferred a certain dignity upon this form of

---

[1] Medical practitioner and psychiatric specialist, Usigliano, Italy.

knowledge, which is not based on cause and effect and runs parallel to "rational" knowledge.

Among the "secrets" divination claims to reveal is naturally the origin of disease; and among the things it claims to see in the future is the course of disease, its prognosis. In the history of medicine divination has actually been used for the diagnosis and prognosis of disease and for deciding upon the most effective remedies for treating it; and it is an instrument which has, in a culturally homogeneous society, the secondary therapeutic effect of making the patient feel that the unseen world is supporting the therapist and is involved with him in the treatment. Divination consequently played a part before the appearance of "scientific" medicine; but it could only exist in cultures open to magical thinking. The practice was swept away by the revolution of the enlightenment. Yet it has continued to exist, although in clandestine forms, even in the industrialized countries, and is at present enjoying a new period of popularity.

In contemporary peasant society in Tuscany (Italy) and elsewhere traditional therapists use a small metal ring hung on a thread; movements of the ring in front of the patient's body indicate the site of the disease, the chances of cure and the effectiveness of the treatment. African healers use a number of cowrie shells, some of them marked with a copper ring, which are washed in water and then shaken between the hands and thrown upon the ground; from the way in which they fall the therapist learns the origin of the disease, the procedures required for its treatment and the prognosis. Another method of divination among healers consists in examining the marks left on the sand by a fox attracted by bait to a particular spot. The *angakok* of the Arctic uses for the same purpose a specially raised bird with clipped wings, which is thrown down on a spot where cabalistic signs have been·drawn in the sand. Lastly, trance is quite often used as a means of divination: the words and gestures of "possessed" people are interpreted by the therapist to reveal the secrets of the disease and its treatment. This type of divination is commonly practised by African healers. Psychodysleptic drugs are not infrequently employed to induce trance or other ecstatic states.

In certain instances, it is difficult to distinguish divination from the general body of phenomena linked with "magical" thinking characteristic of certain cultures. Where the whole of life and all events are interpreted by analogy instead of in terms of cause and effect, divination is an integral part of the system as a whole and practised by everyone on the most diverse occasions. There will then be a host of small signs which make those willing to interpret them sure they are in syntony with the world around them. The same phenomenon occurs in certain psychopathological states described by "scientific" psychiatry.

Divination can thus be regarded as a technique used *also* in traditional medicine by people who have been trained to employ it. Within the complex system of interrelations between therapist, patient and environment, therapeutic divination may be defined accordingly as a practice which makes it possible to call upon the "superindividual consciousness" by means of a culturally codified technique for the purpose of interpreting the origin of disease, indicating the remedies necessary for its treatment and predicting its course.

Exorcism

When a Moslem *malam* in Africa treats mental illnesses especially, he says to the patient: "There are three of us here; me, you and the devil. One of us has to die". So if after the treatment, which may be severe, there is an improvement, obviously the devil must have left the patient's body. While animists have practised exorcism in less dramatic and subtler forms, they often do the opposite and call upon the spirits to enter the patient's body in the rite of possession, a rite at once cathartic and therapeutic.

Exorcism plays an important part in the treatment of certain forms of illness, particularly mental ones, in cultures which have a dominant monotheistic religion. Where there is a clear-cut opposition between an ethereal and benign God and a wicked devil, the embodiment of evil, panic-stricken patients may suffer from fear of madness, and this is one of the essential cultural prerequisites that dictate such therapeutic practices. Known to the most ancient civilizations (e.g., in Assyria), the term "exorcism" and the role of the "exorcist" were codified in the New Testament; and after A.D. 250 a special class of clerics in the Christian church was given responsibility for practising exorcism. In Christianity today baptism still retains certain characteristics of exorcism such as the removal of impediments to grace due to original sin and Satan. Among Roman Catholics, practices still persist which are obviously in the nature of exorcism; a priest may be called upon in some cases of "obsession", and certain popular festivals (in Italy for example) centre round a priest exorcist and a number of "possessed" people.

Several other cultures employ similar practices and newspapers sometimes refer to these when unsuitable treatment given to patients has produced serious complications. Places (e.g., haunted houses) and possessions too, can be the object of these practices. Anybody suffering from an illness the cause of which is incomprehensible to most people may be considered "possessed"; but it is chiefly mental cases that are involved or people engaging in behaviour incompatible with conventional behaviour in the society to which they belong. The psychopathological state most frequently interpreted as being due to diabolical possession is histeroepilepsy or *morbus sacer*. Sometimes even paranormal powers (divination, inspiration, telekinesis, etc.) are attributed to the presence of the devil and so may be an object of exorcism. The commonest exorcism technique is ablution or aspersion of the patient, his house and possessions with water that has been sanctified in various ways: holy water (Christianity), water in which Koranic writings on paper have been soaked, water with which Koranic writings have been washed off small strips of wood (Islam), and water in which powders of vegetable or animal origin believed to possess therapeutic powers have been dissolved (animism). Religious or magical formulae pronounced by the exorcist may precede or accompany the ceremony or ritual. Inhalants (incense or resin smoke) have always been believed to have the power of calling up, repelling or driving out the devil (his elements being air and fire). I once saw a patient being made to inhale smoke from the resin of a particular tree. Fits of coughing, cyanosis and the desperate efforts the patient made to escape from the "assistant's" grasp were interpreted by the physician-priest as signs of a struggle going on inside the patient: "the devil was in pain but still would not leave the possessed person's body". It has frequently happened in the past, and such cases are still occasionally reported, that patients have died worn out by the savage treatment inflicted, not directly upon them, but upon the "devil" possessing them. Toxic substances, beating, burning and tortures of all kinds may be meted out to the devil through the intermediary of the person possessed. Though these extremely cruel practices are now disappearing, traces of them (in ritualized forms) are still sometimes found in traditional medicine all over the world, and in modern medicine too; they are reflected in sayings like "nasty medicine does you good" and "you must get worse before you can get better", and in the idea that illness is due to possession of the patient by evil or external "beings".

In general it may be said that the practice of exorcism is based upon certain beliefs and certain facts. The religious cultural representation of a benign God as opposed to a wicked devil correspond with the distinction between "good" (i.e., socially and culturally acceptable) and "bad" (i.e., socially and culturally unacceptable) human manifestations. Some people, however, consider such beliefs to be just cultural representation ("projections") of socially determined facts. These "bad" human manifestations are attributed to the devil, who is believed to have entered the person, so causing him to fall "ill". Thus illness becomes a sign of that conflict, and the task of the therapist is to restore order by casting out that which lies within the person but which cannot for the time being be integrated into the society or culture he belongs to. The therapist employs practices that, in his belief, invoke the powers of good but may sometimes appear veritably sadistic punishments. Through these practices, which are transformed into rites, the social structure becomes affirmed and cultural cohesion is strengthened.

CHAPTER 13

Hypnosis

Timothy Harding[1]

Hypnosis is " . . . a temporary condition of altered attention, the most striking feature of which is increased suggestibility" (*1*). Its relevance to traditional medicine is threefold. Firstly, it is rather widely used in developed countries as a therapy (*2*) both by physicians and psychologists working within the official health services and by therapists working independently within the area that has been termed "fringe medicine" (*3*); secondly, hypnosis has been the subject of extensive laboratory research which throws light on the physiological and biochemical changes which occur under altered states of consciousness (trance, twilight state) and which may account for the therapeutic effect of a wide range of traditional medical practices; and, thirdly, hypnosis provides a link between modern and traditional medical practices since there are close resemblances between the techniques and effects of hypnosis and several traditional practices such as morita therapy, yoga, meditation of various kinds, dance therapy, or possession as in the Zar cult, Macumba, or revivalist religious practices.

Nevertheless hypnosis is not an easy subject to deal with briefly. Although its principal manifestations were described by de Puységur (*4*) 200 years ago and there have since been extensive studies of its various effects, there is still no comprehensive theory to explain all of the complex manifestations of hypnosis. There are two main theories both of which have wide support: (*a*) the theory which regards the hypnotic trance and related phenomena as reflecting a special, induced state of the central nervous system, i.e., different from, but analogous to, the usual states of sleeping or waking (*5*); and (*b*) the theory which regards the hypnotic state as a normal reaction under unusual conditions of attention, motivation and attitude (*6*). The first theory suggests that the brain is susceptible to being "switched" into different states, e.g., wakefulness, sleep, trance, whereas

---

[1] Medical Officer, Division of Mental Health, World Health Organization, Geneva, 1971–1980; now Faculty Member, Geneva University.

the second theory regards hypnosis as a special, but by no means unique, set of responses to the subject's environment and general psychological state. Hypnosis also presents difficulties because it arouses irrational fears and prejudices among many people, as a result of the fear of "losing control" or coming under the malign influence of the hypnotist. These unfounded fears and prejudices have been further stimulated by stage performers and charlatans who have used hypnosis as a form of entertainment or of unscrupulous treatment. Historically, it is interesting to note that the theory and practice of psychoanalysis derive from Freud's early experimental use of hypnosis in patients suffering from neurotic conditions.

Terminology

The terms *hypnosis*, *hypnotic state*, *hypnotic trance* and *hypnotism* are largely interchangeable. *Hypnotherapy* is used when hypnosis is used as a treatment. *Posthypnotic* refers to phenomena which persist or occur after and as a consequence of hypnosis, including posthypnotic *suggestion* whereby behaviour is influenced. *Susceptibility* is the individual's responsiveness to hypnosis, which also determines the depth of the trance which can be induced. Individuals can be taught to hypnotize themselves, which is termed *autohypnosis*. One specific form of autohypnosis introduced by Schultz is called *autogenic training* (7) and is widely practised in several European countries.

Uses

Hypnosis has been used in a wide variety of conditions and is sometimes used in combination with other forms of treatment, e.g., to induce relaxation in the behavioural treatment of irrational fears or obsessions.

Hypnosis, particularly in the form of autogenic training, is advocated as a way of promoting positive health, a "means to a new, relaxed enjoyment of one's physical existence" (8). It has been used to prepare healthy individuals who face a stressful experience, e.g., athletes, university students, mountaineers. This use of hypnosis as a positive source of health has obvious parallels with several oriental techniques, e.g., yoga. At this point the role of hypnosis in helping individuals to overcome addictive tendencies should be mentioned in view of its possible application to two major public health hazards, cigarette smoking and alcoholism.

The conscious control of certain autonomic functions is facilitated by hypnosis and this has led to its use in various autonomic disturbances such as pathological blushing, irregular or rapid heart beats (technically sinus tachycardia, ventricular ectopics, sinus arrhythmias), appetite loss, excessive appetite, excessive sweating and frequent defaecation or urination (without underlying pathology).

One of the most important uses of hypnosis is in the management of various "psychosomatic" illnesses, i.e., conditions in which pathological bodily changes result from the patient's emotional state (9). These conditions include asthma, migraine, tension headache and various dermatological complaints including warts and erythroderma. Prolonged hypnotic states are sometimes used to control gastric and duodenal ulcers, hypertension and some forms of cardiac disease. Hypnosis has also been successfully applied as a treatment of stammering and of various sexual dysfunctions including vaginismus, impotence and premature ejaculation.

Since subjects under hypnosis are able to ventilate feelings and recall experiences which are normally repressed, hypnosis is used as an adjunct to psychotherapy. It is claimed that by facilitating the ventilation of repressed memories and feelings (sometimes called *hypnoanalysis*), hypnosis can dramatically shorten classical forms of psychoanalysis for the treatment of neuroses and personality disorders. More dramatic and immediately effective is the use of hypnosis in abreactive therapy; i.e., patients suffering from hysterical conversion symptoms (paralysis, blindness, mutism) resulting from an unusually frightening, stressful or painful event can relive the experience under hypnosis and react, in an explosive and cathartic manner, to the feelings which have been repressed. Following such an abreaction, the hysterical symptom usually disappears either permanently or temporarily.

Finally hypnosis is an effective technique for controlling pain and inducing anaesthesia (*10*, *11*, *12*). Autohypnosis can be taught to women during their pregnancy and used to alleviate pain and promote relaxation during labour. Some surgical procedures can be carried out under hypnotic anaesthesia, e.g., dental extractions, mastectomy, Caesarian section, simple gynaecological procedures, and thyroidectomy. Hypnotic anaesthesia is not a suitable method for surgery within the abdomen or thoracic cage. Various forms of chronic pain can be managed by hypnosis, for example in cases of severe burns, trigeminal neuralgia and spinal cord compression, and in the terminal stages of cancer.

To summarize, the uses of hypnosis can be grouped as follows:

(*a*) as a technique promoting positive health and as a prophylactic exercise for individuals subject to stress;

(*b*) as a method whereby a subject can control autonomic functions and thereby overcome troublesome symptoms of autonomic disturbance;

(*c*) as a treatment for a wide variety of psychosomatic conditions;

(*d*) as an adjunct to psychotherapy in releasing repressed memories and feelings, especially in producing abreaction in patients suffering from hysterical symptoms;

(*e*) as a method of relieving pain and inducing anaesthesia.

Technique

This is not the place for a definitive or comprehensive description of how to use hypnosis; such descriptions are available elsewhere (*13*, *14*). The main stages, however, may be outlined as follows:

Selection and preparation

Individuals vary considerably in their susceptibility to hypnosis. Some 20–30 % of the general population have high enough susceptibility for very easy induction of trance and are therefore suitable subjects for repeated treatments or anaesthesia. About 10 % of most populations are found to be insusceptible. Susceptibility is higher among women than among men and is positively correlated with intelligence. The age of maximum susceptibility is usually 9 years and thereafter steadily declines. These factors indicate the need to select subjects carefully before embarking on hypnotherapy. The selection and preparation should include a careful description of the procedure and exploration of the patient's ideas and fantasies concerning hypnosis, and in many cases a trial of hypnosis.

Induction

Treatment is carried out in private, quiet surroundings free from interruption. The therapist gives repetitive verbal suggestions (usually combined with fixing the eyes on a single object) designed to encourage the patient to relax, listen, become drowsy and close his eyes. This is followed by suggestions that arms and legs have become heavy and therefore difficult to move. The therapist then suggests to the patient that he will experience certain sensations, e.g., coldness, tingling, numbness, warmth, and that the patient's arms or legs will move without their control. At this stage a critical point is reached when the therapist challenges the patient by saying that his eyes will remain closed however hard he tries to open them. Beyond this stage, the therapist usually does not have to repeat stimuli to induce suggestions or deepen hypnosis. Individuals may be trained to hypnotize themselves or to respond very rapidly to a simple hypnotic stimulus.

Therapeutic procedures

Once hypnosis is induced the procedure will depend on the therapeutic indication. Analgesia and anaesthesia, for example, are induced by simple suggestion, reinforced by usually painful stimuli (e.g., pinprick). The therapist may also induce profound muscular relaxation, changes in heart rate, respiration, circulation and gastric secretion. It is relatively easy to produce post-hypnotic amnesia for events experienced during or shortly before hypnosis. Finally the therapist may re-establish a complex experimental psychophysiological state from the patient's past, going as far back as infancy.

Termination

The therapist simply tells (commands) the patient to return to his normal state, often by a series of discrete steps. A state of alertness and well-being is usually suggested to follow hypnosis.

Limitations and dangers

Some limitations in hypnosis are already apparent from the above account. People vary in their susceptibility and the range of treatable conditions is fairly narrow. Hypnosis should not be used in patients suffering from psychosis, organic psychiatric conditions or antisocial personality disorders. Response is variable and may not be lasting. Some patients experience anxiety and disorientation following hypnosis. There have been accounts of antisocial tendencies being released by hypnosis. It follows that careful selection of and full discussion with patients is necessary. Repeated treatment may be necessary to ensure lasting improvement.

* *
*

Hypnosis sits astride official and non-official medicine. It illustrates the reluctance of the medical profession to acknowledge a method which is unequivocally effective in certain conditions. Resistance to hypnosis persists among doctors even after careful official reports and inquiries (for example, by the British Medical Association and several ministries of health) have endorsed it as a valid form of therapy. One may conclude that hypnosis is part of a broad range of phenomena and therapies which are used in many forms of traditional medicine and provide possibilities for promoting positive health and for coping with a number of troublesome conditions in a simple, safe and inexpensive manner.

REFERENCES

(*1*) Mason, A. A. *Hypnotism for medical and dental practitioners.* London, Secker & Warburg, 1960.
(*2*) Erickson, M. H. Hypnotic approaches to therapy. *American journal of clinical hypnosis,* **20**:20 (1977).
(*3*) Inglis, B. *Fringe medicine.* London, Faber & Faber, 1964.
(*4*) Puységur, A. M. de *Mémoires pour servir à l'établissement du magnétisme animal.* London, 1785.

(5) HILGARD, E. R. *Hypnotic susceptibility.* New York, Longmans, 1965.
(6) SARBIN, T. R. & COE, W. C. *Hypnotism: a social-psychological analysis of influence communication.* New York, Irvington, 1972.
(7) SCHULTZ, J. H. & LUTHER, W. *Autogenic methods.* New York, Grune & Stratton, 1969.
(8) ROSA, K. R. *Autogenic training.* London, Gollanz, 1976.
(9) MAHER-LOUGHNAN, G. P. Hypno-autohypnosis in treating psychosomatic illness. In: Hill, O., ed. *Modern trends in psychosomatic medicine 3,* London, Butterworth, 1976.
(10) MASON, A. A. Surgery under hypnosis. *Anaesthesia,* **10**:295 (1955).
(11) MASON, A. A. Hypnosis for the relief of pain. *Proceedings of the Royal Society of Medicine,* **49**:481–486 (1956).
(12) CRASILNECK, H. B. ET AL. Special indications for hypnosis as a method in anesthesia. *Journal of the American Medical Association,* **162**:1606–1608 (1956).
(13) WEITZENHOFFER, A. *Hypnotism, an objective study in suggestibility.* New York, Wiley, 1953.
(14) CHERTOK, L. *Hypnosis.* Oxford, Pergamon Press, 1966.

CHAPTER 14
Yoga and meditation for mental health

K. N. Udupa[1]

I. Yoga

Yoga is a traditional science which helps us to coordinate body and mind more effectively. It enables a person to maintain tranquillity of mind and greater calmness in the conscious state and is perhaps the easiest and the safest method to promote mental health. It can also be used as a preventive and curative technique for the management of various psychic and psychosomatic disorders. Although yoga had been described in the Book of Wisdom—the *Veda*—about 4000 years ago, it was presented by Patanjali in an abridged form about 2500 years ago (*1*). Since then a large number of commentaries and books have been written to explain more clearly how one can promote mental health through the different practices of yoga.

More recently, the study of mental health has been given greater importance since conditions of stress in the modern world have greatly increased. Thus, while many people living in the developed countries enjoy great physical comfort, they are experiencing a lack of spiritual enlightenment. On the other hand, most of those living in the developing countries tend to lead more contented lives, even though they have to face starvation and other forms of deprivation as a result of poor economic and technological growth. Because of these difficulties, people all over the world are passing through severe stress and strain, leading to an increased incidence of psychosomatic disorders. In recent years, and in order to overcome such situations, several newer drugs described as sedatives and tranquillizers have been introduced. However, because of the risk of toxicity and habit formation they cannot be used for prolonged periods. On the other hand, the use of yoga, including various types of meditation,

---

[1] Institute of Medical Sciences, Banaras Hindu University, Varanasi, India.

not only prevents the psychosomatic illnesses commonly seen in many countries but also promotes mental health with no harmful effects of any sort. It is therefore considered desirable that everyone should have a basic knowledge of yoga for better physical and mental development. Those who are interested and want to know more about yoga are advised to refer to an advanced treatise on the subject (2).

Integrated yoga

Among all the methods so far described, the sage Patanjali's methods of integrated yoga are the most important. These are (1) *yama* or improvement in our social behaviour; (2) *niyama* or improvement in our personal behaviour; (3) physical postures; (4) breath-holding practices; (5) restraining the sense organs; (6) contemplation; (7) meditation; and (8) attainment of superconsciousness.

(1) It has been stated that improvement in *social behaviour* can be achieved by the following five noble practices: (*a*) non-violence, both physical and psychological; (*b*) truthfulness; (*c*) non-stealing; (*d*) self-restraint in every sphere of life; and (*e*) non-hoarding.

(2) Similarly, our *personal behaviour* can be improved by: (*a*) maintaining a purity of body and mind; (*b*) developing a habit of contentment; (*c*) practising austerity in every sphere of life; (*d*) intensive study of relevant literature; and (*e*) daily practice of dedication to God. These are the ten basic requirements for attaining success in our daily practice of yoga and we are well advised to follow them as much as possible.

(3) *Physical postures.* A large number of yoga postures have been described by various authors. They are mainly meant to improve the bodily health, especially the functions of various organs such as heart, lungs, liver and other organs of the gastrointestinal tract, kidneys, endocrine system, etc. Normally, a person can practise 10 to 15 yogic postures such as cobra posture, plough posture etc. and including stationary types of exercises for all parts of the body for a period of about 15 minutes daily.

(4) *Breathing exercises.* This is an important part of yogic exercise in which one inhales fresh air to the maximum capacity through one nostril, holds it for a while, and exhales it through the other nostril, practising deep expiration. Normally this can be practised 20 times or more daily to improve oxygenation of all the organs and tissues of the body. Through such simple exercises one usually feels much refreshed and relaxed, possibly as a result of better circulation of oxygenated blood in the body.

After the behavioural practices and physical exercises one should continue to practise step by step what may be called the four mental exercises. The first two are touched upon in the next paragraphs; the others are considered later, in the section on meditation.

(5) *Control of sense organs.* In this procedure we have to restrain the

activities of all the sense organs which are the main gatekeepers of our body and mind. This can be achieved by minimizing the chances of having these sense organs stimulated by various external objects, and then by leading as simple a life as possible. Thus, those wise men who practise restraint in life remain much happier and more satisfied than those very rich men who, in spite of having all physical comforts, still remain dissatisfied with life. It is really hard to restrain the mind, but by constant practice with a definite goal one can restrain the sense organs and thereby the mind to a considerable extent.

(6) *Concentration of mind.* In this process one gradually learns how to concentrate on any object by avoiding all distractions. This practice of concentration on an object of one's choice will greatly help to calm any mental excitement and at the same time will induce tranquillity and serenity in the mind. In order to succeed we must have tremendous perseverance and will-power. As much time as possible should be devoted to concentrating on a chosen object and a strenuous, regular and continuous effort should be maintained until the desired goal is achieved.

Prevention of psychosomatic disorders

Studies have shown that the regular practice of the integrated type of yoga can not only prevent the development of various psychosomatic disorders but also improve a person's resistance and ability to endure stressful situations more effectively (*3, 4*). Studies on normal individuals have indicated that a regular practice of yogic postures leads to psychological improvement in the intelligence and memory quotient and a decrease in the pulse rate, blood pressure, respiration and body weight. The biochemical examination of the blood has shown decrease in blood sugar and serum cholesterol, and a rise in the serum protein level. A significant improvement in the functioning of the endocrine glands has also been found, as evidenced by the increased hormonal level of thyroid, adrenal medulla, adrenal cortex and gonads.

By practising breathing exercises alone similar results have been obtained except that the fall in serum lipids was much more marked than was noted in the practice of physical postures. After intensive meditation for 10 days, there was a marked rise of neurohumours and their enzymes such as acetylcholine, catecholamine, cholinesterases and monoamine oxidases; with a fall of plasma cortisol. When all the three integrated yogic practices, namely, physical postures, breathing exercises and meditation, were combined, it was found that there was a decrease in the neurohumours and their related enzymes, and an increase in the plasma cortisol level. Based on these findings, it can be postulated that the regular practice of integrated yoga can promote tranquillity of mind and increase resistance to stress.

Yoga for treatment of stress disorders

The integrated type of yoga has been used for the treatment of about 640 patients with different stress disorders such as hypertension, anxiety neurosis, mucous colitis, bronchial asthma, diabetes mellitus, thyrotoxicosis, migraine and rheumatic disorders of the spine, with gratifying results in about 78% of the patients. In the remaining 22%, when modern drug therapy was added, improvements were much quicker, with lasting benefits. The study of various neurohumoral changes occurring in these diseases before and after the yogic treatment revealed a marked increase in the content of one or more neurohumours in blood and urine. The yogic treatment would produce relief in these patients coinciding with the normalization of their disturbed neurohumoral systems. For example in bronchial asthma an increase in the acetylcholine and histamine contents was observed with a decrease in the serum adrenaline and plasma cortisol level. After a course of yogic and breathing exercises for a period of three months, these asthma patients had much relief along with normalization of neurohumours by a decrease of acetylcholine and histamine and an increase in the adrenaline and cortisol level. Similar results could be obtained in almost all the patients with stress disorders, thus indicating clearly the scientific basis for the mechanism of action of yogic practices in giving relief in such cases.

Promotion of mental health

In addition to the integrated practice of yoga, there are many other methods of yoga that can be used for the promotion of mental health. Among them, the practice of *Kundalini* yoga as described by Gopikrishna is the most important one (5, 6). In this method a person sits on the ground adopting a comfortable posture and meditates for a few minutes on the autonomic nerve centres from below upwards. Thus meditation begins at the inferior hypogastric plexus, then proceeds upwards to the superior hypogastric plexus, the caeliac plexuses, the cardiac plexus, the cervical plexuses, the hypothalamic region and the cerebral cortex. By this process a better voluntary control is gradually obtained over the involuntary functioning of organs and tissues. By reducing the visceral activities supplied by the autonomic nerves, the activity of the psychic centre of the brain can be promoted and enhanced. According to Gopikrishna, who gives his personal experience of *Kundalini* yoga in great detail, there is a remarkable improvement in psychic activity with a feeling of enlightenment in every sphere of activity. Therefore, if this method of yogic practice could be scientifically standardized, it could become an important method for promoting mental health in people all over the world.

Yoga as a rehabilitative measure

There are a number of yogic measures which can be used for the rehabilitation of persons exposed to too much stress and strain in life. These include praying through devotional songs daily for 30 minutes or so (*ghakti* yoga), undertaking missionary service to the poor, sick or deprived people (*karmayoga*), and educating people through philosophical lectures (*jnana* yoga). By following one or more of these measures, all those who are passing through intense mental stress and strain can rehabilitate themselves well enough to lead normal lives and render efficient service to people.

Thus, yoga is truly a very important preventive, curative, promotive and rehabilitative measure for maintaining sound mental health. There is therefore a great need to conduct extensive scientific studies on the subject and to standardize techniques so that many more people can make full use of them throughout the world.

II. Meditation

Meditation is a mental exercise in which we direct our mind to think inwardly by shutting our sense organs to external stimulations. Normally in a conscious state, we use our sense organs freely—seeing pictures, listening to music, eating sweets, smelling scents, or touching the nose with the hand. These sense organs continuously stimulate the brain, thereby producing various responses in the psychosomatic apparatus of the body depending upon the severity and extent of the external stimuli. However, by the constant practice of meditation one can voluntarily reduce these bodily responses to a bare minimum so that the mind can be directed to perform more useful and fruitful functions (7).

By the constant practice of meditation one can also gradually develop voluntary control over various involuntary vital functions of the body, such as the beating of the heart, the digestion of food or the absorption of oxygen from the lungs, which are normally carried out spontaneously under the control of the autonomic nervous system. By meditation a person can also learn to stabilize his emotional changes, thereby restraining abnormal functions of various vital organs of the body. Ordinarily, there are two planes in which the mind functions, the conscious and the unconscious. Yet there can be one more plane which is higher than both, one where the mind goes beyond the level of self-consciousness. This is called superconsciousness. How can this be attained? When a man goes to sleep he enters the plane of subconsciousness; on waking up he regains his consciousness and becomes a normal person. But when a person has attained superconsciousness, usually through the prolonged practice of meditation, on returning to the conscious state he becomes a different person having acquired greater knowledge and wisdom. After practising the *Kundalini* type of meditation for many years, Gopikrishna described his great experience of attaining superconsciousness and the subsequent remarkable events that occurred in his life.

Thus, meditation can be used as a powerful instrument to restrain the sense organs, control the autonomic nervous system and also attain the state of superconsciousness.

Methods of meditation

There are many methods of meditation. The sage Patanjali describes eight steps to achieve the goal of superconsciousness. This cannot be reached suddenly or accidentally. One will have to gradually improve one's social and personal behaviour, by regular practice of yogic exercises, breath control and various mental exercises. Buddha, 2500 years ago, described the *vipasana* method of meditation in which a person sits in a comfortable posture with eyes closed and directs his attention to the tip of his nose to observe his breath continuously. By this simple procedure one learns to practise concentration of the mind. Gradually one can make use of this method for meditation on any noble object to attain peace and happiness. Recently, Maharishi Mahesh Yogi described a simple method popularly known as transcendental meditation. Here again, the person assumes a comfortable sitting position with eyes closed and turns his attention inwards to control his internal environment. Then he repeats certain sacred words called "mantra" and portrays the gods Vishnu, Shiva and Brahma for about 20 minutes. Throughout the period of meditation the person concentrates on prayer and communication with deity and avoids all mental distractions.

Taking into account all these different methods, Benson has described a simple method of meditation for beginners (8), as follows:

(*a*) A quiet environment: For this it is necessary to have a quiet room, one usually kept for worship. This helps to eliminate distraction.

(*b*) A passive attitude: One should not bother about any disturbing thoughts that come to one's mind during meditation but should try to concentrate on the objects chosen.

(*c*) A comfortable position: A comfortable sitting posture is desirable. If this is not feasible, one can also adopt a lying-down posture, but should not go to sleep.

(*d*) A mental device for concentration: In order to shift the mind from external objects to internal thoughts one should repeat silently sacred words known as "mantra" for about 20 minutes, with eyes fully closed.

Such meditation should be carried out twice a day—morning and evening.

In order to study the utility of these methods, and also to know the degree of attainment in each individual case, a biofeedback system has been introduced, using an electronic instrument that can amplify the various psychosomatic changes in the body such as blood pressure, heart rate, muscle tension, skin temperature and brain-wave patterns. By observing one's own bodily functions with this device, one can gradually, through meditation, develop a mental power to control the involuntary functions described above.

Results

Recently a number of studies have been conducted to assess the value of meditation during health and disease. Biochemical studies have indicated that after ten days of intensive *vipasana* type of meditation there was an improvement in mental activity with greater tranquillity of mind as evidenced by a significant increase in the neurohumoral contents of the blood such as catecholamines, histamine, acetylcholine and their related enzymes and with a decrease in the plasma cortisol level. Wallace and Benson, who conducted extensive studies on transcendental meditation (9), observed that the electroencephalograph showed an increase in the alpha-wave activity indicating greater tranquillity of mind. They also observed a decrease in the heart beat and a 20% decrease in oxygen consumption. There was also a marked increase in skin resistance. In several subsequent studies this method has been used clinically in cases of hypertension, drug addiction, alcoholism, etc. with beneficial results. By coupling meditation with biofeedback one can successfully treat a large number of patients with stress disorders.

The promotion of mental health can also be obtained by using other methods of meditation: *Zen* meditation as practised in Japan, Suffism as in the Middle East, and autogenic training as in Western countries. Recently, *Kundalini* meditation has also been used with great benefit not only for improving the level of consciousness, but also in the treatment of certain mental illnesses.

There is great scope for the use of meditation in the preventive, promotive and curative aspects of mental health. However, there is an urgent need to conduct scientific study and to develop standardization of this simple, inexpensive, yet powerful technique for the promotion of mental health, so that people all over the world can use it.

REFERENCES

(*1*) SACHIDANANDA, S. *Integral yoga: the yoga sutras of Patanjali.* Pomfret, CT, USA, Integral Yoga Publications, 1978.

(2) UDUPA, K. N. *A manual of science and philosophy of yoga.* Varanasi, India, Sarvodaya Sahitya Prakashan, 1978.
(3) UDUPA, K. N. *Disorders of stress and their management by yoga.* Varanasi, India, Banaras Hindu University, 1978.
(4) UDUPA, K. N. & SINGH, R. H. *Yoga in relation to the brain–pituitary adrenocortical axis in interaction with the brain–pituitary–adrenocortical system.* London, Academic Press, 1979, p. 273.
(5) GOPIKRISHNA. *The awakening of Kundalini.* New York, Dutton, 1975.
(6) GOPIKRISHNA. *Kundalini—the biological basis of religion and genius.* New Delhi, Kundalini Research and Publication Trust, 1978.
(7) SIVANANDA, S. *Concentration and meditation.* Sivanandanagar, U.P., India, Divine Life Society, 1975.
(8) BENSON, H. *The relaxation response.* New York, Avon, 1976.
(9) WALLACE, R. K. & BENSON, H. The physiology of meditation. *Scientific American,* **226**: 84 (1972).

CHAPTER 15

Traditional midwifery and contraception

Sheila Cosminsky[1]

Every society provides a system of ideas and behaviour for coping with the life crisis of childbirth, a system which includes patterned sets of beliefs and practices concerning pregnancy, delivery, and the puerperium; the social organization of birth; and the mobilization of emotional and social support.

Over two-thirds of births in the world are delivered by local or traditional midwives or birth attendants who are not trained in Western or cosmopolitan medicine but rather in the traditional system of birth.[2] In some rural areas, they are the only source of assistance and care, and deliver over 90% of the births.

Although in some cases, a woman may deliver by herself or be assisted by an older female relative, most societies have specialists whose concern is childbirth. A variety of terms have been used in the literature to denote this specialist, such as "traditional", "lay", "empirical", "native" or "indigenous" midwife, and "traditional birth attendant" (or TBA). Some of the vernacular or local terms used are *hilot* (Philippines); *dai* (India); *daya* (Egypt); *dukun bayi* (Indonesia); *matrone* (Senegal); *bundo* (Sierra Leone); *partera* (Mexico); and *comadrona* (Guatemala). (For a list of local terms, see ref. *1*, pp. 87–89, and ref. *2*). The term "traditional birth attendant" or TBA is used by the World Health Organization and is defined as "a person who assists the mother at childbirth and who initially acquired her skills delivering babies by herself or by working with other

---

[1] Associate Professor, Department of Sociology and Anthropology, Rutgers University, Camden, NJ, USA.

[2] The term "cosmopolitan" is used here to designate what is also referred to as "Western medicine", "scientific medicine" or "modern medicine". For a discussion of the term, see reference *4*.

The term "traditional", as used here, signifies local, folk or indigenous. It is important to recognize that the traditional system is not static but is continuously changing.

traditional birth attendants" (*1*, p. 7), whereas the term "midwife" is used to refer to a person with formal medical education who is officially registered or licensed.

Several studies have shown, however, that the person described as a traditional birth attendant often also provides prenatal and postnatal care and treats maternal and child illnesses. Consequently, the term is too narrow and understates her actual functions (*3*, p. 16). Her role is also increasingly being expanded through participation in other primary health care activities and family planning programmes. Therefore, the term "traditional midwife" will be used in this chapter since it is a more accurate reflection of the role of this type of health worker.

Attempts to improve maternal and child health, to lower infant and maternal morbidity and mortality, and to extend primary health care have led to an increased interest in the traditional midwife and how she can be used as an important human health resource. Many countries have instituted training programmes for traditional midwives in an attempt to "upgrade" their practice on the assumption that this will improve maternal and child health. In some cases, these programmes have also included efforts to expand her role to include related areas of family health, preventive medicine, and family planning. In view of the shortage and maldistribution of official medical personnel and health care facilities, the traditional midwives are seen by several health authorities as being one means of spreading family health care to a majority of people at a reasonable cost in a relatively short time.

One of the major reasons for the lack of success of some of these programmes is insufficient knowledge of the traditional midwives' practices and beliefs. These are often based on assumptions that differ from those of the Western biomedical system, but have a sociocultural basis and are logical and rational within their own context. Another factor influencing a programme's effectiveness is the way in which obstetrical practices are presented by the trainers. It should be realized that the obstetrical practices promoted by official medicine are also shaped by that biomedical system and the values and culture on which it is based. Whereas some of these "modern" practices have been proven scientifically to be more efficacious than alternative practices, others have not and are accepted as a matter of faith by "modern" practitioners.

The purpose of this chapter is to examine the most common patterns of traditional midwifery and contraception and some of their variations, in terms of what would be useful for health practitioners and administrators to know for improved maternal and child health and for more effective health care and training programmes. It is not meant to be an exhaustive catalogue of birth practices. A knowledge of existing childbirth patterns and the role played by local specialists, such as traditional midwives, should be a prime consideration in establishing maternal and child health programmes, and should improve our understanding of the acceptance or rejection of certain practices and the use of certain health resources. In addition, such a comparative view should provide a basis on which to develop safer practices.

Concepts of illness and health

The degree to which pregnancy and childbirth are viewed as medical problems varies. In many societies they are regarded as normal parts of life, whereas in the West, especially in the United States of America, pregnancy and birth are often viewed as a disease or physiological disturbance and treated under the domain of the medical system. Although in some societies childbirth is viewed as a component of the traditional health system and as an illness, in others it is not only considered as a biological event but also viewed holistically with social, ritual, and moral significance. Even in certain societies where illness terms are used to label pregnancy (e.g., *está enferma*, meaning "she is sick", used in Latin America), the emphasis is on the normality of most births; whereas in the biomedical system the emphasis is on the possible complications and abnormalities. On the other hand, even where childbirth is defined as normal, it is usually regarded as a dangerous period creating much anxiety. Various precautions are taken and rituals performed to protect both mother and child. Rituals are also performed as rites of passage to mark their change of status and to provide the mother with support and allay her anxieties.

In many parts of the world, health is considered to be a state of balance or equilibrium, internally and externally. Throughout Asia, Africa and Latin America, this equilibrium is based on variations of humoral medicine, involving balances of the qualities of hot and cold, and wet and dry. The Chinese principles of yin and yang are variations of this theme of balance. Pregnancy and birth are temporary states of imbalance, and care must be taken to restore the balance, usually through proper diet and activity.

The pregnant and postpartum woman is subject to a variety of dietary and behavioural restrictions and prescriptions which are based on this equilibrium principle, and are viewed as preventive as well as therapeutic. For example, a postpartum mother is often considered to be in a cold state because of the loss of blood (which is hot), and must take precautions to avoid cold influences. These precautions may include seclusion, keeping her head covered, not bathing, not eating "cold" substances, but rather eating or drinking "hot" foods and medicines. Cold foods will also make the breast milk cold and the nursing baby ill. The common application of heat in terms of temperature, such as hot baths and teas, is aimed at restoring a healthy balance in the mother. Sterility is commonly attributed to a cold womb and treatment is to "heat" the womb, usually with herbs that have hot qualities or a hot bath or sweat-bath (Guatemala).

Medical personnel should appreciate these classifications and principles, and understand that treatment and advice are more likely to be followed if communicated within the clients' traditions and with respect for their beliefs.

In Indonesia, some kinds of fruit are taboo for women who have just been delivered. The trainers in the Serpong training programme for traditional midwives, "tried to change this attitude, pointing out the nutritional value of the fruit. This proved to be not an easy task, because ancient beliefs cannot be changed overnight" (5). Although the authors of the study quoted did not refer to the hot-cold classification, if that was a relevant factor in why these fruits were forbidden, it might have been more effective to capitalize on these principles and add foods that fit into the belief system (e.g. hot foods) rather than try to change the beliefs, or use the principle of neutralization to accommodate such beliefs (e.g., add a "hot" substance, such as cinnamon, to the fruit).

The concept of heat could be used to teach concepts of asepsis and hygienic practices. The use of boiled water and disinfectants could be viewed in terms of heat, counteracting the harmful effects of cold. The germ theory could be incorporated within this framework and might be more acceptable in such terms.

An extension of the equilibrium principle is the balance of emotions and one's social relations. A common belief is that strong emotions, such as anger or fright, should be avoided during pregnancy and the postpartum period since they upset the body's equilibrium and thus may cause complications, including premature birth, miscarriage, retained placenta, and cessation of milk. Emotional stress might contribute to a difficult or complicated birth, whereas lack of such stress is beneficial. Avoiding stress can be regarded as an element of preventive medicine in these more holistic health systems. The body is a medium used to express particular patterns of social relations. Since most incidents of anger or other stressful emotions involve some type of conflict or change in social relations, the disturbed equilibrium of the social environment must be restored for proper health of the mother and child.

The imbalance caused by the pregnant and postpartum state is viewed in some societies as a dangerous and polluted state. Blood is considered an unclean substance and consequently a menstruating, pregnant, or newly delivered woman should avoid people, cattle and crops.

Concepts of the body, including ideas about the structure and function of different parts of the body, and folk theories of conception and fetal development also form the basis of various childbirth practices and thus should be understood by health practitioners. Certain organs that are recognized by scientific medicine may not be labelled by the traditional system; and, vice versa, units unfamiliar in modern obstetrics may be important in other systems. For example, the Yucatecan Maya consider the *tipté* to be an organ which regulates most internal functions and is located in the centre of the body beneath the navel. The force of labour may dislodge this organ, causing various symptoms, and the traditional midwife massages it back into place (6).

In many Latin American societies, the body is considered to be a tube, in which parts can move up or down or be displaced. Practices such as massage and the use of the abdominal binder are partly based on this concept—the uterus can move; massaging puts it in its proper location, and the binder keeps it there. The placenta is thought to be able to rise in the body and choke the mother if the cord is cut before the placenta is expelled.

Characteristics of the traditional midwife

Most traditional midwives are middle-aged to elderly women, are illiterate due to lack of formal education, and practise midwifery as a part-time occupation. Male midwives have been reported for a few societies, including some in Mexico, Ghana, and the Philippines; however, since most midwives are female, we shall use the feminine pronoun. Although the traditional midwife often has started her practice at a younger age, she is freer to assume midwifery responsibilities when she is postmenopausal. Age and experience usually confer respect and status. The formally trained midwife, on the other hand, is often younger, unmarried, or childless, and is put in a supervisory position over the traditional midwife. Where age confers respect, this can create potential conflict. It can also undermine the value put on age and the respect shown to the elderly by the community. The traditional midwife is usually a member of the local community, familiar with her clients and their family. She speaks their language, and shares the local system of health beliefs and behaviour. She is usually more readily available and accessible. She occupies a respected position within the community, although her status varies in different societies. The *dai* in India occupies a status at the low end of the scale; due to the belief that birth is unclean and polluting, only a person of low caste is allowed to deliver the baby, cut the cord, and dispose of the placenta. In Africa however, the traditional midwife enjoys a high status.

Despite the respect she may command within the community, the traditional midwife tends to be assigned a low status by hospital personnel, medical practitioners and the educated classes who regard her as superstitious, ignorant and dangerous. These attitudes have constituted obstacles to effective programmes and cooperation and need to be overcome. Under the influence of modern medical programmes, the traditional midwife's position becomes ambiguous. In some cases her use of modern techniques and medicines increases her prestige. At the same time, she becomes more dependent on them and on the medical personnel, whose condescending attitudes may undermine her own confidence and subsequently that of her clients.

The relationship between the traditional midwife and her client is usually personalized, informal, supportive and holistic, in contrast with the depersonalized, formal, authoritarian, and segmented characteristics of the Western mode of childbirth. This generalization should be regarded as describing two models which are at opposite ends of a continuum. Societies vary in the degree to which they conform to one or the other model, but most traditional systems of childbirth are more similar to the first one.

"Personalized" means that the midwife usually knows the client and her family, visits her, and operates in an atmosphere of confidence and trust. Care is centred on the client and family rather than practitioner-oriented (7). The traditional midwife is concerned not only with the biological aspects of the birth process, but also with the woman's emotional life, family relations, and spiritual life. During the different phases of childbirth, care is consistent rather than segmented, as happens when a different specialist is concerned with prenatal, delivery, and postnatal care.

In most societies the woman is not isolated from her family but has the support of other family members. In some, the husband is required to assist, whereas in others he is not allowed and only female assistants are present. As Newman has suggested, the social support mode as opposed to the profession-centred mode is characteristic of most traditional birth systems (8). This contrast is also manifested in the locus of decision-making. In the traditional system, the woman retains much of the decision-making power, although she often consults with the midwife; whereas in the Western system, the obstetrician is usually the locus of decision-making and maintains authority over the mother.

The holistic characteristics of the midwife-client relationship are manifested not only in the consistency of care but also the ways in which the midwife's role relates to the larger sociocultural context. In some societies the midwife helps with the household chores of the new mother and washes the blood-stained clothes. She may have godparent or kinship ties with her client. She is often a sacred specialist as well as an obstetrical one and performs various rituals and prayers throughout the birth process (9). Childbirth is frequently regarded as a dangerous period, with both mother and infant susceptible to physical and spiritual harm. Protective rituals, some performed by the traditional midwife, may include prayers, lighting candles, burning incense, animal sacrifices, herbal baths, wearing amulets, and eating special foods.

The contrast between the traditional midwife-client relationship and the authoritarian professionally centred one is illustrated by the following example. During a review class that was part of a training programme for traditional midwives in Guatemala, the midwives were told to bring their clients to the prenatal clinic. Many did not do so, however, explaining that many women refused for various reasons—time, money, embarrassment, etc. The response of the nurse was that the midwives should tell the women that it was an order, and unless the patient went to the prenatal clinic the midwife would not attend the birth nor be responsible if something were to happen. This authoritarian and threatening attitude which the nurse displayed toward the traditional midwife and which she assumed the midwife could show toward the client, reflects the hierarchical, dominant-subordinate control relationships characteristic of the biomedical system rather than any "scientific" purpose of improving health. The nurse could have explained the reasons for going to the prenatal clinic for the detection of risk factors, which the midwife could have conveyed to her client, but she did not. Instead, she acted in an authoritarian manner which is contrary to the type of relationship in that society between the traditional midwife and her client, whom she can advise, warn, or scold, but not command. The locus of decision-making remains primarily in the hands of the client, not the midwife (*10*).

The reaction of the nurse also reflects a lack of understanding of the midwife as a ritual specialist. Many traditional Amerindian midwives believe that they are supernaturally selected and that to refuse to help a woman is a sin for which they might be punished by God.

The traditional midwife is sometimes also feared because she is believed to have the power to harm the mother or child. For example, in parts of Ghana some local midwives can inflict an illness called *asram*, which can cause a fetal death, neonatal death, or puerperal illness in the mother (*11*, p. 119).

Recruitment and training

The reasons for becoming a traditional midwife include inheritance from a female relative, supernatural calling, a dream experience, or a personal decision. Inheritance is the most commonly reported path of recruitment. A variation of the inheritance pattern occurs in India, where the *dai* comes from the lowest castes and caste membership is inherited.

Recruitment through supernatural channels includes signs such as being born with a caul, having dreams or visions, suffering a serious illness, or encountering special objects such as oddly shaped stones, a knife, scissors, a shell, a carving or a statue. These signs are interpreted by a diviner, who indicates the traditional midwife's destiny or calling. It is commonly believed that if a person refuses to take the calling, she or her family will be punished by God or some supernatural agency. The supernatural source and validation of her skills increases the midwife's confidence and protects her by minimizing her liability. Inheritance and supernatural training may be combined. For example, in parts of the Philippines knowledge of midwifery reportedly comes from visions of third-generation relatives, such as one's parents' grandparents (*12*).

Apprenticeship to another midwife, often a relative, is the most common pattern of training. The traditional midwife learns informally by watching and doing. While acquiring skills, she also picks up knowledge of herbs and other medicines. Even when the traditional midwife claims to receive her knowledge from dreams or visions, she has often also assisted another midwife. Sometimes the midwife has learned from watching her own births. In some cases she has begun practising by being called to an emergency birth when no one else was available. Because of her successful delivery, others then began to request her services.

Accountability is often believed to be to God or to some supernatural force. That is, the traditional midwife may believe that the outcome of the birth is in God's hands and that she is only His agent. However, she is also accountable to the community. As a member of the community, she is exposed to various social pressures and sanctions. Her reputation, and consequently the number of her clients, will be influenced by her manner and treatment of them as well as by the number of her successful deliveries.

Prenatal care

The amount and type of prenatal care varies widely. The traditional midwife may be requested to examine the woman at any time during the pregnancy, the most frequently reported times being between the fifth and seventh months.

The prenatal examination usually begins with an informal visit, during which inquiries are made concerning the health of the mother and her family. The traditional midwife usually palpates the abdominal area to determine the position and age of the fetus, and massages the woman, often using some kind of warmed oil or grease. The massage is thought to make the birth easier, to prevent pains during pregnancy, to keep the uterus in place, and to reposition or manipulate the fetus if necessary by external version (*13*).

Many medical personnel consider massaging as potentially harmful because it might be done too vigorously and cause premature separation of the placenta. However, rather than condemning massaging *per se* by the traditional midwives, gentle massaging could be suggested since this may relax the mother and make her feel better as well as giving her emotional support through the physical contact. In several societies, the women feel that massaging is a necessary part of prenatal care. In some African societies, the midwives manually dilate the passages during the last month to prevent obstruction (*14*). Among the Luvale of Zambia, intravaginal application of herbal medicines is the most common mode of treatment for a variety of female conditions and illnesses, including pregnancy and parturition; Spring suggests that this contributes to infection and infertility (*15*).

Prenatal examinations, as well as the actual delivery, are performed in accordance with local standards of modesty. Often the woman keeps fully dressed, exposing only the area necessary for the massage or examination. This is especially the case in many parts of Latin America, Asia, and the Middle East, where much value is placed on modesty, and women feel shame or embarrassment both when questioned concerning pregnancy and sex and when examined by a male physician or even a strange female. The lack of privacy and the nudity involved during examinations at health centres or during hospital deliveries can provoke much anxiety. Medical personnel should be sensitized to the importance of this value and adjust conditions accordingly.

Herbal teas and baths may be administered to the pregnant woman to ease pains, to "heat", fortify, and protect her. The traditional midwives often provide advice on diet and activity, reminding the pregnant woman of the various proscriptions and prescriptions which are intended to guard against spiritual and physical dangers.

A common restriction in groups that adhere to the humoral theory is that foods classified as "cold" should be avoided. Also, very "hot" items like chili should be avoided. The restricted foods sometimes include foods considered nutritious and recommended by Western medicine, such as eggs, which are thought to lead to prolonged labour in such different societies as Nigeria and Guatemala. On the other hand, nutritious foods may be recommended by tradition, such as chicken, which is recommended for pregnant women in Guatemala. In contrast, chicken is tabooed for women in certain African societies, such as the Mbum Kpau of Chad, who believe women will suffer reproductive failure for breaking the taboo (16). Other restrictions are based on the principle of "sympathetic magic", such as not eating rabbit meat or the woman will have multiple births (Guatemala), or not eating armadillo and conch because they retreat in the shell and might cause the child to do the same in the womb, causing a difficult birth (Black Carib or Garifuna).

Food cravings should be satisfied, as it is believed by many groups that the denial of such cravings will result in either deformation of the baby or miscarriage.

Wide variations exist in behavioural restrictions. Some are related to the state of susceptibility of mother and fetus while others are related to the dangerous force of heat or pollution of the pregnant woman. In some societies, the woman is supposed to exercise and work to avoid suffering during birth and so as not to have a large baby. However, she must take care while washing clothes and she should not lift heavy objects.

Traditional midwives are often called if a miscarriage is suspected and may administer herbal infusions or plasters to prevent miscarriages.

Delivery

The majority of births, especially in rural areas, are domiciliary, with the traditional midwife coming to the mother's home. In some parts of Africa, where the traditional midwives now have their own maternity centres, the mother goes there for the delivery. The mother may be secluded in a special hut or partitioned part of the house. In parts of India, birth is secretive, the house is shut, and the woman is not supposed to cry out.

Shouting or crying are disapproved. No admiration or compliments are given after the birth for fear of attracting the evil eye. In a few societies, birth is more communal, there is no seclusion, and relatives and neighbours may attend.

One or more persons usually attend the birth, most often elderly female relatives, in addition to the midwife. Ford's survey of 64 cultures indicated that in 31, men are forbidden to attend the delivery (17). However, in Mexico and Guatemala, the husband is supposed to be present and his assistance is regarded as his responsibility. It is felt that he would then know what the woman has to go through. In some societies (e.g., Carib), this identification goes even further with the practice of *couvade*, in which the husband's behaviour parallels that of his wife's; he either takes to bed or has to refrain from certain activities.

The emotional and social support given at the time of parturition is provided by these assistants and is probably important in allaying anxiety; whereas, in hospital deliveries, the woman is usually isolated from her family.

Patterns of management of labour range from *laissez-faire* to speeding up labour by various forms of interference. As with prenatal care, the most commonly reported pattern is abdominal massage and pressure, often rubbing on some type of oil or herbal mixture. Surgical interference is rare, but episiotomies have been carried out by village midwives in the Sudan because of labour difficulties due to female circumcision (18). In the Punjab, India, a particular type of manipulation known as heeling is reported. The midwife (*dai*) exerts pressure and counteraction with each labour pain with her feet on either side of the birth canal. The midwife also lubricates the vaginal canal with clarified butter or oil (19). In some societies, the traditional midwife also practises vaginal dilation as well as vaginal lubrication.

Chemical interference by administering herbal teas is more common and frequently used to ease labour pains or to speed up labour. Research has shown some of these herbs to be oxytocic, such as the Mexican herb, *cihuapatle* or *zoapatle* (*Montanoa tomentosa*) (20). Some of these plants may also be used as abortifacients because they can produce uterine contractions.

Most medical personnel consider the use of herbs as harmful and condemn the practice. Cases have been reported of women coming to the hospital with tonic uterine contractions or even rupture after having taken too much of certain herbs. Such practices are obviously harmful and attempts should be made to modify or eliminate them. However, the wholesale condemnation of the use of herbal medicines is unjustified. An underlying assumption is that the traditional midwife uses these herbs indiscriminately and ignorantly. In many cases, part of the traditional midwife's special knowledge is the proper amounts of such herbs to be used for various purposes and the effects of these amounts. It is ethnocentric and potentially dangerous to condemn indigenous herbal medicines while promoting other oxytocic agents, analgesics and anaesthesias, some of which may be beneficial while others have been shown to be harmful to the mother or fetus and still others have unknown effects (21). A blanket condemnation of the utilization of all herbs is not warranted in the present state of our knowledge.

More research on and analyses of these plants should be made. Whereas both herbs and pharmaceutical medicines may be harmful in excess or have side-effects, they may be medically effective when used in proper amounts. Rather than denigrate traditional practices, appropriate dosages and preparations of herbal medicines might be scientifically determined, thus enabling them to be employed for the certain benefit of mother and child.

A survey of 76 non-Western societies showed that 62 used an upright delivery position, such as kneeling, sitting, squatting, or standing (22). A rope may be tied to a roof beam for support, or a chair or edge of a bed used, or another person may hold the woman with arms around her, sometimes from the front, sometimes from behind, and help her push down on her abdomen. In some parts of Africa, the child is supposed to be born on the soil, the source of fertility (23).

The supine or horizontal position is being advocated and imposed by many Western trained personnel, while the traditional vertical position is condemned. The supine position makes it easier for the obstetrician or midwife to view the baby, but may be more difficult for the mother since she must push against gravity. Moreover, the vertical position is usually accompanied by gradual stretching of the tissues, whereas the supine position promotes the use of various forms of chemical or instrumental interference, such as induction of labour, episiotomies, and use of forceps. It has also been shown that one exerts maximum intra-abdominal pressure in a squatting or vertical position (11, p. 128). In rural households, where the technological aids and facilities that are used in a hospital delivery are non-existent, the horizontal position may lead to a more anxious and difficult birth.

Where modesty is a strong value, the traditional position is more appropriate than the horizontal position which exposes the lower part of the body. Verderese and Turnbull suggest:

> New methods or practices to be demonstrated should be adapted to traditional ones rather than vice versa. For example, if the trainer could adapt her methods of delivering a baby, and allow delivery in the native traditional position—kneeling or sitting up position it might reduce emotional tension in the traditional birth attendants and their clients. (1, p. 65).

Nevertheless, most medical personnel and most training programmes emphasize the supine position. This is reinforced through audiovisual aids. For example, a recent manual for training traditional midwives used by the Guatemalan Ministry of Public Health (24) shows a drawing of a woman lying down on a bed giving birth. In some rural houses, there is no bed and people sleep on mats or in hammocks. Care must be taken not to eliminate a beneficial and appropriate position in favour of one whose advantages have not been scientifically proven and are now being strongly questioned.

In cases of prolonged or difficult labour, various techniques are used to induce gagging or contraction of muscles, such as putting the woman's braid in her mouth, putting fingers down her throat, using snuff, making her sneeze, giving her oil to drink, and making her blow in a bottle. Unlocking bolts and locks, opening drawers, untying the mother's hair, or using charms made from moults of animals, are techniques based on sympathetic magic that may be employed to hasten labour. The traditional midwife may also perform rituals, say prayers, and listen to confession. A *shaman* or diviner is sometimes consulted to divine the cause of the difficulty, which may be attributed to adultery (usually blamed on the mother) or to witchcraft, and to perform the appropriate ceremony. Shaking the mother or other rough treatment is reported in some groups for dealing with difficult or prolonged labour.

Delayed delivery is based on some concept of a normal rate. What is regarded as the normal rate in a specific group? Are the different stages of labour recognized, and what is considered the normal length of each? In some societies women are exhorted to bear down from the onset of labour or too early, and this may lead to damage to the mother and child or to exhaustion and uterine inertia (*18*).

Traditional midwives usually deal with abnormal presentations by external manipulation of the fetus. If a part of the body is extended, they first push it back in with lubrication. More rarely do they attempt internal manipulation.

In most societies, the traditional midwives offer encouragement and emotional support, allay anxiety, and relieve pain. In a few groups, certain practices seem to increase discomfort and anxiety. The actual effects and efficacy of the various practices and the attitudes of the traditional midwives and their clients need more extensive research.

The placenta and umbilical cord

According to Ford's crosscultural survey (*17*), the usual practice is to delay cutting the umbilical cord until after the delivery of the placenta, although in a few societies the cord is cut before the placenta is expelled. The placenta is commonly believed to have a special relation to the infant, sometimes referred to as the second child, and it is believed that the child will die if the cord is cut before the placenta is expelled. As mentioned earlier, traditional midwives in Guatemala also believe that the placenta will then rise up within the mother's body and choke her.

Some scientists advocate waiting until the cord stops pulsing in order to allow more blood and oxygen to circulate to the baby. However, many of the training programmes tell the traditional midwives to cut the cord immediately after the birth on the grounds that the child may be neglected and overexposed, resulting in pneumonia or bronchitis (25).

Cutting tools include bamboo, shell, broken glass, knife, sickle, trowel, razor, and scissors. These are rarely cleaned in an antiseptic manner before their use. Dressing of the cord includes such substances as salt, talcum, ground shells, clay, palm oil, dried dung, ash, soot, juice of banana shoots, spider webs, and a variety of herbs. The main risk from either a contaminated cutting instrument or a contaminated dressing is tetanus neonatorum. In parts of Africa and Central America, the midwife cauterizes the cord with either a hot blade or candle flame and applies hot candle wax. This leaves the cord dry and sterile and prevents tetanus (26). Where it is difficult to ensure aseptic conditions, such a practice may be beneficial. Some traditional midwives combine practices. One Guatemalan midwife cauterizes the cord with a candle flame, then uses alcohol, thiomersal, and talcum powder on the cord.

In some groups, spider webs were used for dressing the cord. Most physicians initially viewed this as a dirty and dangerous practice, but it was later shown that spiders' silk has antibiotic properties—"a fact that TBAs had apparently recognized for years" (27).

The umbilical cord is usually tied with thread, string, or plant fibre, at a specific length which varies widely. Certain signs of the mother's future, such as the number and spacing of children may be read from the cord.

Because the placenta is often believed to affect the future life of the child, its disposal is important. The placenta and cord are usually buried; sometimes they are burned first. This burial is supposed to keep the child to the land. Sometimes the cord is guarded and used in medicines. Proper disposal may be a cause of anxiety to the mother in hospital deliveries. To avoid this possibility, the placenta and cord could be given to the mother or husband to dispose of as they wish.

For a retained placenta, many of the practices and techniques are the same as those that are used for delayed labour: massage, gagging, and administration of herbal teas. Manual extraction of the placenta is done rarely.

Treatment of the newborn

The baby's eyes may be wiped with a rag or cotton, treated with a drop of lemon juice, oil, onion, boric acid, zinc oxide, silver nitrate or patented eye drops. In India, khol is put around the eyes, which is believed to strengthen them. Purgatives are sometimes administered to clean the meconium. If the baby is not given the colostrum of the mother, substitute liquids such as sugar water or water with anise or some herbs may be given for the first two or three days, until the mother's milk begins to flow. The traditional midwife may clear the baby's throat and nose of mucus and blood with her fingers, which could be a source of infection. The newborn baby may be cleaned with oil or washed in lukewarm water. Usually the midwife visits and checks the umbilicus several times during the first week or until the cord drops. Various amulets may be used and the midwife may perform various rituals to protect the baby from illnesses such as those induced by the evil eye. Sometimes the baby's head, nose and limbs are shaped by being bound or manipulated. Swaddling of the infant is very common. Sometimes the baby is wrapped in several layers of covers in order to keep it warm, with the result that it sweats from being overheated.

Postpartum treatment of the mother

Alcohol, salt, and various herbs are sometimes used to treat wounds of the birth canal and prevent infection. Massaging the abdominal area to ease afterbirth pains and cause retroflexion of the uterus is very common (28). Breasts are also massaged, which is believed to stimulate the flow of milk. Special herbs or mixtures may be taken to increase the milk flow. Herbal teas are also commonly administered as remedies for postpartum pains.

Heat is often applied. In parts of Guatemala and Mexico, the sweat-bath is used; in other areas, hot herbal baths or sitz-baths are given. In South-East Asia, the practice of "mother roasting" or "lying by the fire" is common. In some societies, postpartum food restrictions are stressed more than those during gestation because they are believed to affect the quality and quantity of the mother's milk.

The use of an abdominal binder is also a common practice. Among the Mayan Indians it is used to keep the uterus in place and to close the bones, which are believed to open during delivery (6, 29).

In some communities, the father must also follow postnatal restrictions, which are a form of the *couvade*. For example, among the Black Carib or Garifuna of Belize, the father should avoid strenuous work activities, sex and the use of weapons or sharp instruments until at least the umbilical cord has dropped, or else the baby's navel will bleed. These practices have been interpreted by some investigators as being related to the belief that the child receives its body and blood from the mother but its soul or spirit from the father.

The mother is usually confined and her activity restricted for a period that varies from 8 to 40 days, depending on the society, but is also affected by the mother's economic status and household help. This set of proscriptions and prescriptions is referred to in China as "doing the month" (30). Various rituals may be performed at the end of the convalescent period, such as the *xe ch'at* on the twentieth day among some Guatemalan Mayans (31) or the *Sebau'* on the seventh day in Egypt (32). These rituals mark the end of the midwife's duties, restore the mother's relationships with relatives and neighbours, and mark the return of the mother to normal activities and reintegration into the larger social group.

Contraception

Some means of contraception or birth control exist in most societies. The specific measures vary widely in their effectiveness and their rationale. The most widespread and most reliable method is abstinence. This is often combined with certain taboos, perhaps the most common one being the taboo against sex during lactation. This practice is based on the belief that intercourse or pregnancy will change the quality of the mother's milk and make the infant sick or force it to be prematurely weaned. This has the effect of spacing births, even though this rationale may not be verbalized or be a conscious one. Prolonged breast-feeding by itself is said to suppress ovulation; it depends on a number of factors including the frequency and intensity of suckling. Increasing westernization and urbanization have led to the shortening and in some cases the abandon of lengthy postpartum abstinences and in the decline of the length of breast-feeding, resulting in shorter birth intervals.

Abstinence during special rituals, before certain activities such as hunting, or on specific days of the month, is practised in several societies. Sometimes these practices are related to beliefs about pollution, supernatural influences, economic activities and sexual roles. Periodic abstinence (or the "rhythm" method) is often practised during what is believed to be the fertile period. This period may be defined erroneously as during menstruation or five days before or five days after. Such misconceptions may promote intercourse during the actual fertile period, although they still reflect people's desire to limit births. In India, abstinence is supported by beliefs that intercourse and semen loss are weakening and conserving semen is strengthening.

Other types of "social" methods involve variations of intercourse, such as withdrawal or coitus interruptus, pseudocoitus (interfemoral), and coitus obstructus (manual obstruction of the urethra) (33).

Turning of the womb or retroflexion by external massaging has been reported in several societies. In the Philippines it is referred to as "tipping the matrix" or "bending the tubes" (34). According to Ascadi (35), this measure as practised among the Yoruba in Nigeria is not very effective. Other physical means, such as the woman lying down on her belly or jumping up after intercourse so that the sperm runs out, are mentioned occasionally.

Mechanical methods include sheaths or condoms, which have been made out of fish skin, animal skin, bladders and intestines, and pessaries or obstructive plugs or caps placed over the cervix. The latter have been made out of herbs, gum arabic, honey, dung, rock salt, or other absorbent or impervious material inserted in the vagina. Some of these, such as salt, gum arabic and certain herbs may be effective chemically by changing the pH of the vagina and acting as a spermicide. Precoital insertion of patent medicines such as crushed aspirin or quinine pills is an adaptation of this principle. Similarly, precoital and postcoital douching, using such substances as salty water, vinegar, lemon juice, and boric acid, may change the pH of the vagina and thus affect the mobility or vitality of the sperm.

Many reports exist of indigenous plants used for contraception. Most of these are taken as herbal teas; others are inserted vaginally or used as douches. Some of the plants may contain active principles that inhibit or neutralize gonadotrophic pituitary hormones (36); others are abortifacients and provoke uterine contractions; and still others are of unknown effectiveness. In some groups, the use of these herbs is accompanied by various rituals and incantations which are believed to be necessary for their effectiveness.

The use of charms, beads, amulets, rings, belts and various magical objects are other traditional methods. Some of these are believed to block the passage of the semen and sperm. Others are related to concepts of conception, such as the action of spirits being necessary for conception and being preventable by these charms.

Although technically not a form of contraception, abortion is one of the most common types of birth control. Even where abortion is illegal or strongly disapproved of, various abortion techniques are commonly known. The extent to which it is practised, however, is often unknown. Chemical means of abortion include herbal teas, drugs such as quinine and ergot, and various types of poison such as laundry blue, lime or potash, some of which may have fatal effects. Mechanical means include insertion of sticks, herbs, roots, and irritants. Physical methods include jumping from a tree or other activity, hard, deep massage, and pressing weights on the abdominal region.

Knowledge about abortion methods may be denied where it is socially disapproved of. In some cases, however, when asked for herbs or methods used as emmenagogues, to bring on menstruation, the traditional midwife or lay person would mention several. Some of these herbs may also be abortifacients.

The opposite problem, barrenness or infertility, is an important concern among many women, especially in groups where a woman's status depends on her having offspring. Infertility may be attributed to the coolness of the womb and treated with heat, as in the form of a sweat-bath, and with "hot" quality herbs; misplacement of organs is treated by massage; misbehaviour of the wife is treated with rituals and confession; for witchcraft or supernatural sanction, the treatment may involve pilgrimages to shrines or participation in special groups or cults, such as the Aladura sect among the Yorubas in Nigeria, or the Tigari sect in Ghana.

Research

Much of our knowledge of birth customs and related cultural institutions is derived either from research done by anthropologists and sociologists or from reports by physicians and other health professionals. The anthropological reports are usually part of a general ethnography of a particular group, derived from interviews, case studies, and participant observation. Few observations of actual births have been made, however, and usually what is reported are the ideal rules—that is, what people say they should do and what they say they do, but not necessarily what they actually do. More recently, several studies have focused specifically on childbirth and the role of the traditional midwife within the health system and within the community, and have utilized more rigorous research designs and observations of childbearing. There is still a need for more studies of behaviour—for example, when and how frequently people follow the culturally prescribed dietary rules.

Medical professionals, on the other hand, often see only the complications brought into the health centres and hospitals, some of which they attribute to traditional practices. They also become aware of other traditional practices when they conflict with their Western obstetrical ones. As a result, they emphasize what they consider to be the negative aspects of traditional practices and rarely mention positive ones.

Some pilot projects for maternal and child health and family planning programmes[1] have carried on interdisciplinary field studies with surveys of traditional midwives, their characteristics and activities in order to utilize the midwives more effectively. These studies, as well as a few others (*37*) have focused on evaluating the potential effectiveness of the traditional midwife as a family planning worker.

Other types of research have reviewed official policies concerning traditional midwives and training programmes through questionnaires sent to the health ministry personnel running the programmes (*1*, *2*).

A few cross-cultural reviews of the literature have been made which show both the range of variation and the most common patterns of midwifery practices (*2*, *18*, *28*, *38–40*). These and other investigators have suggested classifying birth practices into harmful, beneficial, neutral, and uncertain (*41*). The goal of this classification is to change or eliminate those deemed harmful by the medical personnel and build on or incorporate beneficial ones. The latter has rarely been done, the emphasis being on the negative aspects.

This type of classification, however, entails certain problems. A number of practices are either positive or innocuous in their effects and others have unknown effects, yet they are condemned and denounced by the medical establishment. Classification or evaluation is usually done according to supposedly "objective" or "scientific" criteria, such as infant mortality. Few practices are clearly evaluated; most practices are more or less beneficial or harmless as compared to alternative practices. Verderese and Turnbull consider protective rituals, ceremonies, placenta disposal, and the ritual bath for the mother as harmless practices, but say "they have

---

[1] These projects include the Danfa programme in Ghana, the Serpong family planning project in Indonesia, and the San Pablo Autopan project in Mexico.

positive psychological effects on the TBAs themselves and their clients" (*1*, p. 38).

Jordan (*13*) has shown that for many Western obstetrical practices, inconclusive and contradictory medical evidence exists regarding positive and negative effects. Justification of these practices is often based on insufficient evidence. Consequently, attempts to classify birth practices on the basis of medical criteria are often inconclusive. Nevertheless, many traditional practices are often condemned on little or no scientific evidence. There is a need to develop a broader set of evaluation criteria, including criteria from traditional cultures, as well as to ascertain on a scientific basis what might account for effective practices.

Some research on medicinal plants used in midwifery and contraception has been done (e.g., by the Mexican Institute for the Study of Medicinal Plants—IMEPLAM), but more research is needed in this area to determine the chemical constituents and efficacy of these plants. Research on other traditional practices, such as the use of the sweat-bath or other forms of heat, and massaging, needs to be done before judgments about their benefits or harmfulness can be made. Few controlled studies have been made. One is a study in India of the correlation between the level of training of the midwife, the instrument used to cut the cord, the type of dressing of the cord, and the incidence of tetanus neonatorum (*42*).

Coordination

The traditional midwife is a direct link to women of reproductive age who might otherwise not be reached by the usual clinic and health delivery services. Given the shortage of medical personnel and the goal of expanding primary health care, she is an important human resource. For increased articulation with the official health system, modifications may have to be made in the attitudes of the medical personnel and in the teaching methods employed, rather than following the tendency to emphasize changing the practices of the traditional midwives.

Since the majority of traditional midwives are illiterate, teaching methods must be adapted. Materials and techniques should be simple, inexpensive, relevant to the local culture and literacy conditions, and made of locally available material. Demonstration aids, such as dolls, cords, balloons, flannel-boards, and pictures should be used, but care should be taken with cartoon-like figures that may not be understood. One should also be careful of possible biases in the content of audiovisual aids, such as showing the use of the horizontal delivery position rather than the traditional one. Training should be practical and concrete, rather than abstract, with emphasis on participation and action. It should be behaviourally oriented rather than formal lectures and the verbal mode of knowledge (B. Jordan, personal communication).

The tone and attitude of the medical personnel should be respectful rather than belittling, condescending or condemnatory.

Support services should be provided from the official health system. It is useless to tell traditional midwives to refer patients if health care services are inaccessible. Support also refers to communication and respectful treatment. If the traditional midwife is scolded, ignored, or looked down upon by the medical staff, she will be reluctant to refer her clients again. If kits such as the UNICEF kits are given, instruments and medicines should be replenishable or easily available. Some authority should be designated as responsible for replenishing supplies (3, p. 20).

Training has been primarily unidirectional (43) with emphasis on "upgrading" the indigenous practices. The possibility of reciprocal teaching and accommodation should be considered as a way of learning the viewpoint of the midwives, why they prefer certain practices, what they see as problems and how they handle them. Attempts should be made to understand, build on and incorporate traditional practices (such as the local social support mechanisms) and "upgrade" the Western-based obstetrical system, rather than simply to eradicate or change the traditional one. Trained traditional midwives could also be used in teaching other midwives in future programmes and an adapted apprenticeship system could be developed. In order to achieve a closer and more effective relationship, the official health care system needs to be made more compatible with the sociocultural framework of the traditional midwives and their clients.

REFERENCES

(1) VERDERESE, M. DE L. & TURNBULL, L. M. *The traditional birth attendant in maternal and child health and family planning.* Geneva, World Health Organization, 1975 (WHO Offset Publications No. 18).

(2) *Traditional midwives and family planning.* Baltimore, MD, Johns Hopkins University, Population information program, 1980 (Population Reports, Series J. No. 22).

(3) IMOAGENE, O. Current information on the practice, training and supervision of traditional birth attendants in the African Region. In: *Training and supervision of traditional birth attendants: report of a study group, Brazzaville, 1976* (Unpublished WHO document AFR/MCH/71).

(4) LESLIE, C., ed. *Asian medical systems.* Berkeley, University of California Press, 1976, pp. 6–8.

(5) LUBIS, F. ET AL. *Report of the course for traditional midwives in the Kecamatan Serpong.* Leyden State University and Universitas Indonesia, 1973 (Serpong paper No. 14), p. 12.

(6) FULLER, N. & JORDAN, B. *Maya women and the end of the birthing period: postpartum massage and binding in Yucatan, Mexico.* East Lansing, MI, Michigan State University, Department of Anthropology, 1979 (unpublished document).

(7) KANG-WANG, J. F. The midwife in Taiwan: an alternative model for maternity care. *Human organization,* **39**:70–79 (1980).

(8) NEWMAN, L. F. Midwives and modernization (Introduction). *Medical anthropology,* **5** (1): 1–12 (1981).

(9) PAUL, L. & PAUL, B. The Maya midwife as sacred specialist. *American ethnologist,* **2**:707 (1975).

(10) COSMINSKY, S. *Childbirth and change: a Guatemalan case study*. Paper presented at the American Anthropological Association, Los Angeles, 14–18 November 1978.
(11) AMPOFO, D. A. & ACOLATSE, P. A. The art and science of the traditional birth attendant in Ghana. In: *Training and supervision of traditional birth attendants*. Brazzaville, World Health Organization, 1976 (document AFR/MCH/71).
(12) HART, D. From pregnancy through birth in a Bisayan Filipino village. In: Hart, D., ed. *Southeast Asian birth customs*. New Haven, CT, USA, Human Relations Area Files Press, 1965.
(13) JORDAN, B. *Birth in four cultures*. Montreal, Eden Press, 1978.
(14) GELFAND, M. *Medicine and custom in Africa*. London, E. & S. Livingston, 1964.
(15) SPRING, A. An indigenous therapeutic style and its consequences for natality: the Luvale of Zambia. In: Marshall, J. & Polgar, S. *Culture, natality, and family planning*. Chapel Hill, NC, USA, University of North Carolina, 1976 (Carolina Population Center, Monograph No. 21) pp. 99–125.
(16) O'LAUGHLIN, B. Mediation of contradiction: why Mbum women do not eat chicken. In: Rosaldo, M. & Lamphere, L. *Women, culture and society*. Stanford, Stanford University Press, 1974.
(17) FORD, C. *A comparative study of human reproduction*. New Haven, Yale University Press, 1945 (Yale University Publications in Anthropology No. 32).
(18) JELLIFFE, D. and BENNETT, F. World-wide care of the mother and newborn child. *Clinical obstetrics and gynaecology* **5**:69 (1962).
(19) GIDEON, H. A baby is born in the Punjab. *American anthropologist* **64**:1220–1234 (1962).
(20) ORTIZ DE MONTELLANO, B. Empirical Aztec medicine. *Science* **188**:215–220 (1975).
(21) HAIRE, L. The cultural warping of childbirth. International Childbirth Education Association, *ICEA news*, 1972.
(22) NAROLL, F., NAROLL, R. & HOWARD, F. Position of women in childbirth. *American journal of obstetrics and gynaecology* **82**:943–954 (1961).
(23) JETT, J. *The role of traditional midwives in the modern health sector in West and Central America*, Washington, DC, US AID, 1977 (document REDSO/WA-76-61).
(24) GUATEMALA, MINISTERIO DE SALUD PÚBLICA y ASISTENCIA SOCIAL. *Manual para el adiestramiento de comadronas tradicionales. Guia para la enfermera responsable del programa*. Guatemala City, Dirección General de Servicios de Salud (División de Salud Materno, Infantil y Familiar, Departamento de Enfermería), 1976.
(25) IMOAGENE, O. Some cultural uniformities and gaps in traditional birth attendance: the case of Nigeria. In: *Training and supervision of traditional birth attendants: report of a study group, Brazzaville, 1976* (Unpublished WHO document AFR/MCH/71), p. 100.
(26) SOLIEN DE GONZALEZ, N. & BEHAR, M. Child-rearing practices, nutrition and health status. *Millbank Memorial Fund quarterly* **44** (2, pt. 2): 77–96 (1966).
(27) WORLD HEALTH ORGANIZATION *Traditional birth attendants*, Geneva, 1979 (WHO Offset Publication No. 44), p. 26.
(28) COSMINSKY, S. Cross-cultural perspectives on midwifery. In: Grollig, F. & Haley, H., ed. *Medical anthropology*. The Hague, Mouton Press, 1976, pp. 229–248.
(29) COSMINSKY, S. The role of the midwife in Middle America. In: *Congreso Internacional de Americanistas, Mexico City, 1974. Actas del congreso*, vol 3. Mexico City, Instituto Nacional de Antropología y Historia, 1976, pp. 279–291.
(30) PILLSBURY, B. *"Doing the month": confinement and convalescence of Chinese women after childbirth*. Presented at the American Anthropological Association 75th Annual Meeting. Washington, DC, Nov. 18–21, 1976.
(31) COSMINSKY, S. Birth rituals and symbolism: a Quiche Maya–Black Carib comparison. In: Young, P. & Howe, J. ed. *Ritual and symbol in native Central America*. Eugene, University of Oregon, 1976 (Anthropological papers No. 9), pp. 107–123.
(32) EL-HAMAMASY, L. *The daya of Egypt: survival in a modernizing society*. Pasadena, CA, USA, California Institute of Technology, Cal-tech Population Programme, 1973 (Occasional papers, Series 1, No. 8).
(33) NEWMAN, L. Birth control: an anthropological view. In: *Addison-Wesley module in anthropology*. Reading, MA, USA, Addison-Wesley, 1972.

(34) RUBEL, A., LIU, W., TROSDAL, M. & PATO, V. The traditional birth attendant in metropolitan Cebu, The Philippines. In: Polgar, S., ed. *Culture and population: a collection of current studies.* Chapel Hill, NC, University of North Carolina, 1971 (Carolina Population Center Monograph No. 9), pp. 176–186.

(35) ASCADI, G. Traditional birth control methods in Yorubaland. In: Marshall, J. & Polgar, S., ed. *Culture, natality, and family planning.* Chapel Hill, NC, University of North Carolina, 1976 (Carolina Population Center Monograph No. 21), pp. 126–155.

(36) COLMEIRO-LAFORET, C. Anticoncepcionales de origen vegetal. *Revista de obstétrica y ginecología,* **21**:179–184 (1962).

(37) ROGERS, E. & SOLOMON, D. *Traditional midwives as family planning communicators in Asia.* Honolulu, East-West Communication Institute, 1975.

(38) SPENCER, R. Primitive obstetrics. *Ciba Symposia* **11**:1158–1188 (1950).

(39) MEAD, M. & NEWTON, N. Cultural patterning of perinatal behaviour in childbearing—its social and psychological aspects. In: Richardson, S. & Gutmacher, A., ed. *Childbearing—its social and psychological aspects.* New York, Williams and Wilkins, 1967.

(40) OAKLEY, A. Cross-cultural practices. In: Chard, T. & Richards, M. ed. *Benefits and hazards of the new obstetrics.* Philadelphia, PA, J. P. Lippincott, 1977.

(41) KELLY, I. An anthropological approach to midwifery training in Mexico. *Journal of tropical pediatrics* **1**:200–205 (1956).

(42) GORDON, J., GIDEON, H. & WYON, J. Midwifery practices in rural Punjab, India. *American journal of obstetrics and gynecology,* **93**:734–742 (1965).

(43) MCCLAIN, C. Traditional midwives and family planning: an assessment of programs and suggestions for the future. *Medical anthropology,* **5**(1): 107–136 (1981).

CHAPTER 16
Selected individual therapies*

H. A. W. Forbes[1]

Anthroposophical medicine

Anthroposophical medicine is a comprehensive system for treating all the disturbances of the whole man. It is an active, well-established therapy with about 2000 European practitioners, mainly in Germany (*1, 2*).

Anthroposophical medicine is based on the working out by a modern mystic, Rudolf Steiner (1861–1925), in Western terms and materials, of the disturbances of the three energies that also form the basis of ayurvedic medicine. These energies are thinking, will and feeling.

Emphasis is placed on using the illness as a lesson and making the necessary self-adjustment. Herbal and mineral remedies are used externally and internally, including homoeopathic potencies. Heat, cold, art and eurhythmics are also employed (*3*).

Anthroposophical medicine is taught only to qualified allopathic medical practitioners at the Lucas Clinic, Arlesheim, Switzerland, but short courses are run in many countries. The remedies are manufactured mainly by two firms, Weleda A. G. and Wala Heilmittelbetriebe.

Autogenic training

Autogenic training is so called because it is self-generated. It is used mainly in Germany where it was developed by Dr J. H. Schulz (1884–1970) following observations by Oskar Vogt. Almost all the literature is in German except a six-volume textbook by Dr Wolfgang Luthe published in America (*4*). It is a form of self-healing.

---

* Further information on alternative medicine will be found in Chapter 23 on traditional practices in the European Region of WHO.
[1] Formerly, Consultant Physician, Plymouth, United Kingdom.

The mind uses relaxation of the physical body in quiet surroundings to gain cooperation with the instincts and emotions. When these three are in harmony they are receptive to positive suggestions. Many practical formulas have been worked out for self-programming to deal with all common conditions and life situations. Autogenic training has great potential for use as self-care.

Bates' technique of visual education

William H. Bates, M.D. (1860–1931) was a New York ophthalmologist. He realized that glasses are like crutches. They allow the user to get about, but make his condition worse. He held that emotional states and relaxation of mind and body had a more rapid and fundamental influence on vision than the action of the eye muscles. He devised physical and mental exercises that cure poor vision. Because the mechanical theory of vision cannot explain his method, his ideas have been rejected. With the advent of the new physics and the Pribram-Bohm theory that the brain is a holographic structure extracting our reality from a holographic universe (5, 6), there is a satisfactory explanation of why his system works. This self-healing method is worthy of further investigation.

Breathing

Few people are aware that there are more energies in the air than oxygen. Among others there is *qi* (Chinese), *ki* (Japanese), or *prana* (Indian). This can be directed mentally for conscious use by the whole man. About 25% of people breathe wrongly, using the abdominal muscles against the action of the diaphragm. Nearly all people breathe too fast because they seldom fill their lungs. *T'ai chi* and yoga teachers correct these faults and show how to use the energies for healthy living in its widest sense. Proper breathing is important in self-care.

Biofeedback

About the mid-1960s researchers using an idea taken from radio-communications began to ask whether an animal could be taught to control its automatic body functions. The answer was yes, and the procedure was called biofeedback. It was soon found to be applicable to man. The autonomic nervous system was shown to be teachable. The mental states that are part of the process of learning can themselves be learnt by biofeedback techniques.

Suddenly a vast new field of practical psychosomatic medicine was opened up. Blood pressure can be lowered, cold hands warmed, migraine and epilepsy controlled, hemiplegias rehabilitated and deep meditative states induced. It seems that any bodily or mental function that can be monitored may be altered.

There is now an annual digest of biofeedback literature (7). Most research comes from Japan and the USA.

Colour therapy

Colour was used by the ancient Egyptians and the Sumerians and has been part of Indian Ayurveda and Chinese medicine for thousands of years. It is little used in the West. In Europe there are about 150 practitioners and several hundred in the USA. Colour therapy works by using light waves of a specific frequency to alter a person's energy fields and the individual cells' vibratory pattern (8). Colour can be used in the form of light-baths, water treated by being kept in coloured glass containers and taken by mouth, colour transmitted radionically or by thought in healing.

Colour therapy is good for altering mental states, but also for some physical conditions such as arthritis. It is best used as an adjunct to other therapies and is not suitable for self-care. The wrong colour combinations can cause sickness. More attention should be paid to the use of colour in decorating and lighting work-places (9, 10).

Flower remedies

In Britain there are three remedies made from water in which flowers have been dipped in sunlight for a few hours. This process has the advantage that the plant is not destroyed.

The first was the discovery of a Welsh homoeopathic physician, Dr Edward Bach (1886–1936), towards the end of his life. Thirty-eight single flowers or buds are used, each being specific for an emotional state or a personality type. The Bach remedies seem to work on the same principle as homoeopathy and herbs—they transmit a pattern of energy. The author has used them increasingly in medical practice for the past 17 years. They work best in the young and those with recent disturbances (11).

The other two flower remedies, Vitaflorum and Exaltation of Flowers, are each made from many flowers in the same way as the Bach remedies. The one remedy treats every person and condition. The use of all these remedies is worldwide on a small scale. They are excellent for self-care, being totally without side-effects and harmless if the wrong remedy is given.

Gerson treatment

In every country people have found that a certain type of diet helps their apparently incurable diseases. Naturopaths, doctors, dentists and lay people have been doing this increasingly for the last 60 years. They make this observation for themselves and do not know that others have done the same. Some have come to the same conclusion by finding out what food keeps their pets healthy and then applying it to their patients. The diet consists of raw fresh vegetables and is low in salt, fat, carbohydrates and meat. The sort of conditions that are said to benefit include migraine, skin tuberculosis, *cancer*, atheroma (hardening of the arteries) and arthritis (*12*).

One man stands out from among these innovators—the late Max Gerson (M.D. Freiburg 1907), who worked in America from the early 1940s. He developed his treatment, which consists of a diet plus mineral and vitamin supplements, to relieve his migraine, but found it relieved skin tuberculosis and cancer fairly quickly and atheroma more slowly. He published his results widely in Europe and in America (*13*), but they have been ignored. A reassessment would be worth while.

Modifications of Gerson's regime are increasingly being used in the treatment of cancer in the USA and Europe by naturopaths and doctors.

Healing

Though healing is a single therapy, because it treats the whole person it is helpful for all conditions. Healing refreshes the parts the other therapies cannot reach. Besides being ancient it is practised worldwide. It cannot, therefore, be considered the monopoly of any religion. According to his or her unique beliefs, every healer has a different way of healing and ideas on how it works. Yet though there is this great diversity there is an underlying common principle (*14*).

Healing is a natural personal thing—mothers heal their children daily when they have a close bond with them. Everyone has the potential to be a healer. But, just as all can learn to play an instrument, few can earn their living as musicians. Because of their delightful natural talent, musicians are held in high esteem by society and no one grudges them their earnings. It should be the same with healers.

We are all from and of one energy that goes by many names—Brahma, Tao, God, Great Spirit, to mention only a few. In this energy we live and move and have our being. When it is apparently moving it travels in waves; when apparently still it exerts fields of force. In healing the knack is to be still and become a channel for this energy. In this state the suction produced by a genuine desire to get well draws energy to the person needing healing. The healer does not heal, but only provides a means.

Healing can be passive, performed by one person on behalf of another, or active as in self-healing. It is traditionally used passively because sick people often become too ill to help themselves and because the possibility of self-healing is little known. Autogenic training is a well documented form of self-healing.

The above explanation is too simple; it just gives the basic principle of healing. The world in which we live consists of the universal prime energy formed into patterns of degraded energies and forces. In this complexity people lose their way and, forgetting there are no limits, mistake a fluid situation for a fixed reality and feel distressed when their belief systems are disturbed. Healing using the primary energy is rare. Many other lesser but none the less powerful energies are commonly used. What happens depends on how still the channel can be and the requirements of the person receiving healing.

If the couple of healer and healee are compatible everybody feels better after healing, even if the disease does not respond because the sufferer is incurable. Their ability to cope with their problem is transformed. Estimates of cure rates vary, but a realistic average is that one-third are completely and one-third partially relieved of their condition (*2, 15, 16*).

Healing has the greatest cost-effectiveness of all therapies. It requires no apparatus, only the fees of the healer, and a healer can treat more patients in a given time than any other therapist. There are also the additional advantages of its use in self-care both for prevention and treatment, and there are more healers in every country than all the other traditional therapists put together. That is why health administrators should pay more attention to promoting healing than any other therapy.

Hydrotherapy

In every country there are springs that people visit to drink and bathe in because they feel better for doing so. This has been common knowledge for thousands of years. Some springs have a reputation for curing certain conditions. These are much used in continental Europe by the medical profession, but in the United Kingdom the mechanistic outlook of the doctors has led to an almost total decline of their use. In many countries in Europe the state will finance its citizens' treatment in a spa. They know it works.

External applications can take the form of vapour, total or partial immersion, hot or cold baths, douches, jets or sprays. The water may be used internally by drinking or enemas. How the waters work is less certain than that they do so. It may be through their saline content. Many spa waters have a similar composition. This may work on a homoeopathic principle. Maybe it is just good to relax in water in pleasant, caring surroundings and self-healing does the rest, or the negative ions do the trick.

Health administrators should encourage spas which should be available to all, not just the rich.

Negative ions

Air molecules are continually being broken down into positively or negatively charged particles. It is pleasant to sit to leeward of a fountain where the negative ion concentration is high. Some hot dry winds upset people. They increase the positive ion concentration in the air. This raises the serotonin concentration in the body which produces the same physical changes as the winds. A rise in hospital admissions, crime, suicide and accidents coincides with such winds. Compared with country areas, urban areas have a lower negative ion concentration and the positive ions are particularly high in plasticated surroundings full of electrical gadgets that create discharges.

In the 1950s in the USA the early negative ion machines produced ozone and were banned. However, the new generation of machines that work by high voltage discharge are safe and are used in Denmark, Germany, the USSR, the United Kingdom and the USA. In the Federal Republic of Germany and the USSR negative ionization is used on a large scale in public installations.

Negative ion therapy is not considered cranky any longer. It helps people to function better in adverse conditions and improves many diseases. It is a useful therapeutic agent and has considerable public health possibilities (*16*).

Radionics

The word radiesthesia comes from two Greek words meaning radiation sensitivity. To grasp how it works, remember Einstein's remark "the field is the only reality" and the Pibram-Bohm theory that the mind works as a laser beam does on a holographic plate and focuses information from other reality of meaningful pattern that is outside space and time (*5, 6*). The patterns of the energy fields emitted by all forms of matter can be measured by a trained operator reading his own sensations or using an instrument such as a twig or a pendulum. The use of this human attribute is very old and traditional—probably Neolithic. Nowadays a trained water diviner tunes in to water, metal, oil and people.

Radionics is the application of the radiesthetic faculty to the treatment of disease. It was so called by Harold Abrams, M.D. (1863–1924), who was a neurologist and Professor of Pathology in what is now called the Department of Medicine at Stanford University, California. He developed a machine to do this and found that a measure of wave-length was needed to distinguish between different diseases; he called the process radionics after the recently discovered radio. Radionics spread to Britain where Dr Guyon Richards improved the machine and the Horder Committee reported favourably on its diagnostic capabilities in 1924.

The Radionic Association is the professional organization representing those who practise radionics.

Radionics has the same therapeutic range as healing: everybody and every condition. Many different instruments are used, some very sophisticated, and the present consensus is that radionics is an instrumentally tuned form of distant healing (2, 21, 22). As practised at present, it is not applicable to self-care but ways of using it for this could be developed. Since radiesthesia has a predictive aspect, its application to prevention presents interesting possibilities.

Reflexology or zone therapy

Zone therapy, which now tends to be called reflexology, was first introduced in the USA by Dr William H. Fitzgerald about 1907. Whether he got the idea for it from American Indians or from China is uncertain. Something similar was used by some tribes in the USA, and Chinese medicine considers that every organ has a corresponding situation on the hands, feet, face, ears and eyes. The Chinese and Japanese also have a system of massage based on such correspondences and pressure on acupuncture points called *shiatsu* (20).

Fitzgerald taught that the body was divided vertically into 10 zones corresponding to particular organs, that the shoulder was reflexly connected to the hip, knee to elbow and so on, but that it was particularly in the feet that firm massage was effective. All tender points are dealt with, and this seems to work by stimulating the body to deal with the disorder.

Eunice Ingham, a nurse, developed the subject in the USA and lectured widely. Doreen Bayly did the same in the United Kingdom and both formed schools. It is a growing point, for it is easy to learn and use in self-care. Recently Robert St. John in the United Kingdom has found that some mentally retarded children, including those with Down syndrome, can be helped to become gradually normal by the age of about 6 years. Reflexology often produces considerable psychological benefit. It is common in the USA and is spreading rapidly in the United Kingdom.

Shiatsu **and** *do-in*

Though the origin of these therapies is Chinese, they are better known under Japanese names. *Shi* means finger and *atsu* pressure. *Do-in* is the Japanese pronunciation of the Chinese word *tao-yin* and means self-stimulation (17). The latter has two aspects—movement or *t'ai chi* (see below); and 'no-move' which consists of breathing exercises and a sequence of finger pressures on selected acupuncture points that takes ten minutes and leaves one alert and energetic. Finger pressure on acupuncture points is often called acupressure (18, 19). These are valuable techniques for use in self-care and first aid.

T'ai chi

T'ai chi literally means great pole or axis and also supreme ultimate. It is a form of active meditation designed to relate the individual to the universe by concentrating the *qi*, (*Ki* in Japanese and *Prana* in Sanskrit), and regulating its flow. *Qi* is a pre-physical energy existing in air (see "Breathing" above).

T'ai chi is a slow relaxed ballet preceded by breathing exercises. During the movements the breath is taken in as the arms move up and out and exhaled as they are contracted and brought down. The spine is kept straight, but not stiff, and its axis is always over the weight-bearing foot. When it is being performed one becomes aware of an energy that feels like sparkling air flowing between the palms and over the body as the movements are done. It is suitable for everyone at any age.

T'ai chi is a valuable form of preventive self-care but it also has therapeutic applications.

REFERENCES

(1) FORBES, A. *Try being healthy.* Saffron Walden, Essex, UK, Langdon/Daniel, 1976.
(2) HILL, A., ed. *A visual encyclopaedia of unconventional medicine.* New York, Crown Publishing, 1979, & London, New English Library, 1979.
(3) TISSERAND, A. *The art of aromatherapy.* Saffron Walden, Essex, Daniel, 1977.
(4) LUTHE, W. *Autogenic training.* New York, Greene & Stratton, 1969–1973, vols. I–VI.
(5) GLOBUS, G. ET AL., ed. *Consciousness and the brain.* New York, Plenum, 1976.
(6) SHAW, R. E. & BRANSFORD, J. ed. *Perceiving, acting and knowing: towards an ecological psychology.* New York, Halsted Press, 1977.
(7) *Biofeedback and self-control* (An Aldine annual on the regulation of bodily processes and consciousness). New York, Aldine, 1970–1977.
(8) GHADIALI, D. P. *The spectro-chrometry encyclopaedia,* 1933. See also summary in: GALLERT, M. L. *New light on therapeutic energies.* London, Clarke, 1966.
(9) BIRREN, F. *Color psychology and color therapy.* Secaucus, NJ, USA, Citadel Press, 1978.
(10) OTT, J. *Health and light.* New York, Pocket Books, 1976.
(11) CHANCELLOR, P. M. *Handbook on the Bach flower remedies.* Saffron Waldon, Essex, Daniel, 1971.
(12) FINKEL, M. *Fresh hope in cancer.* Saffron Walden, Essex, Health Science Press, 1978.
(13) GERSON, M. *Cancer therapy–fifty cases reviewed.* Los Angeles, Cancer Book House, n.d.
(14) MEEK, G. W., ed. *Healers and the healing process.* Clevedon, IL, USA, Theosophical Publishing House, 1977.
(15) SIMONTON, O. C. ET AL. *Getting well again: A step-by-step self-help guide to overcoming cancer.* Los Angeles, Tarcher, 1978.
(16) STANWAY, A. *Alternative medicine: guide to natural therapies.* London, Macdonald & Jane's, 1980.
(17) DE LANGRE, J. *The first and second books of do-in.* Los Angeles, Tarcher, 1978.
(18) WOOD, D. L. & WOOD, J. J. *First aid at your finger tips.* Saffron Walden, Essex, Health Science Press, 1977.
(19) HOUSTON, F. M. *The healing benefits of acupressure.* New Canaan, CT, USA, Keats Publishing, 1974.
(20) OHASHI, W. *Do-it-yourself shiatsu.* London, Unwin Paperbacks, 1979.

(21) BAERLEIN, E. & DOWER, A. L. G. *Healing with radionics.* Wellingborough, Northants, Thorsons, 1980.
(22) TANSLEY, D. *Dimensions of radiations.* Saffron Walden, Essex, Health Science Press, 1977.

WHO photo: D. Henrioud
This serene image was devised in AD 1027 to show budding doctors the acupuncture points.

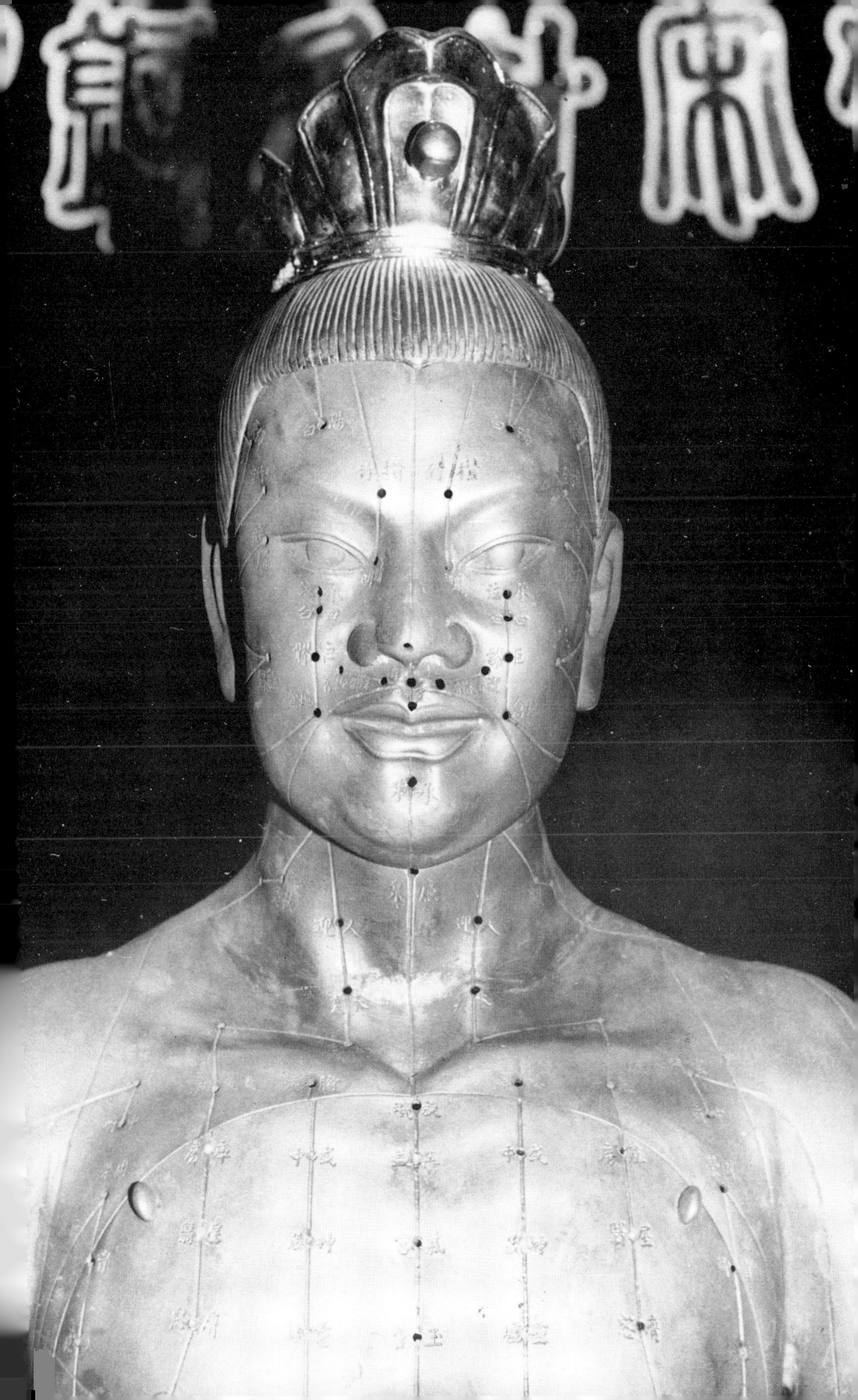

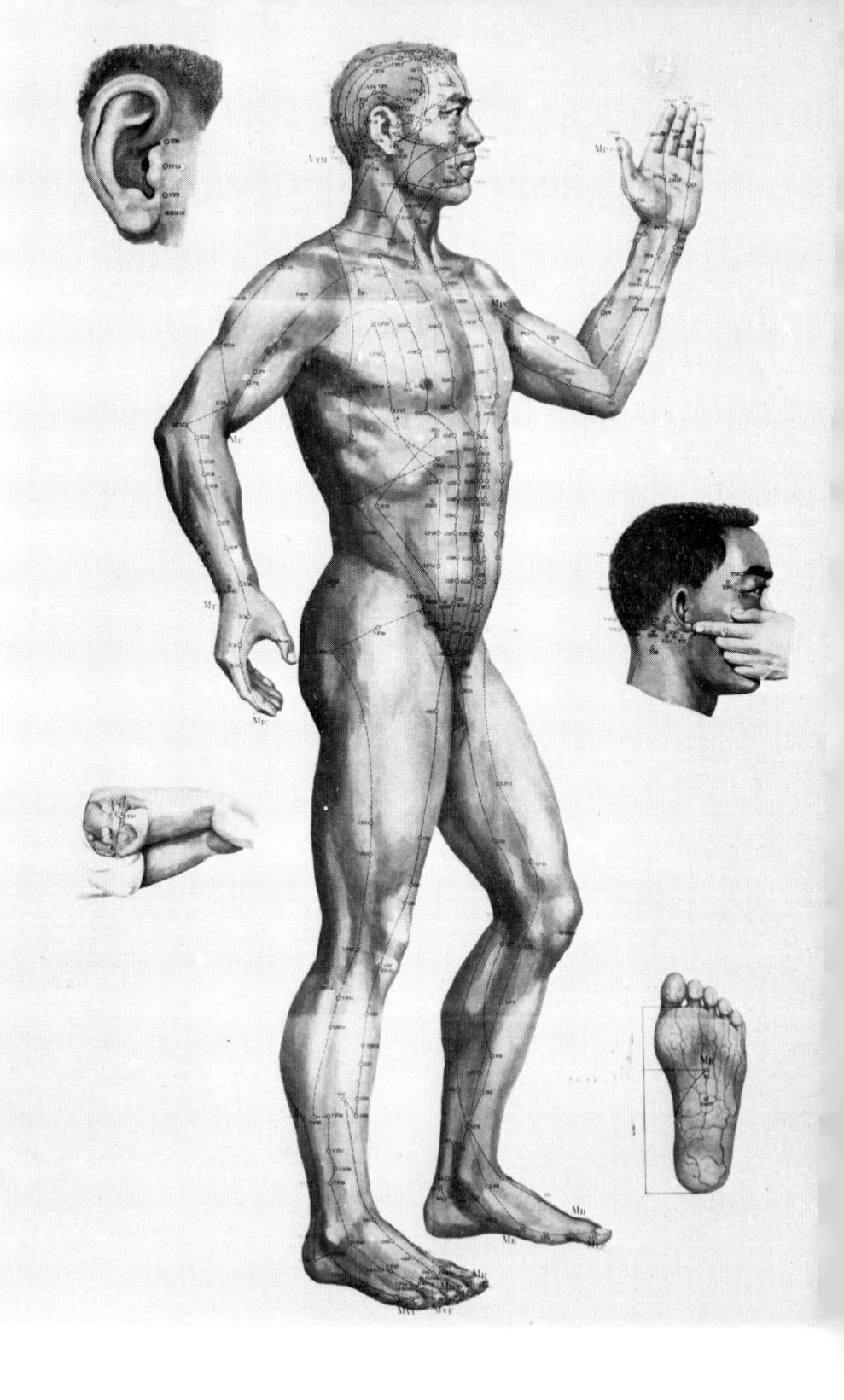

WHO photo
A modern anatomy chart for Chinese medical students shows the acupuncture points and meridians.

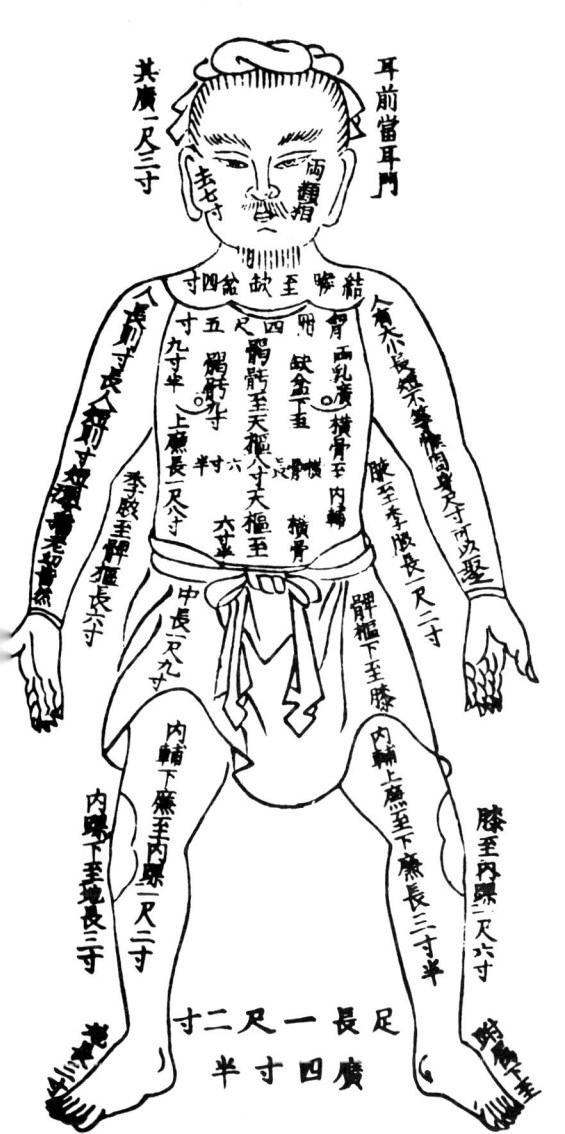

WHO photo

Above: This illustration of acupuncture points is taken from an early Chinese medical textbook.

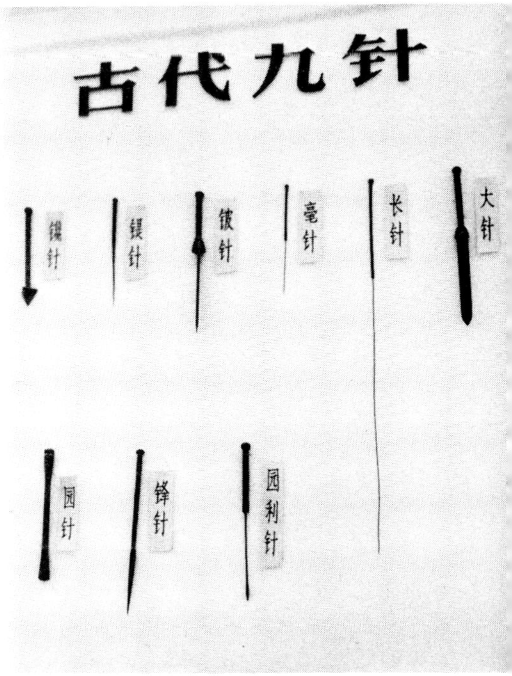

WHO photo: D. Henrioud

Right: A collection of ancient needles, on display at the Institute of Traditional Chinese Medicine, Shanghai.

WHO photo: D. Henrioud

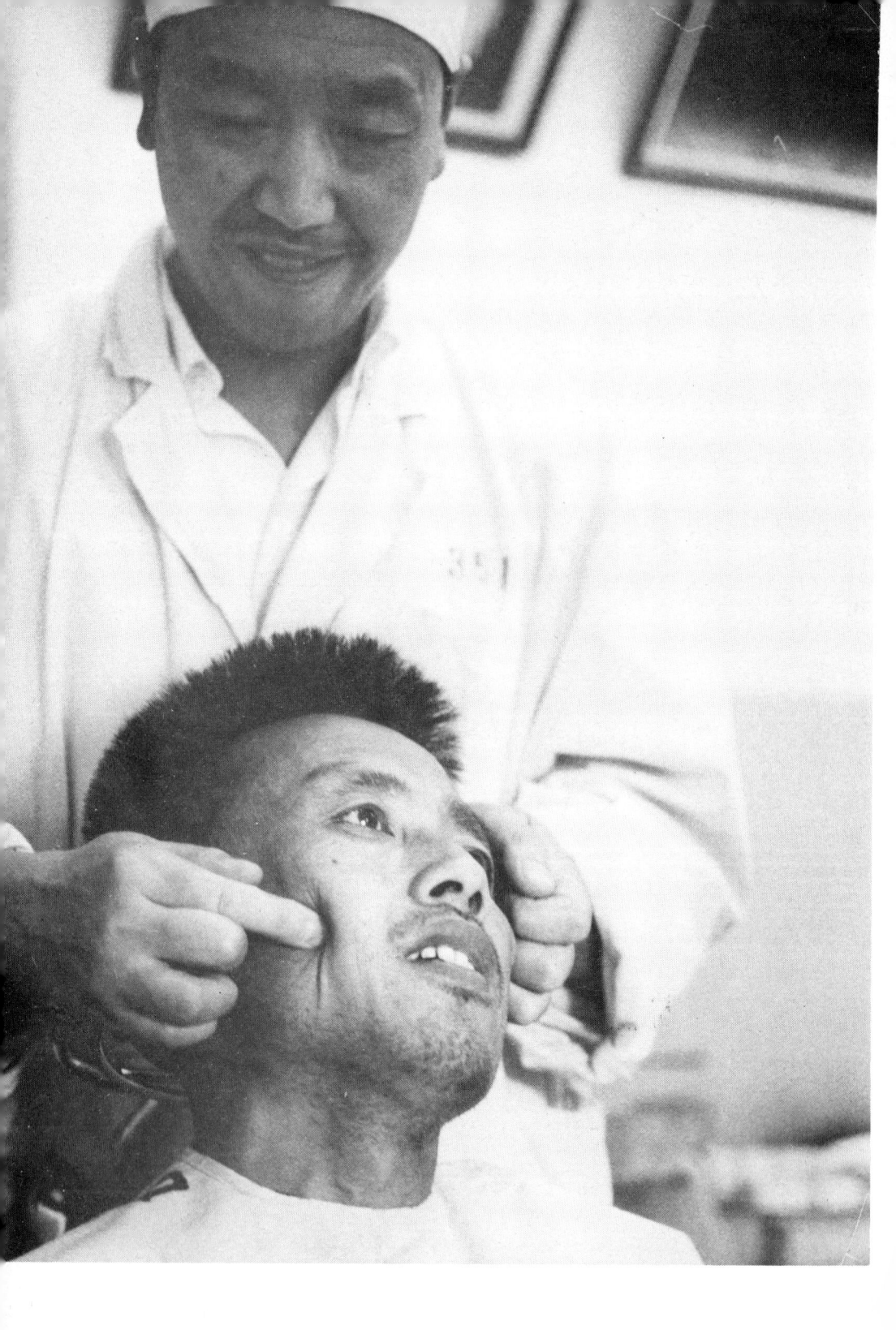

Acupressure. In dentistry, there may even be no need for a needle. Seconds after this picture was taken, the dentist painlessly extracted a tooth.

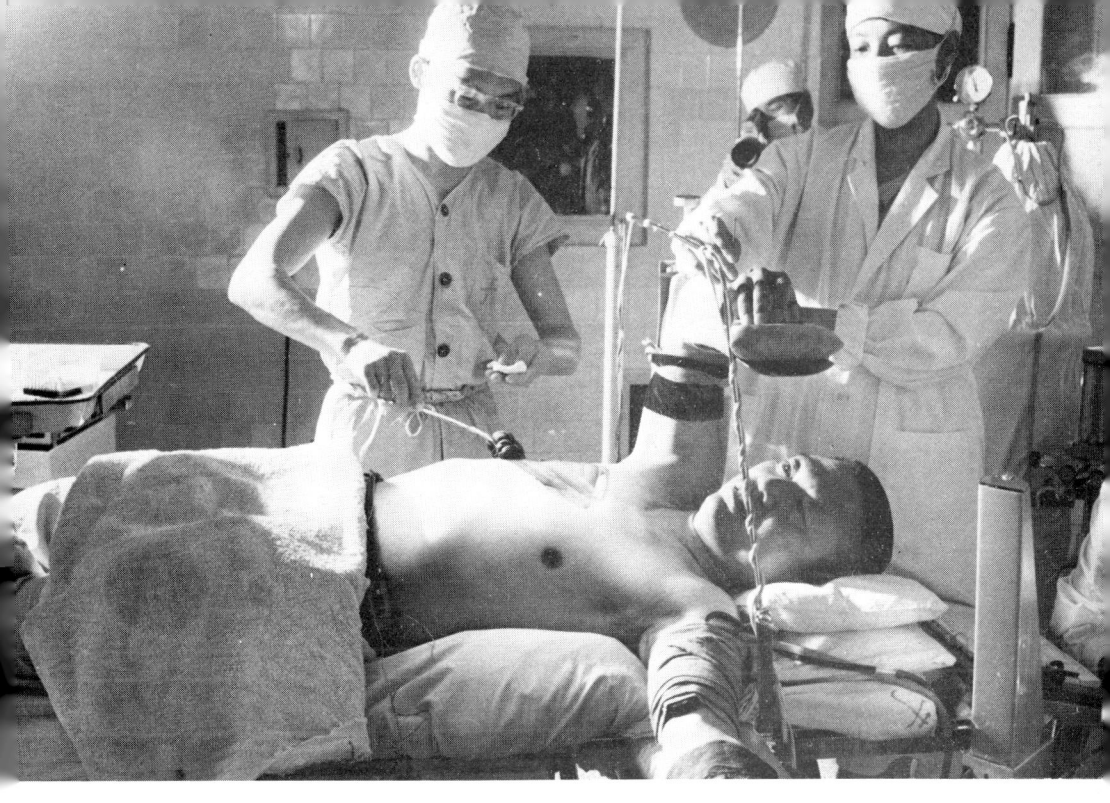

WHO photo: D. Henrioud

bove: Acupuncture analgesia. A nurse swabs the patient's chest with iodine where the first incision will be made, while the acupuncture needle is manipulated incessantly up and down.

WHO photo: D. Henrioud

Below: In China today, the ancient skills of acupuncture are practised in combination with modern medical methods. Here the needles are being electrically stimulated.

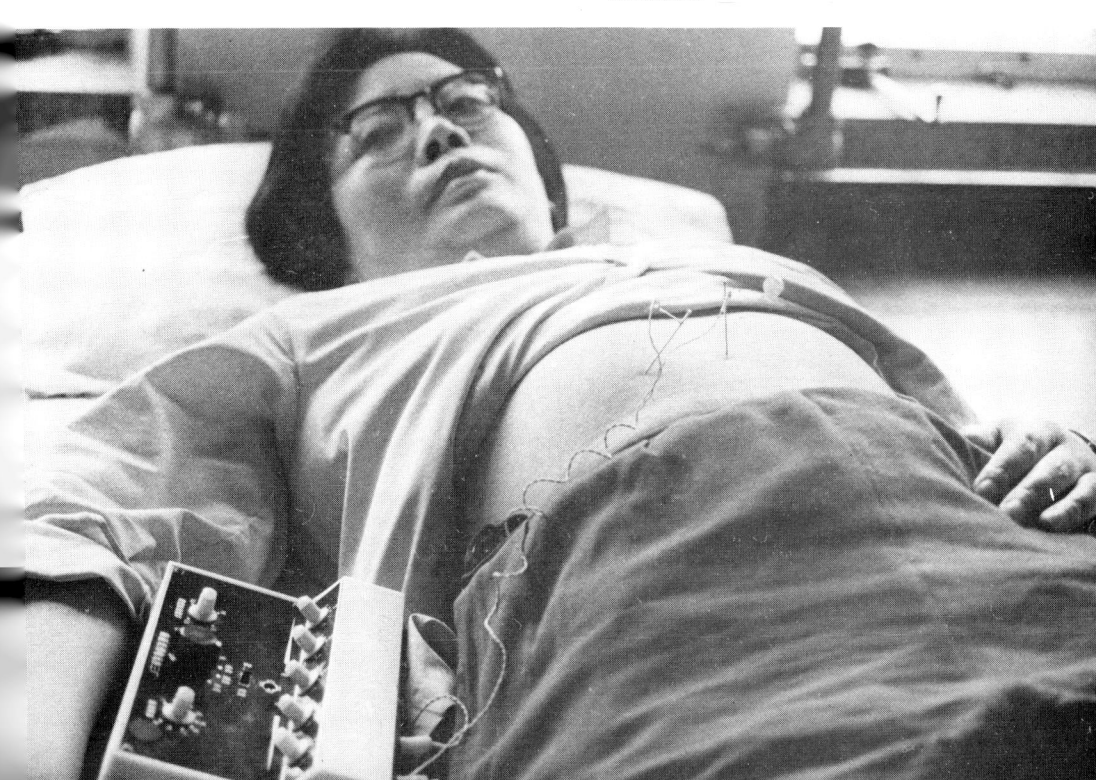

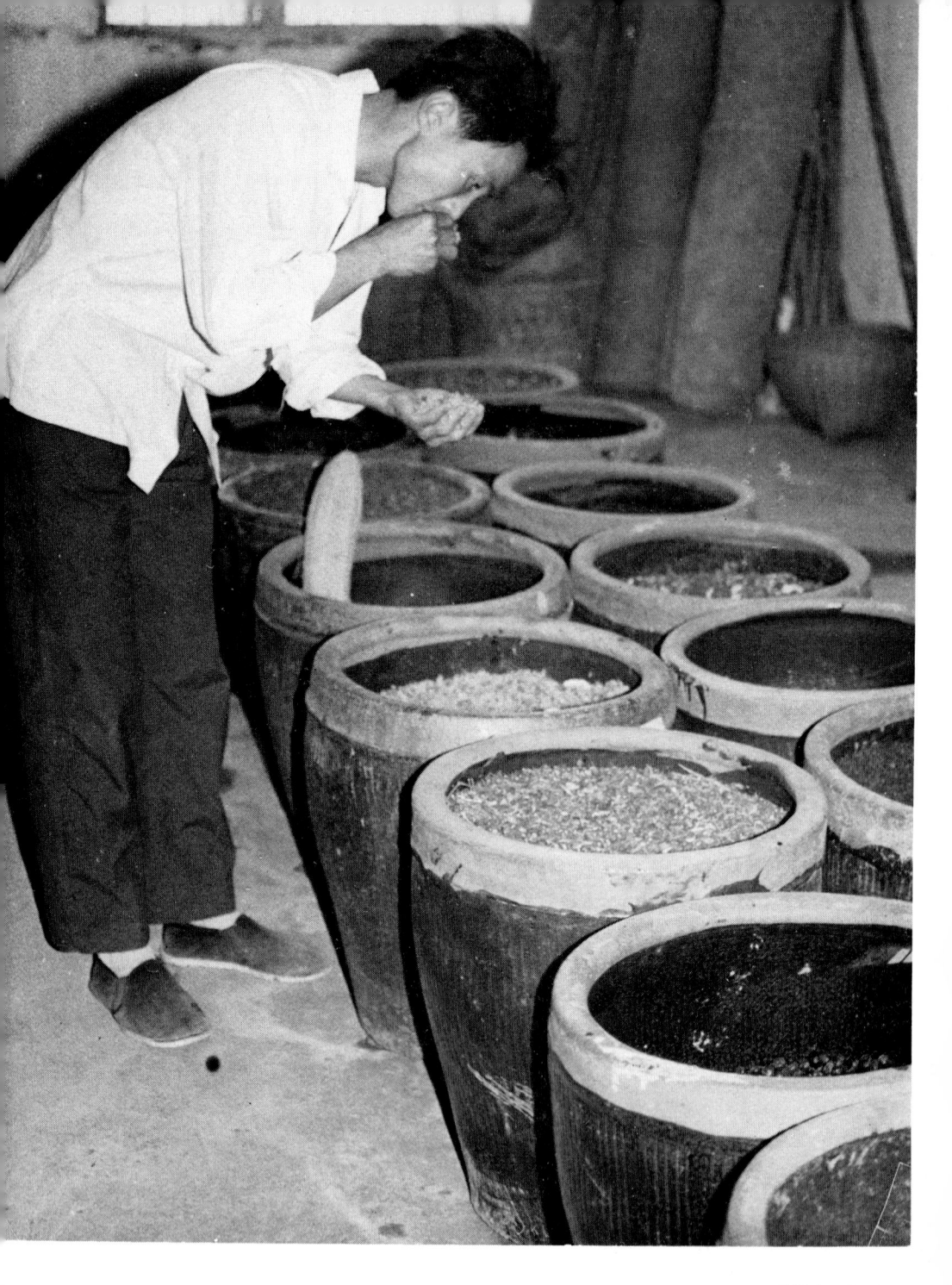

WHO photo: D. Henrioud

The hospital serves as a collection point for herbs, leaves and other ingredients, many of which are cultivated in commune gardens nearby (China).

WHO photo

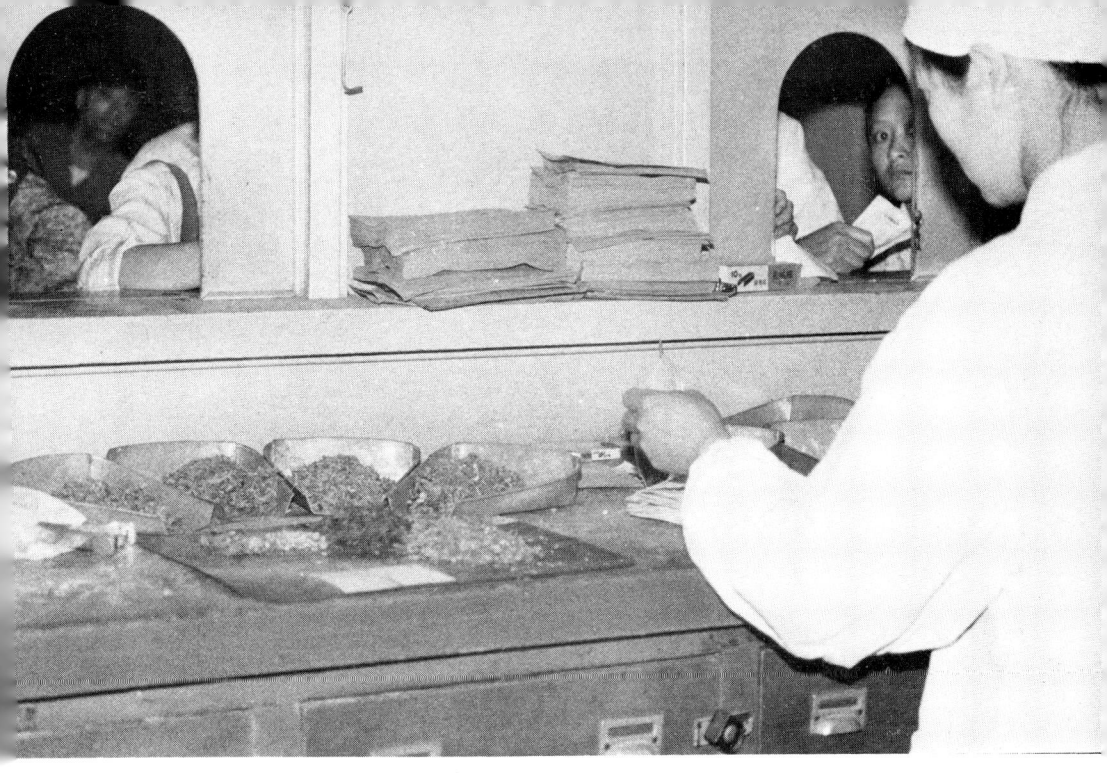

Above: In China eager clients press to the windows of the pharmacy where packs of herbal preparations are being made up.

WHO photo: D. Henrioud

Below: This pharmacy in Beijing specializes in preparing herbal prescriptions while you wait.

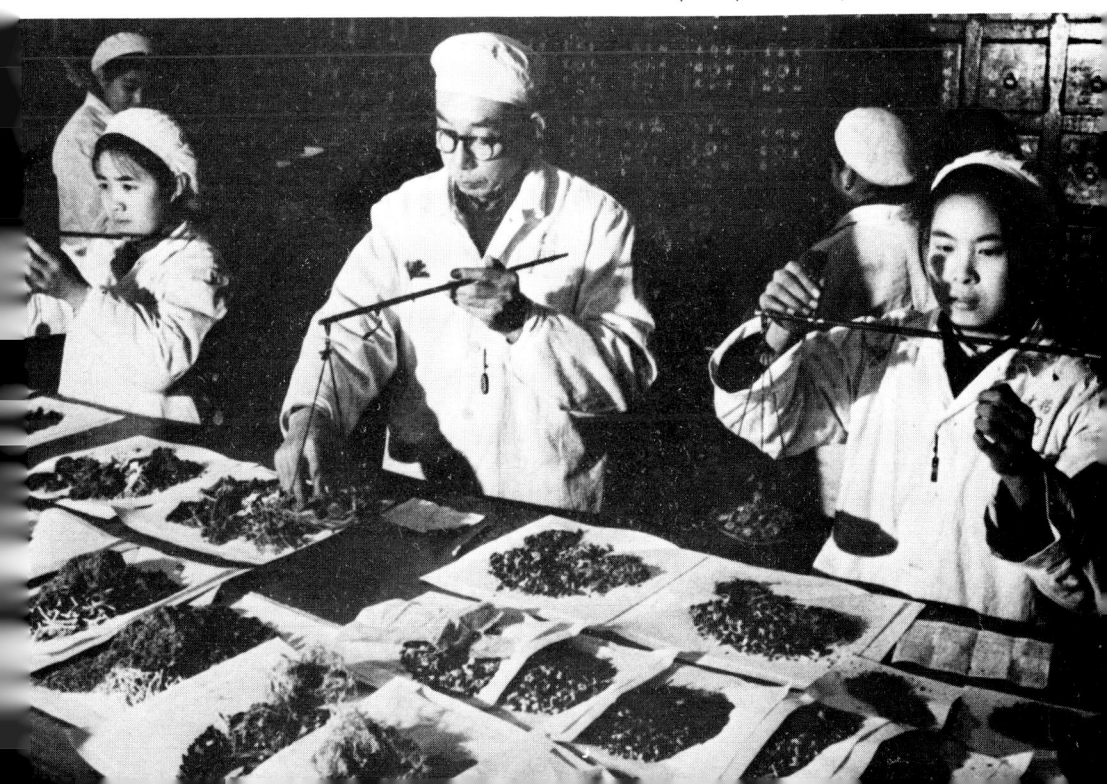

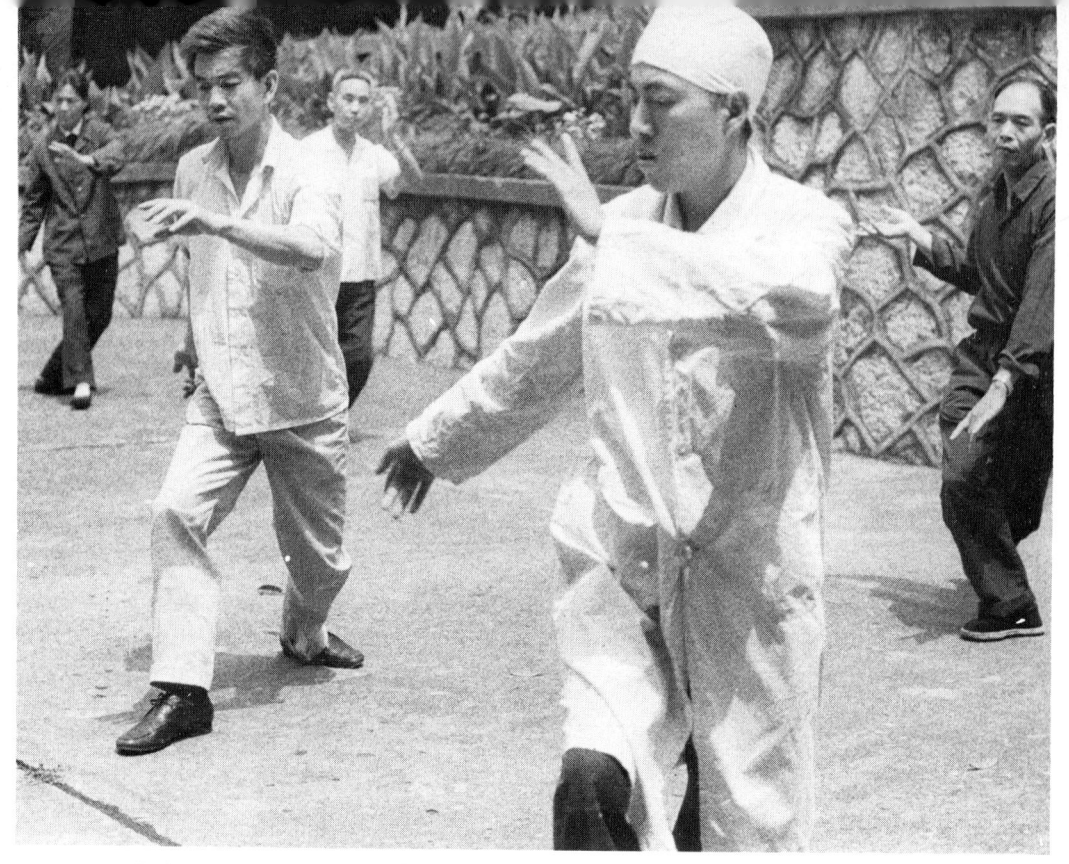

WHO photo: D. Henrioud
Above:
T'ai Chi, a kind of slow-motion martial art, is regarded as a healthy exercise for doctors and patients alike.

WHO photo: R. Bannerman
Right:
The simplest of equipment suffices to prepare traditional Chinese herbal medicaments and roll them into pellets.

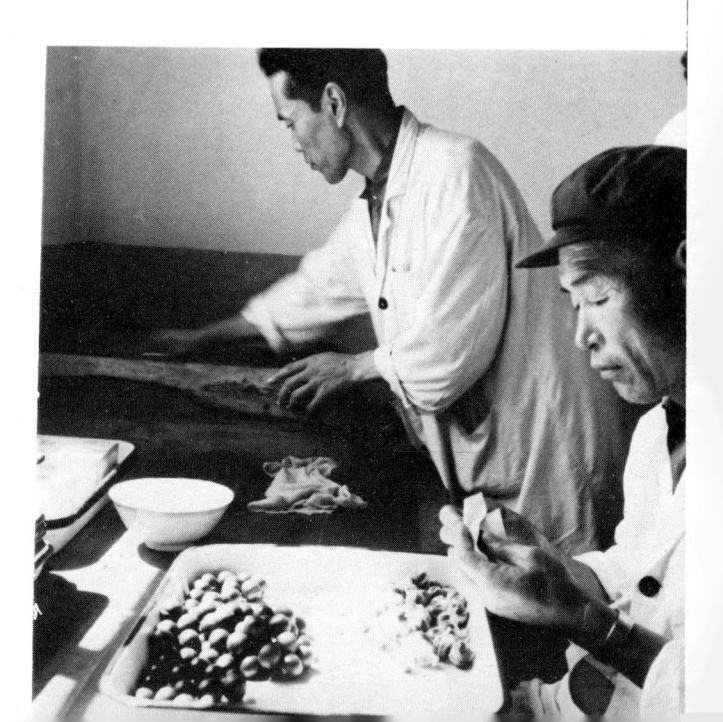

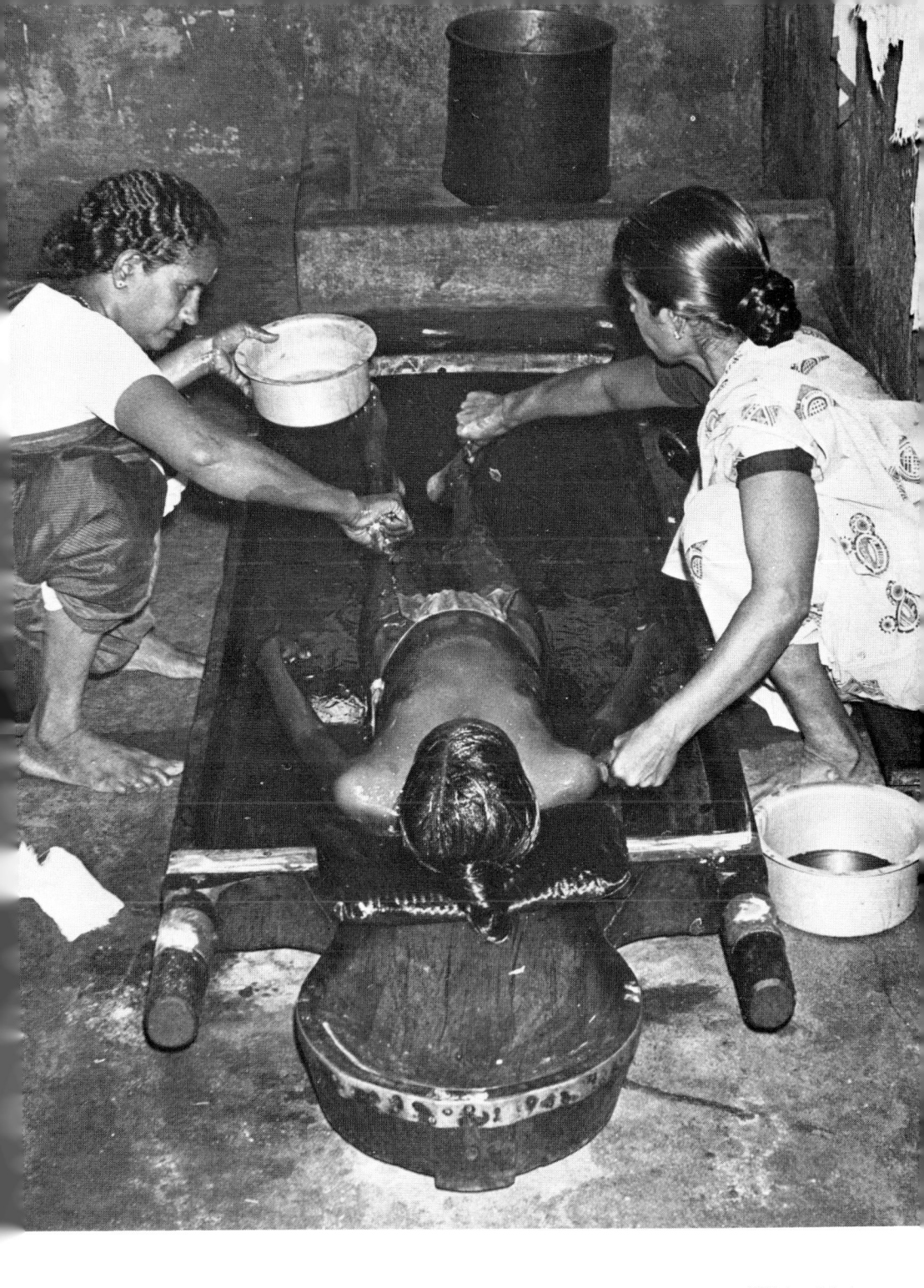

WHO photo: A. Kochar

In India, the Ayurvedic Trust accepted this patient with rheumatoid arthritis as an inpatient, and treated her with oral herbal medicines and external applications of medicated oil and paste.

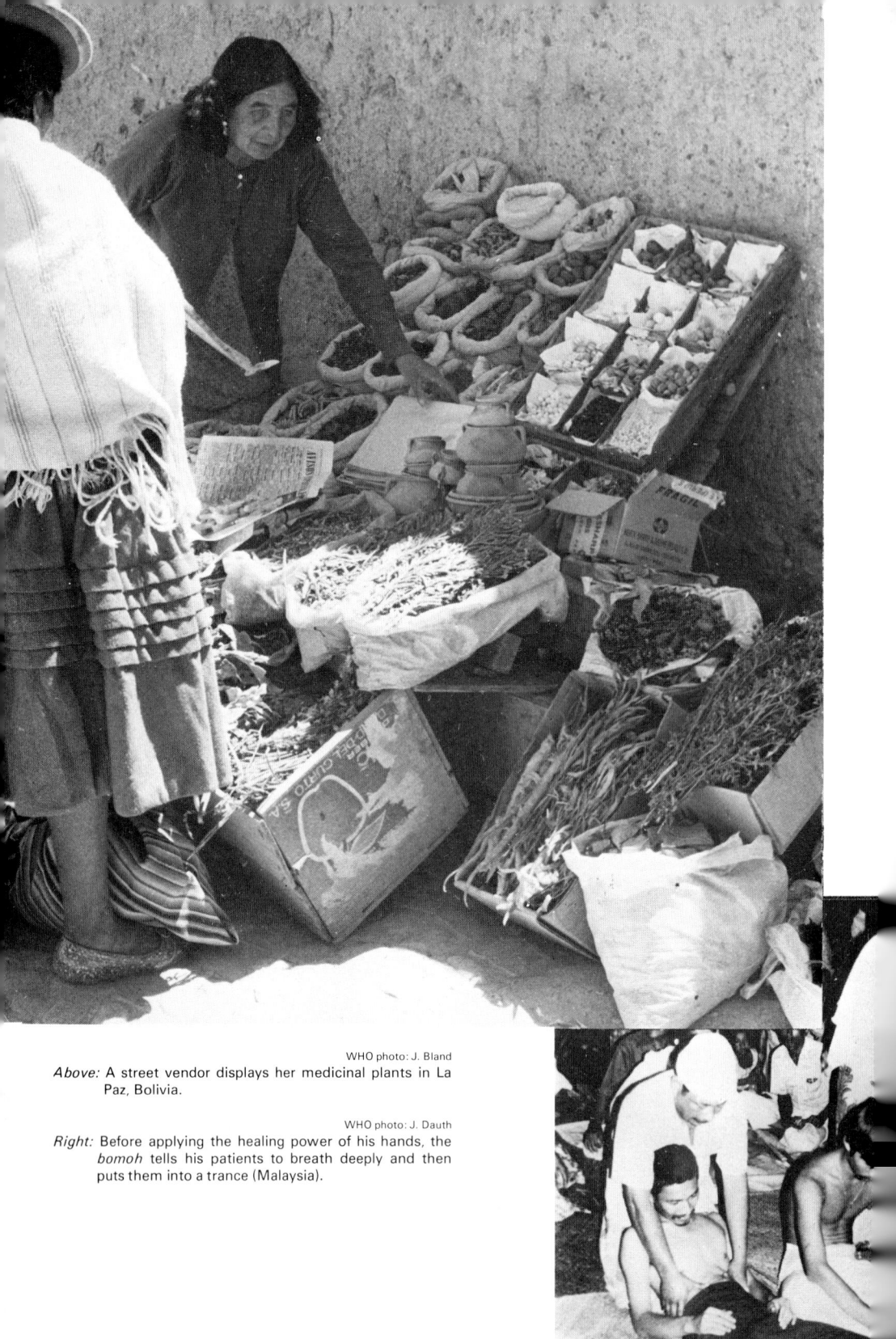

WHO photo: J. Bland
Above: A street vendor displays her medicinal plants in La Paz, Bolivia.

WHO photo: J. Dauth
Right: Before applying the healing power of his hands, the *bomoh* tells his patients to breath deeply and then puts them into a trance (Malaysia).

WHO photo: P. Kurup

A patient undergoing Thirummal treatment, in which his body is covered with medicated oil and massaged delicately by hand or foot: one of the accepted techniques of Ayurveda.

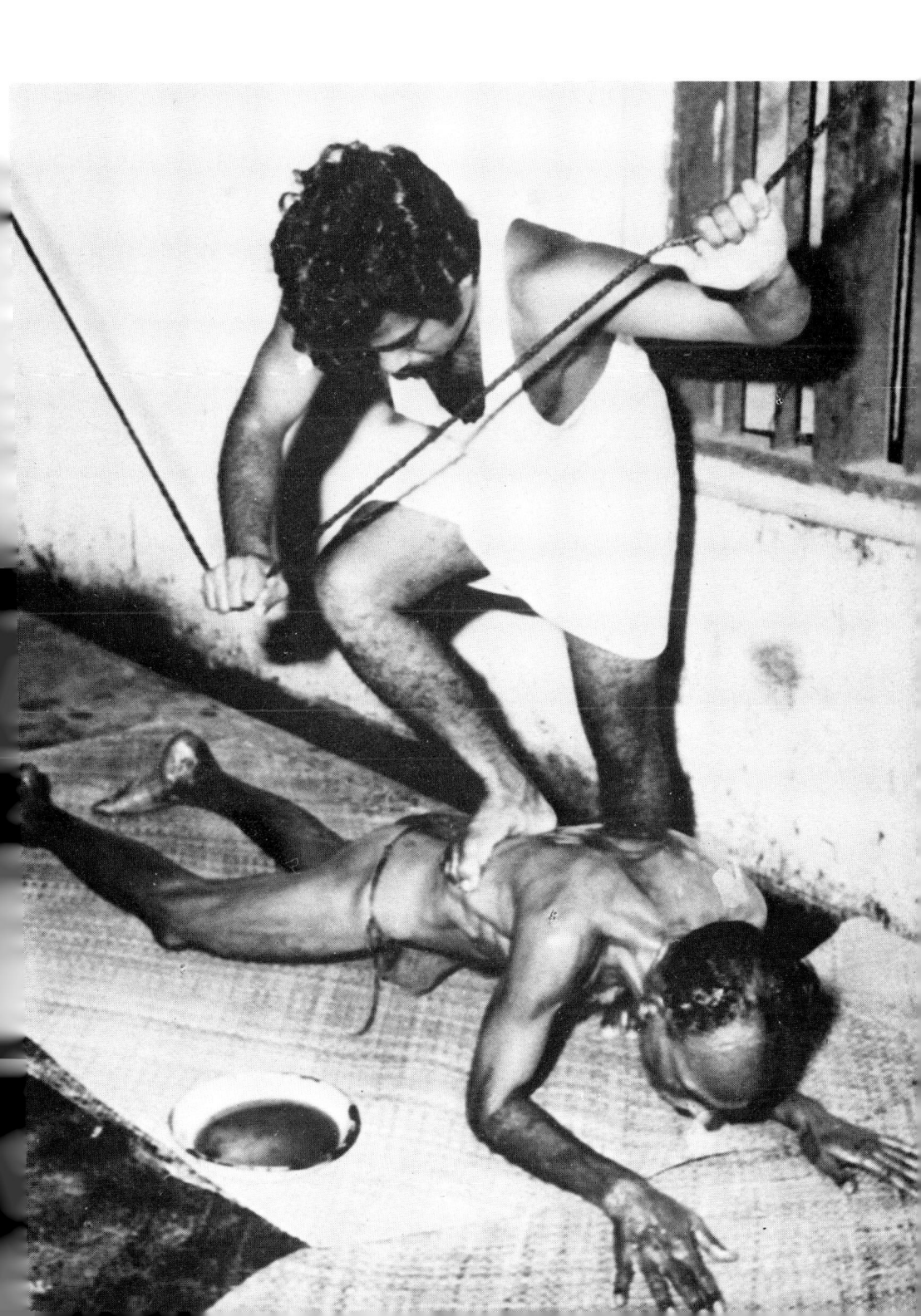

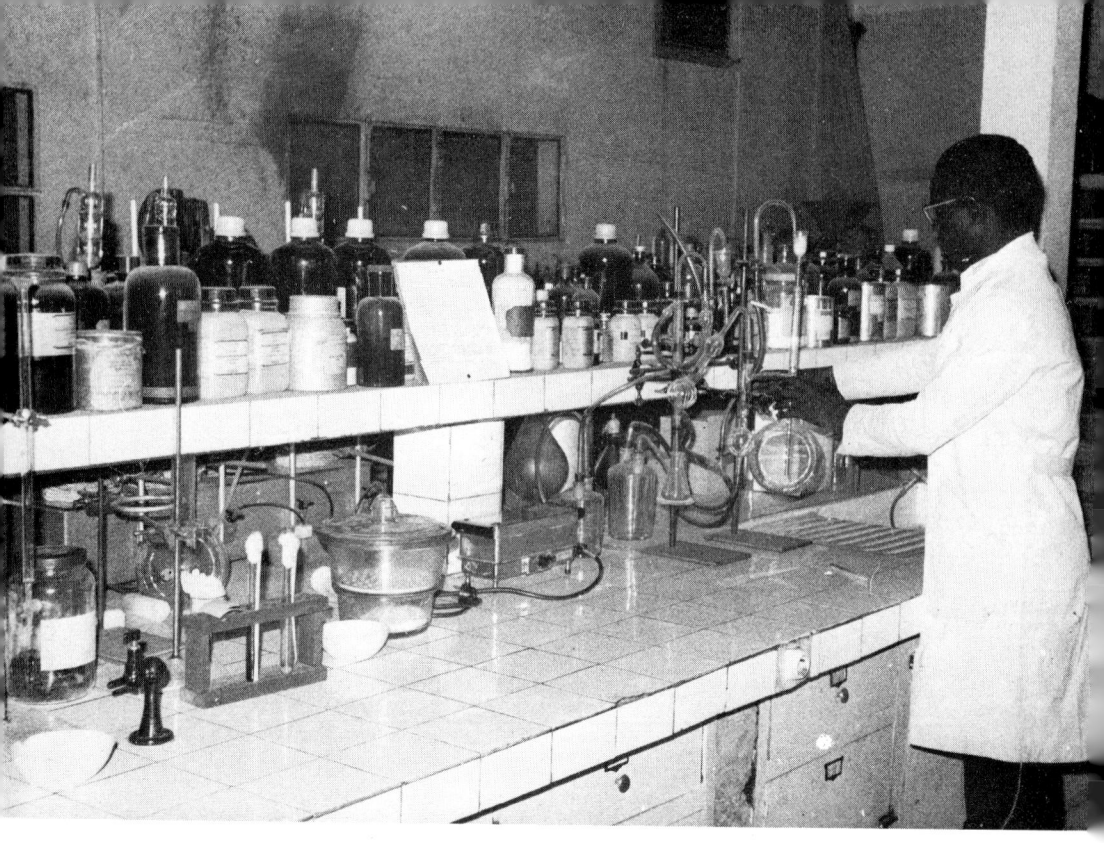

WHO photo: F. Perabo

Above: The laboratory in Bamako, Mali, where herbs are checked before being used in traditional medicine. Knowledge of herbs is integrated into the official medical curriculum.

WHO photo: J. Bla[r]

Below: Plant medicines usually constitute "mild therapy" and have fewer disadvantages than the concentrate[d] substances—whether extracted from vegeta[ble] matter or produced by synthesis (Bolivia).

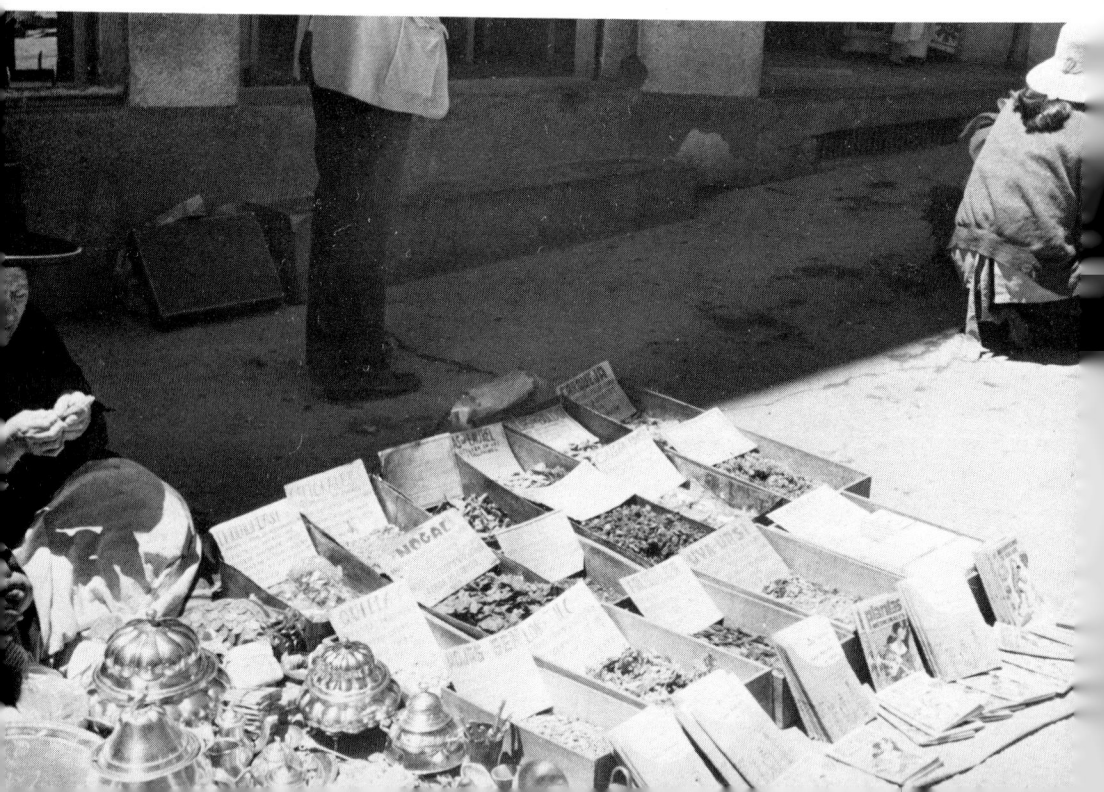

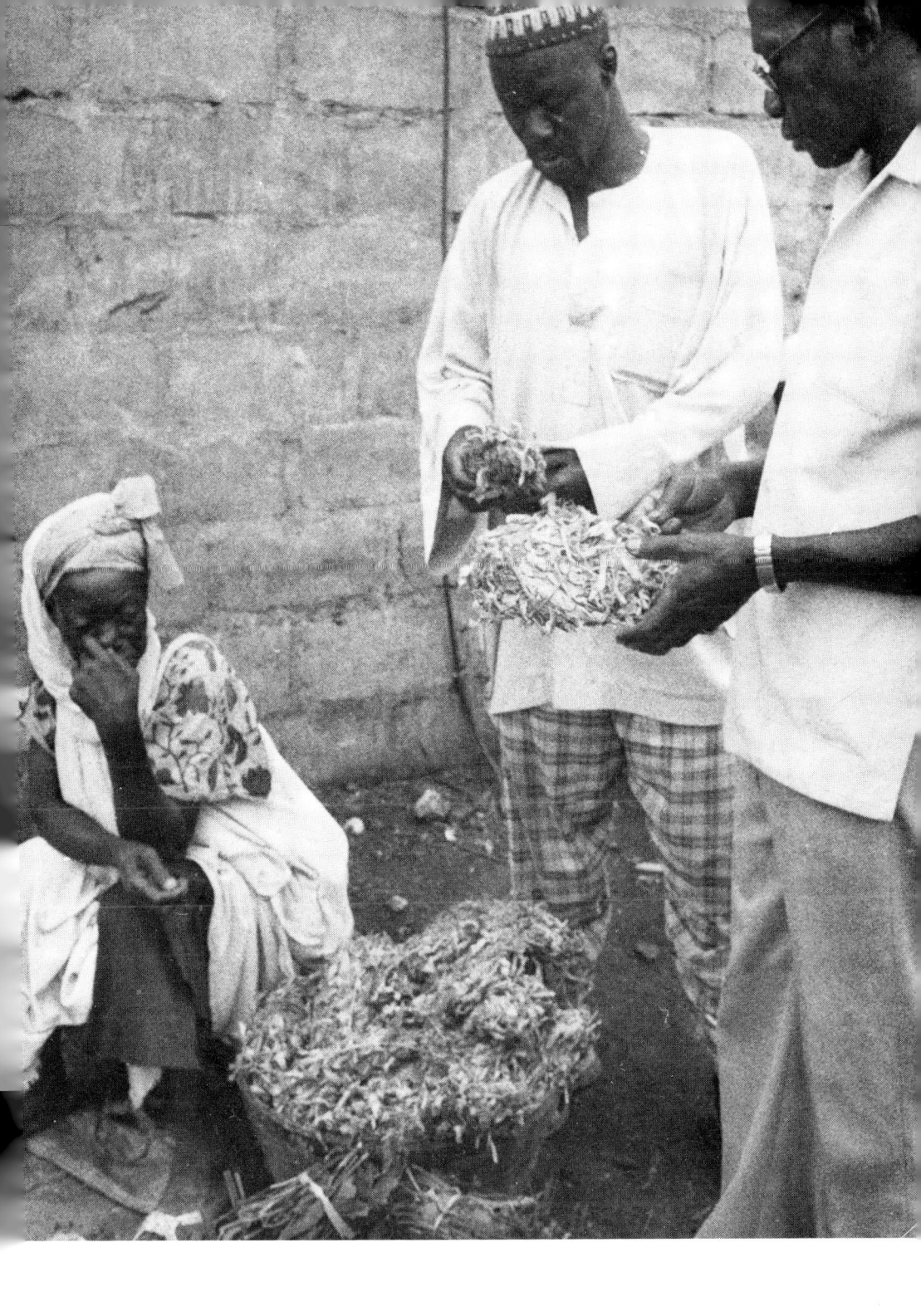

WHO photo: F. Perabo
A pharmacist from the Ministry of Public Health checking herbs on sale in the Bamako markets, Mali.

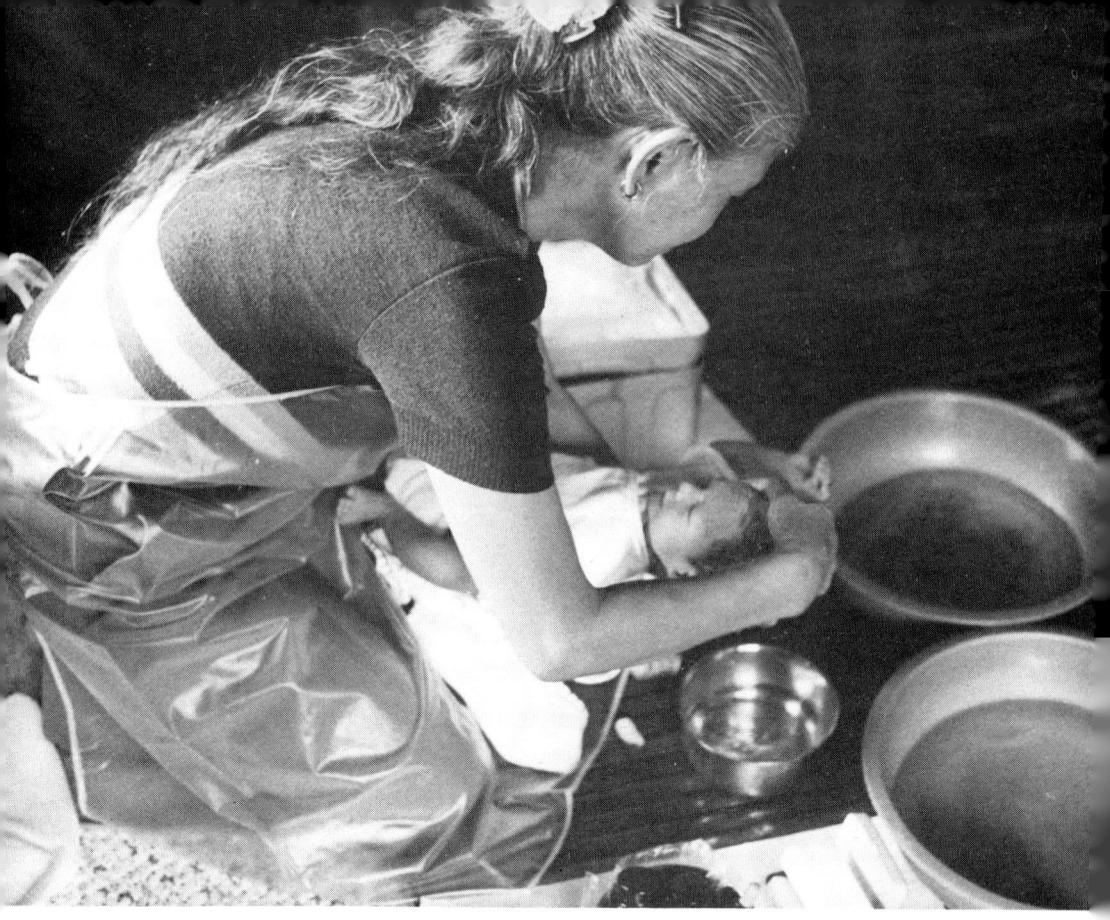

WHO photo: J. Abcede

Above: Mrs Rosa Raymundo, a traditional birth attendant, dons a plastic apron before bathing a newborn child, as she has been taught during special training (Philippines).

WHO photo: R. da Silva

Below: This woman has come to consult a healer at an African centre for traditional medicine. Such healers are respected in their communities for their wide knowledge of plants and diseases as well as for their understanding and wealth of human experience.

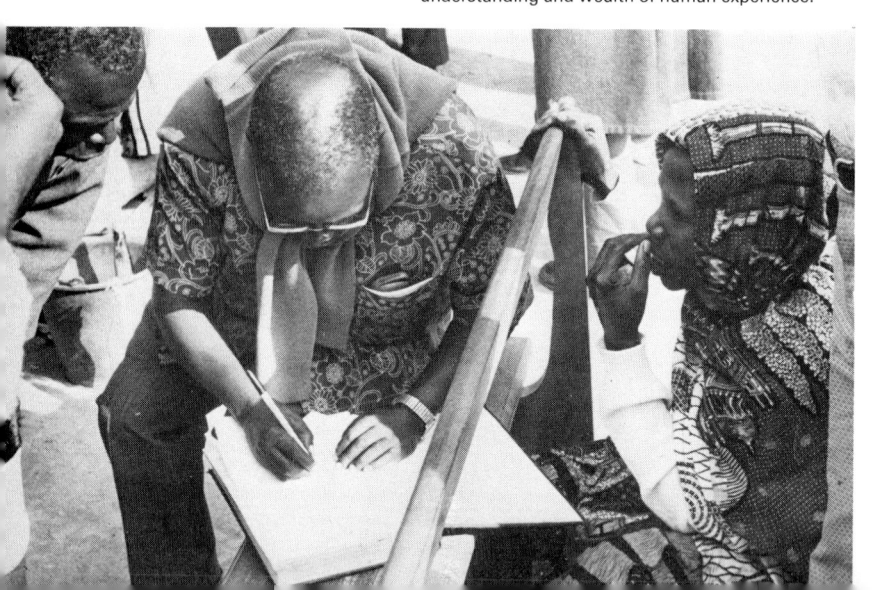

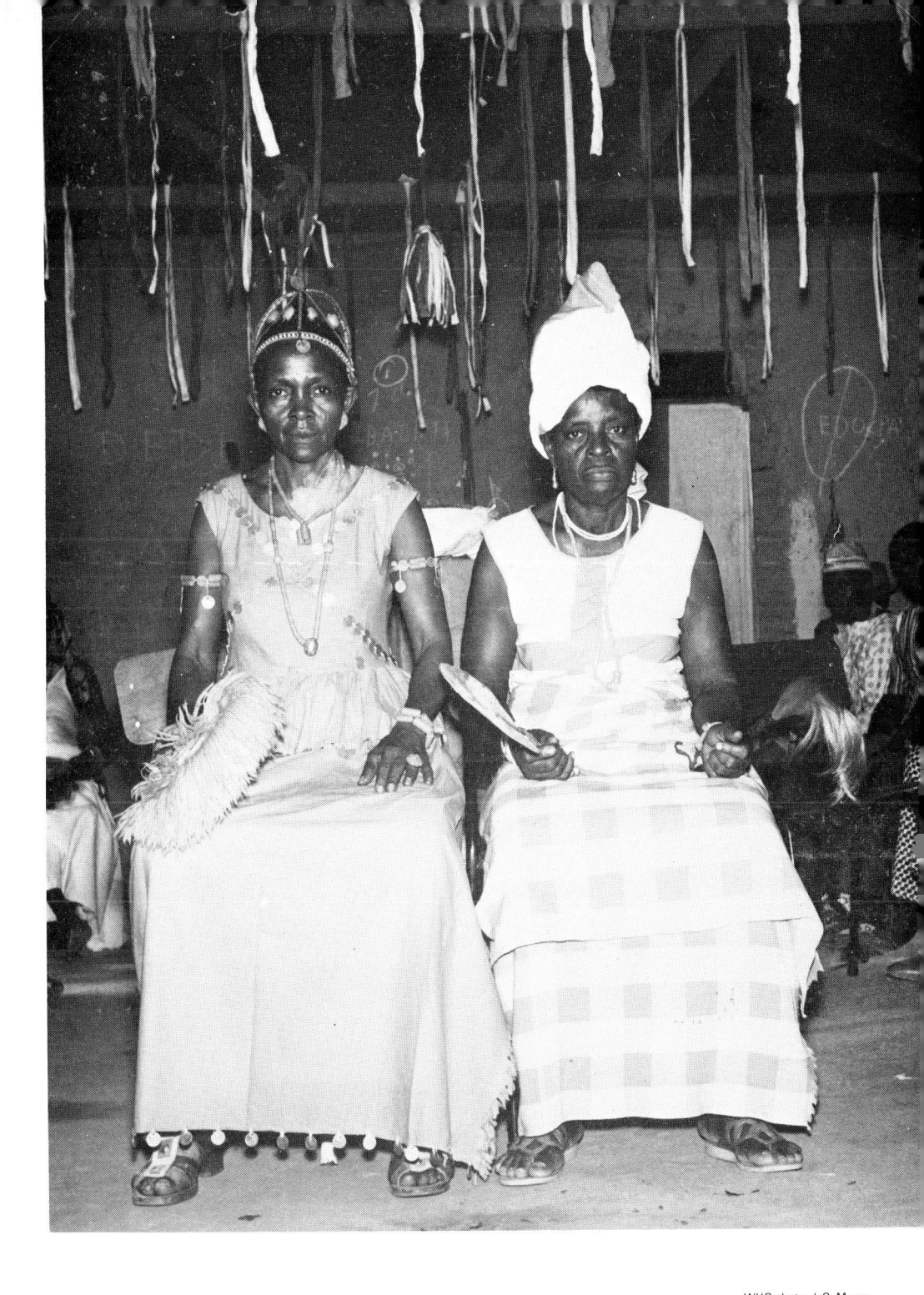

WHO photo: J. O. Mume

Two women who are recognized in their Nigerian community as traditional healers. The woman on the right specializes in problems related to childbirth.

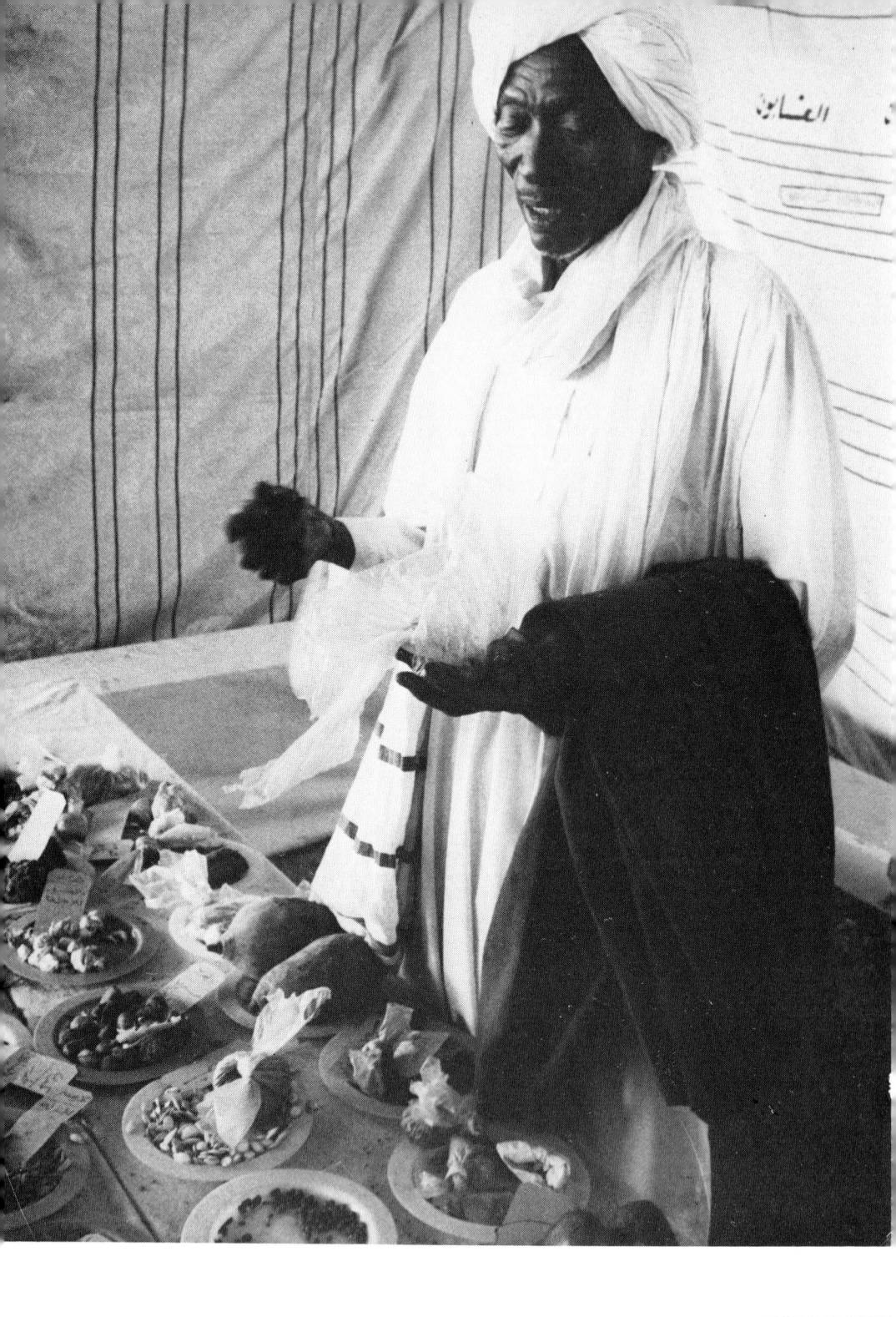

A traditional herbalist sells his wares in a Sudanese market.

Part Two

Herbal medicines and herbal pharmacopoeias

CHAPTER 17
Endangered plants used in traditional medicine

Edward S. Ayensu[1]

Traditional societies have always considered their medical practitioners as influential spiritual leaders who handle both the routine and extraordinary medical problems of the society. Using magic and religion as two pivotal rites in their employ, traditional medical practitioners help to conceptualize the ultimate reality of their culture and all the activities they embody. The concept of disease has always been personified to such an extent that its treatment is effected either by the use of man's hidden spiritual powers or by the application of plants that have been found to contain healing powers or by both.

Generally, we can identify three types of traditional medical practitioners, and the extent of their use of medicinal plants varies. The herbalists are those who enjoy the prestige and reputation of being the real practitioners of traditional medicine. The divine healers are those whose practice depends upon their purported supernatural powers of diagnosis. On occasion they also administer medicinal plants that are supposed to have special spiritual powers. The witch doctor on the other hand is the practitioner who is credited with the ability to intercept the evil deeds of a witch or to exorcize the evil spirit that possesses the patient. Here again plants thought to have exorcizing powers are used as part of the treatment.

In the face of initiatives from various quarters towards the promotion of traditional herbal medicine, the world's forests are being depleted at an alarming rate by business concerns that see no harm in human mismanagement of the environment. Such action is based on the assumption that if man exploits his resources to the limit, he will adapt to new situations or find new resources. The unfortunate reality is that every acre of natural vegetation that is indiscriminately destroyed before it is

---

[1] Director, Office of Biological Conservation, Smithsonian Institution, Washington, DC, USA, and Secretary-General, International Union of Biological Sciences.

explored, may rob mankind of yet another medicinal plant that could be the key to the cure of one of the ailments that still elude our skills.

Lately there has been much concern over the way in which the traditionally attributed values of products from endangered animal species, such as musk deer glands and rhinoceros horn, are causing depletion of the species. The glands of musk deer may fetch US $200 each (*1*), and rhinoceros US $675 per kilogram (*2*); both products are said to cure impotence or have aphrodisiac properties. The possibility that populations of certain primates used in advanced medical research may be endangered has also received much attention.

Little regard, however, has been given to members of the plant kingdom which are potentially or actually useful in traditional medicine, but whose numbers may be declining rapidly due to habitat destruction or over-exploitation. These are the endangered and threatened plant species of traditional medicine. Some species such as American ginseng (*Panax quinquefolius*) are vulnerable due to mass harvesting, while others are congeners (members of the same genus) in highly valuable medicinal groups, such as *Catharanthus*.

Apart from the known plants used in various healing systems, the needed exploration of the field—particularly in the tropics where most developing countries are located—has barely commenced. The tropical regions of the world are believed to contain nearly two-thirds of all organisms. With a rather rich vegetation still awaiting study, special efforts should be made to collect and name the novel species and subject samples to phytochemical analysis to determine the extent of activity and subsequent utility (*3, 4, 5*).

Catharanthus coriaceus

Catharanthus coriaceus, a highly restricted endemic plant of Madagascar, where the flora as a whole is acutely threatened by grazing and burning, is the most endangered species in the genus *Catharanthus* (*6*). Although no phytochemical research has yet been done on *C. coriaceus*, it is a potentially important species since its close relative the Madagascar periwinkle (*C. roseus*) is of well-known value for alkaloids which have actual clinical effect in the treatment of cancer. The alkaloid vincristine, derived from *C. roseus*, which is phenomenally expensive, is a frequent component of chemotherapy programmes which have led to a significant decrease in mortality among young leukaemia patients in the United States, and the compound ajmalicine is used in Europe for the treatment of heart diseases (*7*). This has led to decimation of natural populations of *C. roseus* in areas around the world. *Catharanthus coriaceus* should obviously be conserved in Madagascar and investigated for its medical properties.

Acorus calamus

Acorus calamus, a Eurasian aroid known as *vacha* in India, where it is used in 51 different drug preparations, contains an essential oil in the rhizomes that possesses marked insecticidal and sedative properties. Supplies of this plant in India are becoming scarcer (*8, 9*). Apparently it used to be common in India in the northeastern areas such as Manipur and the Naga Hills, yet it has been imported into Bombay from overseas for its medicinal aromatic rhizomes. Srinivasan (*9*) has suggested that proper use of existing local Indian produce of *Acorus*, including measures to extend the plant's range in India, is desirable lest the local supply become disused or neglected.

A team at the Regional Research Laboratory (CSIR) in Jammu Tawi, India (*10*) has recently isolated a new insect chemosterilant from this species, with antigonadal functions specific enough to indicate that it may represent a new concept in insect chemosterilization. One can appreciate the value of maintaining local stocks of such important threatened species in case they should be required for independent local mass production at short notice.

Ginseng

There has been a dramatic and systematic amalgamation of herbal medicine in the health care programmes of the People's Republic of China. The Chinese have been responsible for the recent upsurge of interest and respect accorded to herbal medicine. Unlike India, Africa and Latin America, China has succeeded in bridging the gap between Western medical systems and the traditional practices that have managed to keep many rural and urban populations in a reasonable state of health for many generations. The fact that charlatanism has often characterized traditional herbal practices did not deter the Chinese from exploiting the very best elements of herbal medicine in their attempt to improve the health situation of their country. There are several plants whose continuous use by the Chinese and other peoples has often been called in question, because phytochemical analyses have not identified the active principles that often give credence to the potency of commonly used plants. One example is the ginseng, comprising a North American (*Panax quinquefolius*) and an Asiatic (*P. ginseng*) species. These are perennial herbs with fleshy, often bifurcating roots, stems bearing a single whorl of three palmately compound leaves, and a solitary, terminal umbel of flowers.

Scientific analysis has substantiated the presence of relatively inert compounds, such as a β-sitosterol and oleanolic acid, in ginseng. Chinese and Soviet scientists have reported physiologically active compounds of a glycoside nature that have not been structurally characterized. One such glycoside is panaquilon, which is claimed to stimulate endocrine secretion.

Another is panaxin, which is reported to act as a brain stimulant and serve as a cardiovascular tonic. Panaxic acid is said to help the heart and blood vessels in the endless task of keeping man alive. Panacen has been hailed as an effective analgesic and a tranquillizer. Finally ginsenin is claimed to be an antidiabetic substance. Despite the various purported medicinal properties of ginseng, it is no wonder that most Western medical practitioners attribute the drug's supposed effectiveness to its "power of suggestion". It is, however, possible that the plant does have curative powers when all the glycosides in it act in concert.

The world demand for ginseng is so high that the wild American species has been depleted. *Panax quinquefolius* has been placed on Appendix I of the Convention on International Trade in Endangered Species of Wild Fauna and Flora (CITES). An export permit from the country of origin and an import permit from the country of destination are required for legal trade in ginseng roots, subject to the satisfaction of the proper authorities that each transaction will not be detrimental to the survival of the species in the wild.

The vast majority of cultivated American ginseng comes from plantations in the State of Wisconsin. However, wild ginseng, which accounts for only about 25% of United States production, receives much higher prices because its less uniform roots are believed to have greater potency.

Most American ginseng is exported to the Far East, notably to Hong Kong, whence it is redistributed to other parts of Asia. Conversely, the growing domestic market for ginseng in the United States is satisfied by products derived from cultivated Asiatic *Panax ginseng* imported from the Republic of Korea.

Wild American roots are sold at approximately US $110–130 per pound to dealers, and an estimated 65 000 pounds of wild roots were exported in the 1975–1976 season. Thus we encounter a case where the demand by herbal practitioners has caused depletion of a product in nature, fortunately counteracted to some extent by a commercially propagated supply, yet not enough to obviate the need for state-by-state quotas for export of the wild ginseng roots.

Rauvolfia serpentina

If Western science had taken the proponents of ancient works such as the Vedas seriously, we would have reaped much earlier the benefits of such plants as *Rauvolfia serpentina*. An examination of the ancient systems of Ayurveda and Unani will indicate that *Rauvolfia serpentina* was well known and in use by medicine men of India, Sri Lanka, Nepal, Burma and other oriental countries for the treatment of insanity.[1]

---

[1] Possibly associated with hypertensive encephalopathy—RHB, ED.

The first Western scientist who published the uses to which the plant was put in India was Garcia de Orta in 1563. Most European physicians were very sceptical of the purported properties of the plant. However, in 1952 the alkaloid reserpine was isolated, thus confirming the plant's value. Since then the alkaloidal extract, as well as purified alkaloids of *Rauvolfia serpentina*, have become very important in the treatment and control of hypertension.

The administration of the extract brings about a lowering of the blood pressure in hypertensive states, lowering of the pulse, and exhibition of a general sense of euphoria. The alkaloids in the plant have been shown to be phenotropic, and to influence the functions of the mind and behaviour. It is no wonder that the medicine men of India consistently administered this plant to the insane. Today the plant is cultivated in commercial quantities in many parts of the world, notably India and Thailand.

According to Santapau (*11*), before 1952 *Rauvolfia serpentina* was used in the indigenous systems of medicine, but the demand was not great; the plant was common and abundant in forest areas all over peninsular India. However, after the publication of the various papers extolling the medicinal powers of the plant, a ruthless search was started all over the country, a search that only came to a halt when *Rauvolfia* was found to have disappeared from forest areas.

The species is now consistently indicated by various other authorities as becoming very rare in nature (*8, 9, 12, 13*). When an important species such as this is over-collected, there is always the potential for disappearance of important, discrete gene pools of infraspecific variation which may be useful in further research on the chemical properties of the entire genetic composition of the species.

Two distinct ecotypes, i.e., basically subspecies that grow in different environments due to characteristics that are probably physiological but genetically controlled, have been recognized in *R. serpentina*. Various stocks from Kerala, Dehra Dun (Himalaya), Karnataka and Goa are being explored for reserpine and alkaloids at the National Bureau of Plant Genetic Resources, New Delhi (*14*). Thus we may hope to have more valuable data from wild variant populations of the species before its decline to mere remnants of its original abundance.

Species on Appendix II of CITES

Two threatened species utilized by traditional medical practitioners are listed on Appendix II of the CITES (see above). One is *Saussurea lappa*, the source of *kuth* roots; the other *Dioscorea deltoidea*, a steroidal hormone source. In order for trade in these species to be legal pursuant to the Convention, an export permit is required from the country of origin, and a complementary documentation certificate must be obtained from the country of destination.

Locally, the export of *Saussurea lappa* is restricted in Kashmir. The roots are utilized in a multitude of ways, among others as a tonic, and carminative; as an antispasmodic in bronchial asthma, cough and cholera; and as an ointment for ulcers. They are also smoked as an opium substitute. The present scarcity of this valuable plant has been indicated by various Indian botanical authorities (*8, 9, 12, 15*).

Dioscorea deltoidea has been much sought after by private agencies and pharmaceutical firms, having been continuously collected in India, except perhaps in the more inaccessible areas of the Himalayas (*11, 13*). Its natural range includes parts of Afghanistan, Pakistan, India, Nepal, Bhutan, China and Viet Nam. The roots yield cortisone, a steroidal hormone used in treating rheumatic diseases and ophthalmic disorders. The plant is cultivated in Punjab and Kashmir for the edible roots. Investigations of its genetic variability are being undertaken by the Regional Laboratory in Jammu Tawi, India (*16*), and tissue cultures are under way in Calcutta (*17*).

India

India unquestionably occupies the topmost position in the use of herbal drugs, utilizing nearly 540 plant species in different formulations (*19*). For centuries a great majority of India's population has depended on crude drugs and drug extracts for the treatment of various ailments. In fact India was one of the pioneers in the development and practice of well-documented indigenous systems of medicine—the most notable being Ayurveda and Unani. The materia medica of these systems contains a rich heritage of indigenous herbal practices that have helped to sustain the health of most rural people of India.

Today about 75% of the population consult mainly traditional physicians and the sales turnover of indigenous medicines is about one and a half times that of modern drugs (*18*).

The first three Indian orchids discussed below are of potential or actual use in traditional medicine and at present endangered or vulnerable (*6*).

Paphiopedilum druryi is native to Kerala but is endangered or extinct in the wild due to forest fires and excessive collecting. There are indications of its use in ayurvedic medicine and it may have useful alkaloids. Though known in cultivation around the world, only about a dozen individuals are being grown in India. Various authorities have indicated its decline in the wild state (*20-22, 24*).

Dendrobium pauciflorum is endangered, possibly extinct, and known from West Bengal and Sikkim in areas open to tree felling. It may likely be found to have alkaloids of potential value, if rediscovered in the wild. Its precarious situation has been noted by U. C. Pradhan (*21, 22, 25*).

Diplomeris hirsuta, which possibly contains useful alkaloids in the tubers, is restricted to a tiny population in West Bengal that is vulnerable to landslides. Its decrease in numbers has been pointed out by G. M. Pradhan

(20), U. C. Pradhan (21, 22, 25), Kataki (23), and Varmah and Sahni (26). Another species, Dendrobium nobile, deserves mention. Occurring in the Himalayan regions of India and China, it is a source of dendrobine, a principal alkaloid, and is exported from China by the ton in a dehydrated condition (27). The abundance of this species in India is seriously decreasing as various botanists have warned (11, 21-23, 25).

The Indian National Orchidarium at Shillong has brought approximately 350 indigenous orchid species into cultivation for conservation purposes.

Various endangered and threatened plants that have been indicated as of potential or actual use in traditional medicine are listed in Table 1.

Table 1. Endangered plants of actual or potential use in traditional medicine

Species	Common name	Family	Threatened range	Use
Acorus calamus	Vacha	Araceae	India	Sedative
Alpinia galanga	Khulanjan	Zingiberaceae	India	Drug
Arbutus canariensis	Madrono	Ericaceae	Canary Is.	Vitamin C
Artemisia granatensis		Asteraceae	Spain	Infusion
Catharanthus coriaceus	Periwinkle	Apocynaceae	Madagascar	Alkaloids
Commiphora wightii	Guggal	Burseraceae	India	Drug
Dendrobium nobile		Orchidaceae	India	Dendrobine
Dendrobium pauciflorum	Picotee dendrobium	Orchidaceae	India	Alkaloids
Dioscorea deltoidea	Kins	Dioscoreaceae	Afghanistan to Viet Nam	Cortisone
Diplomeris hirsuta	Snow orchid	Orchidaceae	India	Alkaloids
Dracaena draco	Dragon tree	Liliaceae	Canary Is., Cape Verde Is., Madeira	Gum resin
Gentiana kurroo	Kadu	Gentianaceae	India	Drug
Lodoicea maldivica	Double coconut	Arecaceae	Seychelles Is.	Drug
Nelumbo nucifera	Lotus	Nymphaeaceae	India	Drug
Paeonia cambessedesii		Paeoniaceae	Balearic Is.	Epilepsy
Panax quinquefolius	American ginseng	Araliaceae	United States	Tonic Tea
Paphiopedilum druryi		Orchidaceae	India	Alkaloids
Pelagodoxa henryana	Enu, Vahane	Arecaceae	Marquesas Is.	Endosperm
Podophyllum hexandrum	Indian podophyllum	Berberidaceae	India	Drug
Rauvolfia serpentina	Sarpagandha	Apocynaceae	India	Drug
Rheum rhaponticum	Wild rhubarb	Polygonaceae	Bulgaria, Norway	Medicine
Rumex rothschildianus		Polygonaceae	Israel	Medicine
Ruta pinnata	Tedera salvaje	Rutaceae	Canary Is.	Balsam-like properties
Santalum album	Sukhad	Santalaceae	India	Drug
Saussurea lappa	Kuth roots	Asteraceae	India	Various
Sisymbrium cavanillesianum		Brassicaceae	Spain	Mustard-like properties
Toxocarpus schimperianus		Asclepiadaceae	Seychelles	Pharmacology

* * *

The present critical situation regarding the loss of gene pools for parental and related strains of a number of the world's important food crops is now becoming generally understood and appreciated by many (*28, 29*), and attempts are under way to locate even more potential food species from among the under-exploited plants suited to tropical regions (*30*).

Loss of varieties and strains useful to food-plant breeding, as well as massive tropical deforestation, desertification, and the firewood crisis, have reached proportions of global concern. Research must now be intensified on the chemistry and proper conservation of endangered plants of use in traditional medicine, for the fact that people have taken traditional medicinal plants for granted over the years has led to a failure to develop any real professional attitude towards usage of these plants, particularly in the rural parts of the world.

REFERENCES

(*1*) PUTMAN, J. J. India struggles to save her wildlife. *National geographic*, **150** (3): 299–343 (1976).

(*2*) INSKIPP, T. & WELLS, S. *International trade in wildlife*. London, International Institute for Environment and Development/Fauna Preservation Society, 1979 (an Earthscan publication).

(*3*) AYENSU, E. S. *Medicinal plants of West Africa*. Algonac, MI, USA, Reference Publications, 1978.

(*4*) AYENSU, E. S. Plants for medicinal uses with special reference to arid zones. In: Goodin, J. R. & Northing, D. K., ed. *Arid land plant resources*. Lubbock, TX, USA, International Center for Arid and Semiarid Land Studies, 1979, pp. 117–178.

(*5*) AYENSU, E. S. *Medicinal plants of the West Indies*. Algonac, MI, USA, Reference Publications, 1980.

(*6*) LUCAS, G. & SYNGE, H. *The IUCN plant red data book*. Gland, Switzerland, International Union for Conservation of Nature and Natural Resources, 1978.

(*7*) VIETMEYER, N. The greening of the future. *Quest*, September 1979: 25–31.

(*8*) MAHESHWARI, J. K. *The need for conservation of flora and floral provinces in South-East Asia*. Morges, Switzerland, International Union for Conservation of Nature and Natural Resources, 1970 (IUCN publications, new series, No. 18, vol. 2, pp. 89–94.

(*9*) SRINIVASAN, K. S. Protection of wild (plant) life. *Bulletin of the botanical survey of India*, **1**: 85–89 (1959).

(*10*) SAXENA, B. P. ET AL. A new insect chemosterilant isolated from *Acorus calamus* L. *Nature*, **270**: 512–513 (1977).

(*11*) SANTAPAU, H. *Endangered plant species and their habitats*. Morges, Switzerland, International Union for Conservation of Nature and Natural Resources, 1970 (IUCN publications, new series, No. 18, vol. 2, pp. 83–88.

(*12*) SAHNI, K. C. *Protection of rare and endangered plants in the Indian flora*. Morges, Switzerland, International Union for Conservation of Nature and Natural Resources, 1970 (IUCN publications, new series, No. 18, vol. 2, pp. 95–102.

(*13*) QURESHI, I. M. & KAUL, O. N. *Some endangered plants and threatened habitats in South-East Asia*. Morges, Switzerland, International Union for Conservation of Nature and Natural Resources, 1970 (IUCN publications, new series, No. 18, vol. 2, pp. 115–126.

(*14*) GUPTA, R. & MITAL, S. P. Exploration and improvement studies on some important medicinal plants. In: *Advance notes on symposia and discussions, section of botany*. Gauhati, 67th Session of Indian Science Congress, 1980, pp. 18–20.

(*15*) SUBRAMANYAM, K. & SREEMADHAVAN, C. P. *Endangered plant species and their* habitats—a review of the Indian situation. Morges, Switzerland, International Union for Conservation of Nature and Natural Resources, 1970 (IUCN publications, new series, No. 18, vol. 2, pp. 108–114.

(16) SOBTI, S. N., PUSHPANGADAN, P. & ATAL, C. K. Cytogenetical improvement of medicinal and aromatic plants. In: *Advance notes on symposia and discussions, section of botany.* Gauhati, 67th Session of Indian Science Congress, 1980, pp. 22–23.

(17) MITRA, G. C. Role of tissue culture in medicinal plants research. In: *Advance notes on symposia and discussions, section of botany.* Gauhati, 67th Session of Indian Science Congress, 1980, pp. 25–27.

(18) RUSTOGI, R. P. Search for new medicinal plants from Indian flora. In: *Advance notes on symposia and discussions, section of botany.* Gauhati, 67th Session of Indian Science Congress, 1980, pp. 16–17.

(19) KAPOOR, S. L. & MITRA, R. *Herbal drugs in Indian pharmaceutical industry.* Lucknow, India, National Botanical Research Institute, 1979.

(20) PRADHAN, G. M. Habitat destruction of Himalayan orchid jungles. In: *Proceedings of the Eighth World Orchid Conference, Frankfurt, 1975.* Frankfurt, 1976, pp. 331–334.

(21) PRADHAN, U. C. Conservation of eastern Himalayan orchids: problems and prospects, parts I, II & III. *The orchid review,* **83**: 314–317, 345–347 & 374–375 (1975).

(22) PRADHAN, U. C. Conserving Indian orchids. *American Orchid Society bulletin,* **46**:117–121 (1977).

(23) KATAKI, S. K. Indian orchids: a note on conservation. *American Orchid Society bulletin,* **45**:912–914 (1976).

(24) MAMMEN, V. & MAMMEN, O. Rediscovering *Paphiopedilum druryi* in southern India. *Orchid digest,* **38**:31–36 (1974).

(25) PRADHAN, U. C. Conservation of eastern Himalayan orchids: problems and prospects. In: *Proceedings of the Eighth World Orchid Conference, Frankfurt, 1975.* Frankfurt, 1976, pp. 335–340.

(26) VARMAH, J. C. & SAHNI, K. C. Rare orchids of the northeastern region and their conservation. *Indian forester,* **102**:424–431 (1976).

(27) PEMPAHISHEY, K. T. Orchid eaters of "Shangri-la". *American Orchid Society bulletin,* **43**:716–725 (1974).

(28) WILKES, G. Breeding crisis for our crops—is the gene pool drying up? *Horticulture,* **55** (4): 52–59 (1977).

(29) WILKES, G. The world's crop plant germplasm—an endangered resource. *Bulletin of the atomic scientists,* **33** (2): 8–16 (1977).

(30) *Underexploited tropical plants with promising economic value.* Washington, DC, National Academy of Sciences, 1975.

CHAPTER 18

The NAPRALERT data base as an information source for application to traditional medicine

Norman R. Farnsworth[1]

It has been estimated that from 250 000 to 750 000 species of higher (flowering) plants exist on earth; some of these have not yet been botanically described. Although there is no way to determine accurately how many of these species have been used in traditional medicine, a reasonable estimate would be about 10% or from 25 000 to 75 000 species. However, perhaps only about 1% of these (250–750 species) are acknowledged through scientific studies to have real therapeutic value when used in extract form by humans. Virtually all such plants have been "discovered" and put to widespread use in orthodox medical systems, based on information derived from their use in (a) folk medicine, (b) ethnomedicine, or (c) traditional medicine.

Identification of additional useful plants within the group of 25 000–75 000 species that have been used in traditional medicine for more widespread consideration as elements of health care systems throughout the world will be a monumental task. Some of these plants undoubtedly owe their action to (a) ritual associated with their use (psychotherapeutic), (b) a placebo effect, or (c) the presence of one or more chemical substances whose pharmacological action is responsible for the effect claimed in humans.

The problems attendant on attempts to verify the value of plants as real therapeutic agents through controlled human studies are enormous. As a starting point in such an exercise it would seem logical to draw on the rather vast published literature on the pharmacological evaluation of plant extracts as reported in *in vitro*, *in vivo* or controlled human experimental studies. Correlations can often be made that provide greater confidence that a plant alleged to be effective in traditional medicine would indeed be so. Both positive and negative data can be used; however, it must be

---

[1] Head and Professor, Department of Pharmacognosy and Pharmacology, University of Illinois, Chicago, IL, USA.

emphasized that *in vitro* and *in vivo* test results need not necessarily correlate with effects in humans.

The use of retrospective experimental data on plant extracts in assessing the claims made for them in traditional Chinese medicine can be cited as a model for the type of analysis that will be required in the global assessment of plants used in traditional medicine (*1*). A book intended for use by the "barefoot doctors" in the Beijing area was analysed. The book lists 248 plant and animal drugs which enter into 796 polyprescriptions. Each prescription in the book is indicated for one or more uses. For purposes of evaluating the potential effectiveness of the drugs it was considered of prime importance to determine whether the prescription (one or more of its components) had a valid pharmacological basis of action. This was done by searching the periodical literature for reports on the results of pharmacological evaluation of all 248 plant or animal substances entering into the prescriptions, as well as any "folkloric" claims for each of the drugs. All chemical compounds reported to be present in each of the drugs were noted together with the pharmacological effects for each of these constituents. Thus, if a polyprescription contained one or more drugs whose reported pharmacological effects correlated with the alleged use in traditional Chinese medicine of the prescription, or if any of the chemical compounds present in any of the drugs was known to elicit a pharmacological effect that correlated in the same way, it was presumed that the polyprescription most likely had a rational basis for use. Additive to the analysis was the application of a technique based on convergent evolution, which presumes that the fact of peoples geographically distant or with dissimilar cultural backgrounds using a given plant for the same purpose constitutes impressive *prima facie* evidence that the putative use is valid. The likelihood of such a phenomenon being due to mere chance would appear to be statistically remote.

The analysis showed that 44.7% of the 796 polyprescriptions utilized in traditional Chinese medicine presented a valid rationale for the alleged uses. Predictions could not be made on 48.7% of the polyprescriptions since there was a lack of scientific data in the periodical literature which could be applied to the analysis.

An analysis of this type requires an inordinate effort and attempts to correlate and evaluate plants alleged to have a therapeutic effect on a global basis would be an impossible task using conventional methods. On the other hand, such an exercise would be entirely realistic given an appropriate data base which could be weighted and analysed by means of computer technology.

The NAPRALERT system

A computerized data base on the chemistry and pharmacology of natural products is available, and has been used by the Special Programme on

Research, Development and Research Training in Human Reproduction of the World Health Organization. The data base is maintained in the Department of Pharmacognosy and Pharmacology, College of Pharmacy, University of Illinois, at the Medical Center, and has been given the acronym NAPRALERT (Natural Products ALERT). A systematic surveillance of the world literature on the chemistry and pharmacology of natural products has been in progress since 1975. In addition, a substantial amount of retrospective information has been acquired and computerized on selected genera of plants and on the pharmacological activities of natural products. These retrospective searches extend back into the mid-1700s. The NAPRALERT system is maintained on a Computer Corporation of America (CCA) model 204 data management system. During the period 1975–1979, we have produced a data base from some 32 000 scientific articles and abstracts, covering information on 4595 genera of plants, microorganisms and animals (including 5145 records pertaining to monocotyledons, 57 168 pertaining to dicotyledons, 2861 pertaining to fungi, 1790 pertaining to bacteria, and 1278 pertaining to marine organisms). In addition, the data base contains 135 255 pharmacological entries and 141 149 compound records.

The NAPRALERT data base uses the following as sources of information: *Chemical Abstracts*, *Biological Abstracts* and more than 200 current scientific periodicals that are regularly reviewed. The current periodicals have been selected on the basis of a regular review of the data base to determine those journals in which a majority of articles of interest to the system are found. Every attempt is made to computerize information only from original articles; abstracts being used only in cases where articles are difficult to acquire. Articles selected for entry into the data base are those containing information on the presence of secondary chemical constituents in natural products, or those containing results from testing natural products (extracts or pure compounds) for any type of biological activity. Reports on folkloric, ethnomedical or traditional uses of plants are also acquired and computerized. The following major data fields are covered in the NAPRALERT system.

I. Organism record

A. Major class of organism, e.g., monocotyledon, dicotyledon, gymnosperm, bryophyte, pteridophyte, lichen, fungus, bacterium, alga, invertebrate or vertebrate, with the capability of recognizing the class if it is of marine origin.
B. Family of organism (including subfamily, order, tribe, etc.).
C. Latin binomial of organism studied (including the genus, species, subspecies, variety, form cultivar, etc., with appropriate author citation).
D. Latin binomial synonym (including the author citation).

E. Vernacular name given for the organism.
F. Organism part studied, e.g., root, stem, leaf, bark, tuber, aerial parts, whole plant, venom gland, scent gland, whole cells.
G. Organism part modifier, e.g., fresh, dried, lyophilized, fungus-infected, virus-infected, callus, suspension culture, crown gall, tumour on.
H. Geographic areas.

The geographic area where the organism under study was collected is noted (in the case of recording ethnomedical uses, the geographic area where the preparation was *used* is computerized). Provision has been made to enter (*a*) the country, (*b*) the state or province and (*c*) other identifying geographic area. In the case of marine organisms, the major body of water is entered as the "country", e.g., Pacific, and the land mass closest to the collection area is noted as the "province", e.g., Pacific-Hawaii.

Geographic modifier.

A provision is available to note whether the plant has been collected from (*a*) wild-growing indigenous plants, (*b*) cultivated plants, (*c*) naturalized plants, etc.

II. Work types

A large number of selective work-type codes are available for use, depending on the need to be specific or general. Examples are:

—(*a*) isolation from, (*b*) identified in by thin-layer chromatography (tlc), (*c*) identified in by gas-liquid chromatography (glc), and (*d*) isolated from following saponification (the work type is linked to the organism name and the compound record);

—(*a*) *in vitro* pharmacological effect of an extract from, (*b*) *in vivo* pharmacological effect of an extract (the work type is linked to the organism name and the pharmacology record only);

—(*a*) mass spectral data reported, (*b*) proton magnetic spectroscopy (pmr) spectrum reported, (*c*) ^{13}C nuclear magnetic spectroscopy (cmr) spectrum reported; (*d*) tlc data reported (the work type is linked only to the compound record);

—a large number of additional work types that allow retrieval of data relating to some of the following: plant tissue culture, microbial transformations, chemotaxonomy, synthesis, partial synthesis, or agronomic studies.

III. Compound record

For each secondary chemical compound reported isolated from or identified in an organism or for which a biological activity is noted, the following elements are computerized:

A. Compound name (see also IV below)
B. Structure category coding
C. Substructure coding
D. Functional group codes
E. Quantitative yields

The starting weight of plant (or other organism) material from which substances are isolated is recorded (in grams), as well as the weight of substance isolated in pure form. A percentage yield is automatically calculated and stored with the record by the computer.

If a substance is specifically looked for, and is found to be absent, such negative data are also computerized. This type of information is usually restricted to analyses of materials by means of glc, e.g., safrole may be reported as absent in the analysis of an essential oil when, on chemotaxonomic principles, it may normally be expected to be found.

IV. Pharmacology record

The pharmacology record contains the following major elements:

A. Major pharmacological effect.

Each type of biological effect is initially given a major code designation corresponding with the following: (*a*) CNS, (*b*) autonomic, (*c*) haematologic, (*d*) chemotherapeutic, (*e*) toxicologic, (*f*) enzyme modification, (*g*) hormonal, (*h*) cardiovascular, (*i*) effect on plants, (*j*) pheromonal, (*k*) fertility-regulating and (*l*) miscellaneous effects.

B. Specific pharmacological effect.

Within each of the above categories, specific pharmacological effects are assigned. For example, in the CNS category, specific effects can be assigned as follows: CNS stimulant, CNS depressant, analgesic, anticonvulsant, convulsant, hypothermic, euphoriant, emetic, anti-emetic, hallucinogenic, local anaesthetic, neuroleptic, barbiturate potentiation, barbiturate antagonism, etc.

C. Test species used.
D. Sex of test species.
E. Dose employed.
F. Dosage frequency.
G. Route of administration.
H. Quantitative results, e.g. active, inactive, weak activity, strong activity and equivocal activity.
I. Quantitative expression of results, e.g., per cent increased life span, per cent tumour regression, Effective Dose$_{50}$ (ED$_{50}$), Lethal Dose$_{10}$ (LD$_{10}$), LD$_{50}$, LD$_{90}$, LD$_{100}$, Minimum Lethal Dose (MLD), minimal inhibitory concentration (MIC).

J. Substrates, cell lines, test organism, tissues, organs, etc. (used primarily in conjunction with *in vitro* testing).
K. Modifying data, e.g., when alterations to standard testing models are made, these are expressed in written form; or when more detailed information than the coding system provides is required, such information can also be expressed completely in written form.
L. Type extract, e.g., when extracts of organism are made, the type solvent used to prepare the test extract is entered (boiling water, ethanol, methanol, benzene, chloroform, etc.).

V. Demographic record

The demographic record for each citation includes the following elements.

A. Full title of article (translated into English if necessary).
B. Author(s) name(s) (last name, initials of first names).
C. Journal name.
D. Volume, issue number, full pagination, year.
E. Secondary source of information, e.g., from *Chemical Abstracts*.
F. Type of article, e.g., research paper, review article, note, abstract.
G. Language of the original article.
H. Address (of the first author listed on the article), including the department, college, university, city, state or province, postal code number, and country.
I. Grant support designation (country of agency, agency name, grant number(s).

Application of the NAPRALERT data base to traditional medicine

Even though the NAPRALERT data base is incomplete relative to total coverage of the chemistry and pharmacology of plants, experience to date has shown that in many instances important information on plants used in traditional medicine can be obtained. As our capability to enrich the data base with retrospective literature increases, utilization of the system will naturally be enhanced. If one studies the various types of data that are computerized (see above) and realizes that queries linking any of the available data fields can be effected, one sees that the types of problems that can be solved through the use of the data base are almost unlimited. However, without going into the complexities of the data base, there are two major areas in which traditional medicine can be served through the use of NAPRALERT.

Data retrieval

We have found that the greatest number of inquiries from the NAPRALERT data base relate to (*a*) determining all published information on a given plant, e.g., *Matricaria chamomilla*; (*b*) identification of a given chemical compound (or class of chemical compound) in all members of a stated taxon; (*c*) biological effects for a stated chemical compound (or class of compound) known to occur in nature; and (*d*) plants which have been shown to elicit a specific pharmacological effect.

Whereas the NAPRALERT system has so far been used primarily for simple data retrieval, the major application intended for this data base is to solve problems.

Problem-solving pertinent to traditional medicine

Since most problems in traditional medicine are regional ones, it is possible to program the NAPRALERT data base to respond primarily to questions concerning plants of a specific country, e.g., Nigeria; of a specific region within a continent, e.g., West Africa; or within a given continent, e.g., Africa. Eventually, we will be able to analyse published data on the basis of other geographic parameters, for instance, data on plants restricted primarily to arid, mountainous, tropical, subtropical or temperate zone habitats.

Thus, one can query the data base to determine the names of all plants within a specific geographic area which have been reported through pharmacological tests to have antitumour, hypoglycaemic, abortifacient or other types of activity, depending on national priorities within the country, or the interests of the investigator.

Another type of analysis that is possible would be to determine all plants that have a reputation for being used in traditional medicine, for example, to treat arthritis following oral administration. The query can be restricted to a given geographic area or be global in nature. Introduction of a second parameter such as identification of plants, extracts of which have shown *in vivo* antiinflammatory activity, with the computer recognizing only plants having both of these properties, would then produce a list of plants claimed in traditional medicine to be efficacious against arthritis, and shown by available experimental evidence to have a rational basis for this effect. One can then proceed to select, from an enormous number of candidate plants, a selected few having the desired biological effects, for further evaluation.

The WHO Special Programme on Research, Development and Research Training in Human Reproduction recently initiated a Task Force on Indigenous Plants for Fertility Regulation. Primary emphasis in this task force has been a selection of promising plants to investigate for the presence of orally effective and safe substances intended to be used as fertility regulating agents in the male and female. These plants are then assigned to one or more of several collaborating research centres for scientific studies. All of the plants assigned to the centres were identified as promising candidates through an analysis of the world literature pertaining to fertility regulating plants by the NAPRALERT data base. Space does not allow a detailed description of how this was done, but the interested reader may consult the several reports that have been published to date on this subject (2–4), with much of the data being derived from recent reviews on the subject (5–6).

Although it is not possible to state at this time whether the computer analysis approach to selection of plants to investigate for fertility regulating activity is realistic, preliminary experimental evidence from the programme seems to indicate that the method has predictive capabilities.

It would then appear that the NAPRALERT system of analysis could, with appropriate modifications in the computer programs, be applied to virtually any category of biological effect for which a reasonable amount of retrospective literature exists.

Many other problems pertinent to plants used in traditional medicine can be approached in a similar manner, with a more scientific investigational plan than has been possible previously.

Current status of access to the NAPRALERT data base

We have recently been able to make the NAPRALERT data base available to individuals, industrial firms, academic institutions and government agencies, with a modest fee calculated on the basis of actual computer time required to generate data output, the cost of photocopying the material and the mailing costs. We are now working on a plan to have requests from developing countries directed to a single coordinator within a country, who would then relay groups of requests to us at stated intervals. This, hopefully, will reduce the amount of correspondence required to meet individual literature requirements, and hence lower costs.

Future plans for the NAPRALERT data base relative to traditional medicine

The NAPRALERT data base must be considered to be in its infancy as a comprehensive representation of the world scientific literature on the chemistry and pharmacology of natural products, even though we have conducted more than 500 generic literature searches on higher plants (representing thousands of species), with all data on plants in the 500 genera now completely computerized. We feel that NAPRALERT represents a unique data base, specifically of greatest value to scientists in developing countries. For this reason, our future plans will be aimed primarily at serving the needs of interested scientists, institutions, industry and governmental agencies in those developing countries that are interested in exploring their own unique flora and fauna to discover biologically active and useful substances, as well as aiding in the clarification of the status of plants used in traditional medicine within those countries.

We shall be approaching international funding agencies to enlist their cooperation in financing a ten-year programme that will allow us to computerize all of the world literature on natural products, as far back as the year 1900. This will be an enormous effort, which cannot be effectively accomplished without the direct cooperation of interested scientists and institutions in developing countries. Our stepwise plan for attaining this objective is as follows.

1. Explore the mechanisms for making the data base available via satellite to any country in the world having a computer terminal.

2. Initiate an "International Symposium on Establishment of a Global Network of Collaborators on NAPRALERT".

3. Identify scientists in every country who will be willing to work with us:

(*a*) in a training programme on computer programming, data retrieval and full comprehension of the capabilities of NAPRALERT;

(*b*) in coordinating the use of the data base within his or her own country and interacting with users within that country for effective use of the information; and

(*c*) in establishing a network of collaborators within each country to collect information from traditional practitioners on the exact use of herbal medicines, and computerizing this information for subsequent application in order to establish the safety and efficacy of those preparations. We have already initiated plans to carry out such work with certain African states, in collaboration with Professor Sofowora in Nigeria.

(*d*) in making a scientific approach to establishing the safety and efficacy of traditional medicines through evaluation of work on the plants contained in these medicines as published by scientists in any country of the world. This will involve construction of computer programs that will be appropriate to solve the problem at hand taking into account the national priorities of any specific country, the available local flora and any pre-established framework of standards.

4. Utilize the NAPRALERT data base to construct distribution maps of plants of interest to a given country for the purpose of establishing the extent of raw material for industrial or conservation needs, and for many other practical or basic research purposes. Solving of problems of a chemotaxonomic nature would seem to be particularly well suited for application of the NAPRALERT data base.

The scientific applications of a complete data base as described herein are endless, but the few mentioned above should serve to alert interested parties to the practicality of carrying out this work on a global cooperative basis, with each country having perhaps a small but significant input into the system, and all countries having full utilization of the efforts of the team.

REFERENCES

(1) AMERICAN HERBAL PHARMACOLOGY DELEGATION. *Herbal pharmacology in the People's Republic of China. A trip report.* Washington, DC, National Academy of Sciences, 1975.
(2) SOEJARTO, D. D. ET AL. Fertility regulating agents from plants. *Bulletin of the World Health Organization*, **56**:343–352 (1978).
(3) FARNSWORTH, N. R. World Health Organization: programme on indigenous plants for fertility regulation. In: *IUPAC 11th International Symposium on Chemistry of Natural Products, Bulgaria.* Oxford, International Union of Pure and Applied Chemistry, 1978, pp. 475–489.
(4) SOEJARTO, D. D. Plants to control fertility. *World Health*, August–September 1978, pp. 16–19.
(5) FARNSWORTH, N. R. ET AL. Potential value of plants as sources of new antifertility agents, I & II. *Journal of pharmaceutical sciences*, **64**:535–598 & 717–754 (1975).
(6) BINGLE, A. S. & FARNSWORTH, N. R. Botanical sources of fertility regulating agents: chemistry and pharmacology. In: Briggs, M. & Corbin, A., ed. *Progress in hormone biochemistry and pharmacology.* Lancaster, MTP Press, 1981, vol. 1, pp. 149–225.

CHAPTER 19

Phytopharmacology and phytotherapy

Michel A. Attisso[1]

I. Medicinal plants and plant drugs

The decline of phytotherapy in the industrialized countries at the end of the first half of the 20th century was no more than an episode in the application of medicinal plants in the service of health worldwide. In the developing countries, however, phytotherapy has remained the principal therapeutic resource.

In the industrialized countries, a new style of applying phytotherapy has been developed during the last two decades, accompanied by an upsurge in the consumption of medicinal plants as reflected in the volume of international trade. According to the official figures given by the International Trade Centre, the total value of imports of starting materials of plant origin for the pharmaceutical and cosmetics industry rose from US $52.9 million in 1967 to US $71.2 million in 1971, and the annual growth since that date has been of the order of 5–7%.

In this context, impressive amounts of certain plant drugs have been consumed in the form of pharmaceutical preparations throughout the world since 1974:

—3000 tonnes of aloes
—10 000 tonnes of fresh artichoke leaves
—5000 tonnes of chinchona bark
—1000 tonnes of belladona, henbane and datura leaves
—1000 tonnes of foxglove leaves
—5000 tonnes of senna, etc.

Another point of note is that despite the current vigorous expansion of

---

[1] Professor, Faculty of Pharmacy, and Head Pharmacist, University Hospital Centre, Montpellier, France.

organic synthesis, the proportion of medicinal plants to synthetic chemicals going into the manufacture of medicaments is about one to three.

In addition, the consumption of herb teas has been rising steadily in the industrialized countries. The figures for 1974 are as follows:

—150 tonnes of lime blossom
—250 tonnes of mint
—100 tonnes of camomile
—200 tonnes of verbena
—30 tonnes of orange blossom
—30 tonnes of star anise
—45 tonnes of eucalyptus leaves

There is thus a genuine interest now being taken in phytotherapy and medicinal plants throughout the world.

When the reasons for this situation are examined, however, they are found to be quite different for industrialized countries and for developing countries.

The situation in industrialized countries

The situation in industrialized countries has two aspects: the high level of consumption of pharmaceutical products and its consequences; and the demand for raw materials of plant origin.

The consumption of pharmaceutical products in the industrialized countries is steadily increasing. In addition to the drugs that are essential for the treatment of genuine pathological conditions, there is a far from negligible consumption of "convenience" drugs by healthy people, who tend increasingly to make such consumption a part of their life-style. Such drugs include painkillers, various so-called tonics and, more particularly, various psychotropic agents (stimulants, euphoretics, sedatives, tranquillizers and hypnotics), together with anorectics and, to some extent, oral contraceptives.

The prevalence of chemotherapy by synthetic drugs in these countries has led to a true *drug-related chemical pollution*, superimposed on environmental pollution.

This continual chemical bombardment of the human body and its long-term harmful results could be what has triggered the search for and use of therapeutic agents with much less harmful side-effects wherever possible. The desire for a "return to nature", is undoubtedly the reason why people in the industrialized countries are now turning to phytotherapy.

The principal feature of this new therapeutic approach is the association of plant medicine with specific chemotherapy, although chemotherapy may at times be completely replaced by phytotherapy. This new style of phytotherapy is gradually gaining ground and receiving increasing support from the medical profession in many countries. The practical repercussions of the changing situation may be seen in the national pharmacopoeias and the pharmaceutical industries.

As far as national pharmacopoeias are concerned, the principal point to note is the interest that many countries are taking in the preparation of monographs on medicinal plants and plant drugs, regardless of whether these already appear in official lists or are less well known and thus require further scientific investigation.

The situation in developing countries

In regard to the Third World, the distinctive feature of the present status of phytotherapy is the persistence of the practice of traditional medicine, which is its main source of strength. It is based on a series of motivations that are common to all and which explain the desire for a new approach.

While phytotherapy in Europe had by the 19th century begun to cast off its sociocultural and metaphysical aspects, had become more systematic and had eventually developed into a specific chemotherapy based either on chemical substances of plant origin or on the semisynthetic derivatives of such substances, in the Third World the art of restoring and preserving health by means of plants remained firmly established.

In its present form, traditional medicine has a certain universality that springs from its origins, as well as a true diversity that arises from the distinguishing sociocultural characteristics of the peoples of the Third World. Thus, there is a single traditional medicine, branching off into a number of systems rather than several traditional medicines.

The present-day practitioners of traditional medicine ought to be referred to as traditional practitioners and not as healers or herbalists. They are not magicians, sorcerers or witch doctors.

Compendiums of traditional medicines and the starting materials from which they are obtained, as well as all treatment formulas used in traditional medicine, may be regarded as pharmacopoeias in the widest sense of the term. On this basis, they are referred to here as "traditional pharmacopoeias".

Traditional pharmacopoeias in non-codified esoteric systems are oral, but in codified systems of traditional medicine they are true formularies or codes of medicaments, i.e., written pharmacopoeias.

Traditional medicaments do not consist exclusively of phytotherapeutic preparations. Generally speaking, they are very complex preparations composed of vegetable drugs in association with animal and mineral drugs. The raw materials are generally taken from the natural resources of the locality or region. Non-local ingredients are rare or restricted and are found only in some written traditional pharmacopoeias.

Traditional medicaments are also distinguished by their large number of components. From this point of view they recall some of the formulas for compound powders, tinctures, electuaries, conserves, syrups, etc., found in the first European pharmacopoeias and in some modern formulas for phytotherapeutic preparations.

The complex composition of traditional medicaments is explained by the fact that frequently they were not only expected to remove the symptoms of disease but were also supposed to help the sick body support the somewhat aggressive action of the drug itself and to meet a number of sociocultural demands.

Traditional medicaments come in a relatively large number of dosage forms, and in order to produce them a genuine mastery of pharmaceutical techniques is required. Such dosage forms include:

(i) *compound preparations* intended for the extemporaneous preparation of herb-teas, lotions, fomentations and baths;

(ii) *various compound powders* for administration by mouth, by intradermal scarification or by direct application to the skin or certain mucosa;

(iii) *multiple-dose, sweetened paste-like preparations*, for administration by mouth; many of these preparations may contain up to 30 or more components;

(iv) *single-dose solid preparations* for oral administration (boluses and pills, or even tablets in some modernized traditional pharmacopoeias);

(v) *various liquid preparations for oral administration*; the composition of these preparations is generally very complex but they may be classified as infusions, broths, syrups, aqueous solutions or suspensions compounded as required;

(vi) *ointments, salves and liniments* for application to the skin or for the treatment of skin lesions; and

(vii) *eye washes*, often made from fresh plant juices, and powders and aqueous solutions for ophthalmic purposes.

To obtain these medicinal forms the solvents most frequently employed are water, ethyl alcohol, oils and fats. Generally speaking, traditional medicine makes little use of enemas. Injectables as such do not exist but suppositories are available in the form of vegetable tampons.

Here there is no question, as in the industrialized countries, of going "back to nature" or of wanting to combat the chemical pollution of the body provoked by inopportune chemotherapy or by the misuse of convenience drugs of chemical origin. Third World countries are primarily concerned with providing their peoples with adequate coverage of their essential drug needs. In this context, it should not be forgotten that for these peoples health in the immediate future does not mean "a state of complete physical, mental and social well-being" but merely the "absence of disease or infirmity".

II. The utilization of local plant resources in primary health care

In view of the difficulties experienced by developing countries in meeting their needs for essential drugs, the following measures might be taken to encourage utilization for primary health care of their vast local resources:

(i) a real health policy option at national and regional level;

(ii) determination of priorities regarding health problems and definition of possible solutions;

(iii) goal-oriented applied scientific research on medicinal plants, incorporating properly planned programmes;

(iv) effective implementation of these programmes with regard to technical and financial resources and appropriate personnel.

Health policy option

The will to make use of available local resources, in particular traditional medicaments, in primary health care exists in practically all Third World countries.

It is important, however, that it be given concrete expression at national level through effective mobilization of the rural masses, and the provision of information necessary to enable them to accept phytotherapy based on local resources. This may be achieved through the collection of all available information on the empirical treatments by means of plants practised in the country and by encouraging ethnomedical and ethnopharmacognostic surveys.

Meetings should be organized in order to encourage collaboration between modern physicians and traditional practitioners.

Applied research on medicinal plants should also be encouraged and provision made for adequate technical and financial resources.

Goal-oriented scientific research

In many developing countries, appropriate utilization of local resources to cover drug needs is dependent on preliminary scientific study to determine the efficacy and safety of the preparations based on plant drugs that are used on an empirical basis in traditional medicine.

There are two possible approaches to such a study: new-style phytotherapy, and chemotherapy based on the active principles obtained in a pure form from plant drugs as starting materials (molecular therapy).

These two approaches differ in conception, methodology and the means used to put them into practice. There are two main prerequisites regarding research on traditional medicaments—collection of all available objective information by means of ethnopharmacognostic surveys; and the acquisition of an effective knowledge of the resources offered by the local flora, and the opportunities for applying it, by means of an agrobotanical survey.

Preliminary ethnopharmacognostic and agrobotanical research. Ethnopharmacognostic surveys are particularly important in the case of all non-codified systems of traditional medicine. They are the only means of finding out not only the plant species used but also the part of the plant that represents the drug, the time and conditions of harvesting, any preliminary treatment (use in the fresh state, mode of drying, conversion to a stable form), the dosage form actually given to patients, the procedure for obtaining it, treatment formulas, dosage, and mode of administration to the patient.

Hence the technical organization of such surveys, the choice of survey workers, the sources of information and the conduct of the work all merit careful study from the sociocultural point of view.

The standard index cards recommended for use in this field are extremely helpful, but an ability to adapt them to meet each particular situation is essential.

In the case of codified systems of traditional medicine, the sources of information are already available in the form of written traditional pharmacopoeias.

Agrobotanical research should be directed towards the accurate identification of the plant species revealed by ethnopharmacognostic surveys, identification and evaluation of their natural distribution in the country or region, and determination of the feasibility of making use of wild species in ways compatible with maintaining the plant balance, and of the conditions under which such species might be cultivated.

New-style phytotherapy

The basic objective of new-style phytotherapy is to produce phytotherapeutic preparations for immediate use in modern medical practice from the resources of traditional medication. Applied scientific research on the subject consists in evaluating, systematizing, standardizing and improving empirical medicaments based on local vegetable drugs.

These local vegetable drugs fall into two categories—those whose botanical features, chemical composition and pharmacological properties are already universally known and most of which already figure in modern pharmacopoeias (medicinal plants proper); and those that are still unknown or only partially known and for which further scientific investigation is required before they can be incorporated into modern therapeutics (plants considered to be medicinal).

There are consequently three different aspects or scientific approaches to be distinguished in new-style phytotherapy:

(i) proven and established medicinal plants;
(ii) plants considered to be medicinal;
(iii) traditional ready-to-use medicaments.

Appropriate methodology for established medicinal plants. Appropriate research methodology for established medicinal plants presents very few problems. Since the local agrobotanical parameters have already been determined, and the pharmacological properties are known, all that is required is to verify that the locally produced drug (plants picked in the wild or grown as an experimental crop) meets the specified standards. Simple phytochemical studies aimed at producing complete extracts, purified extracts and fractionated extracts corresponding to specific groups of chemical compounds (total alkaloids, total glycosides, flavonosides, various glycoside fractions, etc.) are made in order to arrive at dosage forms; then pharmacotechnical studies are also made to determine the most appropriate dosage form and the formulation for manufacture on an industrial or semi-industrial scale, as well as to develop quality control methods.

Clinical trials should aim only at determining dosage and finding new therapeutic indications, if any. Another useful research aim would be to produce compound preparations that combine a number of vegetable drugs in this category.

These first steps to promote utilization of local resources could be initiated now, under the conditions defined above, in most developing countries. All that is required is to make a preliminary selection of essential vegetable drugs in the light of the health and economic situation of the country concerned.

Appropriate methodology for plants considered to be medicinal. The ultimate aim is to arrive at a scientific assessment of the data on which the empirical use is based. The investigations consequently demand close cooperation between traditional practitioners and all members of the scientific and medical team when non-codified systems of traditional medicine are under investigation. The first two stages are as follows:

(i) a phytochemical study directed towards determining the main chemical groups to which the constituents of the drugs to be tested belong and producing complete and fractionated extracts for pharmacological testing, rather than a sophisticated phytochemical study aimed at isolating and identifying a pure chemical compound;

(ii) pharmacodynamic experiments on animals to verify a drug's pharmacological properties, test that its empirical use is valid, and determine its acute and subacute toxicities.

These two series of laboratory investigations should be carried out in parallel, using as a guideline the data produced by the ethnopharmacognostic surveys. In particular, the extracts for animal experiments should initially be produced with the same solvents as are used in the preparation of traditional medicaments. There is thus no question of beginning with the conventional approach of extraction chemistry, which employs a range of solvents of increasing polarity. This would only be appropriate where the traditional dosage form was based on the complete plant drug in powder form.

In the same way, it should be borne in mind in animal experiments that the parenteral route of administration, which gives the best results, is not used in traditional medicine and that the test substances are medicaments that are already in use on an empirical basis in man. Complete pharmacological screening, as employed in the case of new test compounds, is therefore not the way to tackle the pharmacodynamic problem here.

Even when animal experiments have given negative results, a pharmacotechnical study to produce the most appropriate dosage form, and an evaluation of clinical effectiveness by conventional methods could be undertaken.

The results given by the initial pharmacological and clinical trials should enable a decision to be made on whether the vegetable drugs concerned could be used at once in phytotherapy under acceptable conditions of therapeutic safety, efficacy, and cost-effectiveness.

If the answer is yes, further research should aim at setting standards for these new medicinal plants and the preparations made from them (including long-term toxicity and any contraindications arising from knowledge of the pharmacological spectrum of the drug concerned).

If the answer is no, it would at least be useful to continue phytochemical and pharmacodynamic studies in order to find out any pharmacological properties that empirical use had failed to indicate.

Appropriate methodology for use with traditional ready-to-use dosage forms. Such tests can only be considered in the context of clinical trials using the conventional double-blind method and would only apply to dosage forms described in articles in traditional pharmacopoeias or in certain national pharmacopoeias from Asia.

Because of the complexity of the qualitative and quantitative formulas for these medicaments, little of objective value can be obtained from animal experiments and it is preferable to restrict investigation to the scientific evaluation of each plant component separately.

Molecular therapy

In view of the need for immediate satisfaction of essential drug needs, molecular therapy cannot be considered as a primary research requirement in developing countries under present conditions.

The scientific approach which seeks to isolate and identify pure chemical substances from the vegetable drugs used in traditional medicine, or from the local flora, and then to proceed to conventional pharmacological screening on animals in order to assess their therapeutic properties before embarking on pharmaceutical production, is a very costly process with uncertain results and demands a considerable investment in sophisticated equipment and highly qualified staff.

This form of molecular therapy should be the second stage in applied scientific research on medicinal plants and should be extended to cover all available plant resources.

Unfortunately, in many developing countries, molecular therapy features on the priority programmes of specialized institutes and universities, no doubt because of the obvious material advantages that a patent brings to its holders.

Technical conditions for initiating applied scientific research on new-style phytotherapy

These are of two orders:

(i) preparation of research programmes with allocation of priorities;
(ii) organization on a coordinated multidisciplinary basis.

Research programmes and objectives

Research programmes and objectives must, above all, be very realistic and be based on the same criteria as were defined for the selection of essential medicinal plants in developing countries.

Research objectives could be planned on the following lines in the case of phytotherapeutic preparations likely to prove a valuable supplement to chemotherapy, or capable of replacing chemotherapy in certain cases, and in the case of the natural forms of chemotherapy which might arise from it:

(i) Pharmacological groups having first-priority research topics:

—external antiseptics, agents to combat cutaneous fungi, and cicatrizants;
—internal antiseptics: intestinal, respiratory and urinary antiseptics;
—agents for correcting disorders of the digestive system: laxatives and cathartics, mucilaginous regulating agents, antidiarrhoeal substances, analgesics and antispasmodics;
—cardiovascular agents: antihypertensives and vasodilators, cardiac tonics and analeptics.

(ii) Pharmacological groups having second-priority research topics:
—antidiabetics and hypoglycaemics;
—cardiovascular agents: cerebral vasoregulating and oxygenating agents, agents that protect vessel walls, haemostatics, antianaemics, etc;
—diuretics;
—intestinal anthelmintics;
—psychotropic agents.

(iii) Pharmacological groups having third-priority research topics:
—various antiparasitic agents; antiamoebics, visceral filaricides, antimalarials, trypanocides and leishmanicides;
—agents to combat visceral fungi;
—antibacterial (including antileprosy) agents and antiviral agents;
—antitumorigenic agents, etc.

Integrated overall organization

The implementation of national or regional programmes calls for integrated, multidisciplinary, coordinated organization in which traditional practitioners have a real part to play.

The organizational structure would include:

(i) a national coordinating committee with ultimate responsibility for planning and administration;

(ii) a documentation centre;

(iii) laboratory services;

(iv) health centres responsible for clinical trials.

The links between these various centres and their respective responsibilities are summarized in Fig. 1.

This form of organization may be set up on a regional basis with facilities in two or three different countries; it is not essential for all parts of the organization to be in the same locality.

Complete multidisciplinary organizational structures of this type can hardly be said to exist in the vast majority of developing countries and their establishment is a matter of priority.

Technical facilities, staff and operating funds are essential for implementation and national universities with schools of medicine, pharmacy or basic sciences, and institutes or schools of agriculture, would all be involved.

In most cases it would be unnecessary to set up new institutions for the purpose; what is needed, on the other hand, is to create national or regional coordinating committees.

In view of the high cost of equipment, facilities should be built up gradually and in terms of defined priorities. The technical problems posed by the evaluation, choice and maintenance of equipment are far from negligible and call for careful investigation.

Special attention should be paid to the question of staff, who are in short supply in many developing countries.

Developing countries need to review and plan their requirements in terms of their research priorities. Initially, they would call on the industrialized countries for the specialized training of graduate research workers in all the scientific disciplines required by the multidisciplinary form of organization proposed. Once trained, these research workers would in turn provide training on the spot in universities and specialized institutes for other research workers and laboratory technicians.

The major difficulty will undoubtedly be to find funds, which are lacking in most developing countries. Nevertheless, it is important that each developing country should make an estimate of the overall cost of applied research on medicinal plants and make a minimum of operating funds available, given that external bilateral or multilateral assistance will be primarily allocated to equipment and training.

The shortage of scientific and technical staff and the very limited funds available to developing countries makes cooperation essential among developing countries themselves, with industrialized countries, and with the organizations of the United Nations system.

Cooperation among developing countries. Pooling of technical facilities, funds and staff among developing countries would go some way towards solving the problems involved. Such cooperation could be at regional or subregional level.

Cooperation with the industrialized countries. This is desirable for training purposes and for effective participation in research programmes, under conditions giving express guarantees regarding the future use of the results of research. Such cooperation could also take the form of financial assistance. There are various types of cooperation between different developing countries and industrialized countries; accurate information on this subject is not always available.

Cooperation with the organizations of the United Nations system. WHO, UNESCO, UNICEF, UNIDO and FAO could, like the industrialized countries acting individually, assist in the training of scientific staff and laboratory technical staff by granting fellowships for long-term and short-term specialized studies, and for occasional courses of practical training. These organizations could also take part in the establishment and equipment of laboratory services in some countries, collaborate or assist in the selection of research centres capable of training staff at regional level, and take part in the operation of national or regional research projects by making highly qualified scientific staff available to them.

The conditions governing the allocation of international assistance should be carefully defined by the joint committees representing the various organizations.

Requests for assistance should be made by governments, not directly by

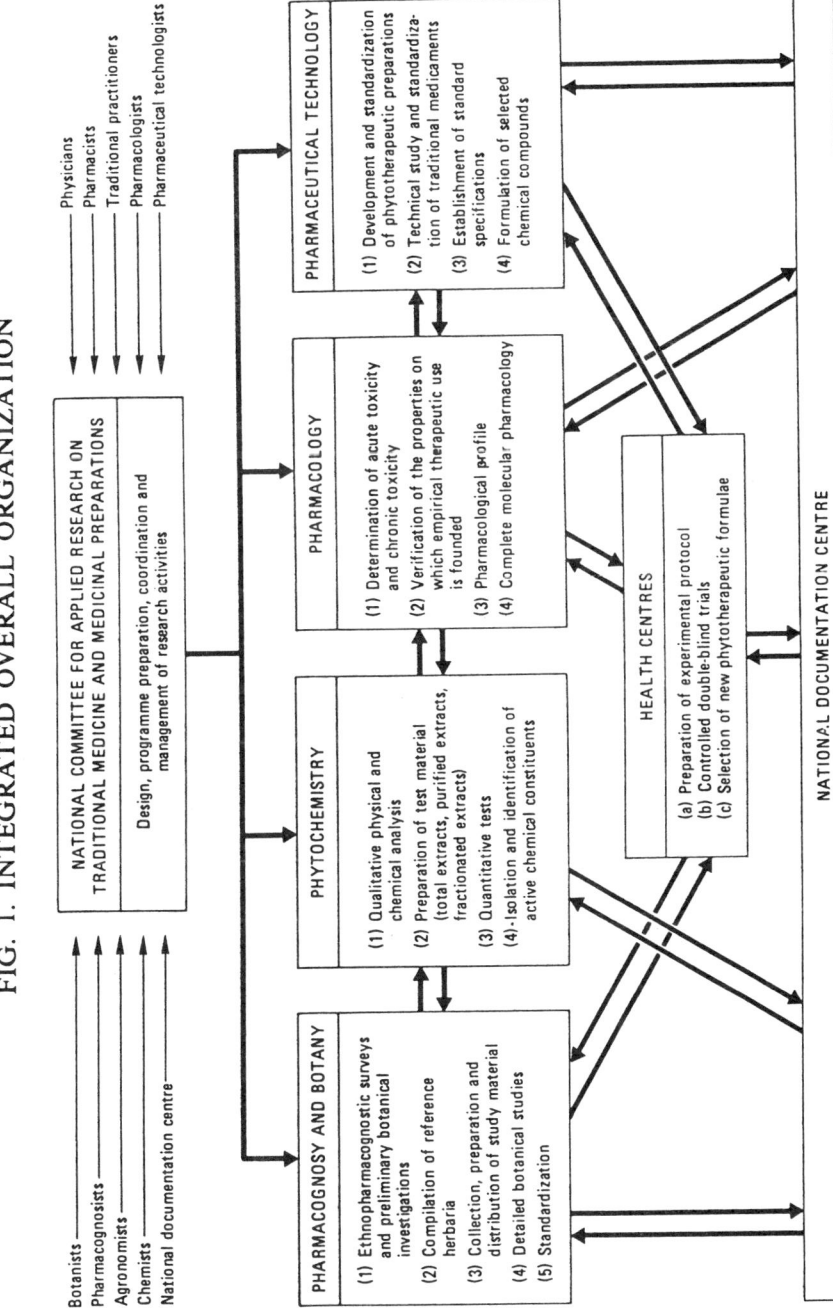

FIG. 1. INTEGRATED OVERALL ORGANIZATION

```
Botanists ─────────────┐
Pharmacognosists ──────┤
Agronomists ───────────┤
Chemists ──────────────┤
National documentation centre ─┤
                               │
Physicians ────────────┐
Pharmacists ───────────┤
Traditional practitioners ─────┤
Pharmacologists ───────┤
Pharmaceutical technologists ──┤
```

NATIONAL COMMITTEE FOR APPLIED RESEARCH ON TRADITIONAL MEDICINE AND MEDICINAL PREPARATIONS

Design, programme preparation, coordination and management of research activities

PHARMACOGNOSY AND BOTANY
(1) Ethnopharmacognostic surveys and preliminary botanical investigations
(2) Compilation of reference herbaria
(3) Collection, preparation and distribution of study material
(4) Detailed botanical studies
(5) Standardization

PHYTOCHEMISTRY
(1) Qualitative physical and chemical analysis
(2) Preparation of test material (total extracts, purified extracts, fractionated extracts)
(3) Quantitative tests
(4) Isolation and identification of active chemical constituents

PHARMACOLOGY
(1) Determination of acute toxicity and chronic toxicity
(2) Verification of the properties on which empirical therapeutic use is founded
(3) Pharmacological profile
(4) Complete molecular pharmacology

PHARMACEUTICAL TECHNOLOGY
(1) Development and standardization of phytotherapeutic preparations
(2) Technical study and standardization of traditional medicaments
(3) Establishment of standard specifications
(4) Formulation of selected chemical compounds

HEALTH CENTRES
(a) Preparation of experimental protocol
(b) Controlled double-blind trials
(c) Selection of new phytotherapeutic formulae

NATIONAL DOCUMENTATION CENTRE

WHO 82619

research agencies and particularly not by individual research workers, and the type and amount of assistance should be assessed in terms of the actual situation prevailing in the country.

The existence of complete multidisciplinary teams should be considered as a *sine qua non* for assistance, although an exception could be made in the case of countries that at first limit themselves to cataloguing the resources provided by traditional medicines by means of ethnopharmacognostic and botanical surveys.

Exploratory missions to consider the establishment of pharmaceutical industries in developing countries should for the present restrict their activity to examining the prospects for local manufacture of a number of simple medicaments or essential, widely used medicaments and should not be concerned with utilization of the resources provided by traditional medicines.

The World Health Organization has already embarked on an inventory of the medicinal plants and plants considered as medicinal that are found in various parts of the world. It would be useful if the Organization could also define the appropriate methodology for assessing the safety and efficacy of vegetable drugs, and prepare texts on general test methods and individual standard specifications for medicinal plants in the form of an international codex or pharmacopoeia.

Specific action by FAO and UNIDO should preferably be taken when research results have reached the application stage. Agrobotanical investigations to determine the best conditions for harvesting plant species and the possibilities for large-scale cultivation could be carried out, on FAO's initiative, by joint field missions representing both organizations. UNIDO could assist in the collection of all information on the economic and technical conditions governing the establishment of pharmaceutical industries primarily designed for the manufacture of simple and new phytotherapeutic preparations from the resources provided by local traditional medicine and the manufacture of some essential, widely used synthetic medicaments. Pilot projects for this purpose could be drawn up by national health authorities and UNIDO.

Part Three

A profile of traditional practices in the WHO regions

CHAPTER 20

The African Region*

The gradual development of traditional medicine activities in the African Region and the decision to encourage them arose out of the political events of the 1960s. With the advent of independence, Africans felt the need to rediscover their sociocultural identity; traditional medicine, an integral part of their heritage, benefited from this return to the fountain-head, particularly because the inhabitants had never stopped making use of it despite the intoduction of modern medicine by the colonial powers. Moreover, economic circumstances made imported techniques and drugs less and less accessible, forcing the authorities to take a fresh look at the problem and study the possibility of using traditional medicine to improve the health situation.

Nevertheless, it was necessary to convince the political decision-makers that traditional medicine had something to offer, for whatever the technical validity of a health programme, the success of its implementation is governed to a large extent by political decisions. We shall not dwell on the resolutions of the World Health Assembly and Executive Board, which are of interest to all Member States, but simply draw attention to the following resolutions adopted by the Regional Committee for Africa which reflect this political will.

In resolution AFR/RC24/R14 the Regional Committee decided that the topic for the technical discussions at its twenty-sixth session in 1976 would be "Traditional medicine and its role in the development of health services in Africa". The inclusion of experts in traditional medicine in the regional expert panels, set up in accordance with resolution AFR/RC25/R8 was further evidence of the wish to bring this heritage back into favour. Finally, resolution AFR/RC28/R3 invited Member States and WHO to take "appropriate steps to ensure the use of essential drugs and medicinal

---

* Regional contribution compiled by Dr C. Ramanohisoa, Regional Adviser, WHO Regional Office for Africa, Brazzaville, Congo.

plants of the traditional pharmacopoeia so as to meet the basic needs of communities and ensure the development of the African pharmaceutical industry".

Following these resolutions, the Regional Office has given strong impetus to the traditional medicine programme at both regional and national levels. Various Member States are endeavouring to set up a mechanism for establishing close collaboration between the traditional and conventional systems, and are making efforts to train and supervise the traditional practitioner so as to improve results and cut out harmful practices.

African traditional medicine in three periods

Three periods can be distinguished in the development of traditional medicine in the African countries. They correspond to very different political and economic situations.

Precolonial situation

This was the prime period for the traditional practitioners, when healers, fetishists, and traditional midwives practised their arts freely and were in any case sole guardians of the people's health. Unfortunately, very little information has come down to us. Knowledge was passed on by initiation within the same family or at most within the same clan. There was no written record of the practices. The techniques of diagnosis and treatment were kept secret. The only information we have comes from the reports of the early missionaries and explorers; inevitably these are fragmentary.

Colonial period

This was marked by the introduction of the colonial powers' own civilization, religion, medicine and technology. The primary aim of this modern or Western medicine was to look after the interests of the colonists in the urban centres or in areas with colonialist enterprises based on agricultural or mining potential. Priority was given to the health of troops, civil servants and native labour. Reference should also be made to the health work of certain denominational missions which in general was more broadly spread.

During this period traditional medicine, which was repressed by the authorities, went underground. By tacit agreement, the practitioners and the users made sure that such activities went on without the knowledge of the authorities. In most countries there were therefore two parallel forms of medicine: an official form to which a small fraction of the population had access (soldiers, officials, company agents, colonists, labourers), and the other used by the bulk of the population in rural areas remote from the towns.

Postcolonial period

The era of independence brought a gradual change in the above situation. Traditional medicine recovered its former status in many countries and there were several attempts to bring about recognition, official status, harmonization and collaboration. A review of the present situation has not been easy because for several countries, precise statistical data have not been compiled and analysed, and the situation regarding traditional medicine is still based on conjecture. However, the collection of relevant information has been initiated by a number of governments. An outline of the situation is given in Table 1. Some recent meetings are listed in Table 2.

Activities at the regional level

In selecting "Traditional medicine and its role in the development of health services in Africa" as the topic for the technical discussions at its twenty-sixth session, the Regional Committee was responding to the wish of Member States to devote all available or usable resources to health development. The aspirations of the peoples, the severe shortage of drugs and the inadequacy of health coverage fully justify this decision. From that time on, the activities of the Regional Office relating to traditional medicine were expanded and intensified.

A Regional Expert Panel on Traditional Medicine was set up at the end of 1975 under the programme for development of comprehensive health services; it now consists of 16 members. Several of these experts have already collaborated with the Regional Office to coordinate study tours, and have undertaken consultantships in certain countries, prepared working documents, and taken part in a variety of meetings.

The first regional expert meeting on this topic was held at the Regional Office in February 1976. The meeting started by analysing the situation in the countries, proposing definitions, and highlighting various aspects of traditional medicine, both favourable and unfavourable; it then outlined approaches for future development, stressed the need for a national political decision, and drafted recommendations on the training of practitioners, the dissemination of scientific information and research to be undertaken in order to promote traditional medicine and integrate the traditional and modern systems. The report served as a basis for the technical discussions in Kampala as reported below.

Technical discussions at the twenty-sixth session of the Regional Committee, Kampala, September 1976

After defining certain terms such as "traditional medicine" and "traditional healer", reviewing diagnostic procedures including methods, techniques and substances used, and highlighting both the favourable aspects and the inadequacies, the participants made recommendations stressing the following points:

—appropriate authorities to take a firm political decision on traditional medicine;
—promulgate laws and regulations reflecting this decision;
—identify and list the *bona fide* healers;
—establish close collaboration between the two systems of medicine;
—motivate traditional practitioners to take part in the work of the health services;
—motivate the members of the health team to accept traditional practitioners;
—promote multidisciplinary activities involving traditional practitioners.

Consultation on traditional medicine, Bamako, Mali, November 1979

This meeting was attended by 32 participants from 7 French-speaking countries of the Region. The problems which received special attention included:

—*Legal status of the traditional practitioner.* In practice the traditional practitioner is tolerated everywhere, even in places where repressive legislation has not been abolished. Some legal status is therefore particularly important for repressing charlatanism and at the same time giving official recognition to the healers. The participants urged WHO to convene a meeting of lawyers and experts to discuss the problem.

—*Harmonization of the traditional and modern systems.* Experience in some countries has shown that this can be of mutual benefit. However, while there was a consensus on the possibility and usefulness of integrating traditional medicine into village primary health care, there was some apprehension that premature integration into the health units without adequate preparation might endanger the usefulness and survival of this precious heritage.

—*The need to safeguard formulas and practices* was discussed and it was stressed that therapeutic and allied substances should be listed and the cultivation of medicinal plants encouraged.

—*The quality control and licensing of drugs* prior to manufacture and sale were also recommended.

—*The need for training* and orientation for healers and traditional midwives was stressed with particular reference to the adoption of appropriate technology and of hygienic and safer therapeutic methods.

—*Orientation in traditional practices for health administrators* and other professional health personnel was considered desirable for effective communication and collaboration between the two health care systems.

—*At the regional level*, the meeting hoped that the intercountry programme would be strengthened and provided with sufficient resources to promote the exchange of information, research workers and traditional practitioners.

Intercountry projects

Since 1979 two intercountry projects have been operating at the Regional Office:

Appropriate technology for health. Traditional medicine has been included in this project, which is perfectly logical in view of the fact that all the techniques of traditional medicine are typical examples of appropriate technologies used by Africans to solve their health problems.

Training programme in primary health care and public health. This project results from the tripartite collaboration between WHO, the United Nations Development Programme (UNDP) and the People's Republic of China and comprises a varied range of study tours and training activities for periods of 3–4 weeks in traditional medicine, community health, environmental health and the control of various diseases. The courses in acupuncture and moxibustion last 3 months with visits to 3 or more major centres such as Beijing, Nanjing and Shanghai.

National activities

As regards the present position in the countries of the African region, Table 1 lists the information it has been possible to collect for 25 countries with respect to the supervisory authorities, the implementing institutes and the areas of interest. The following conclusions can be drawn.

Supervisory authority. The Ministry of Health is responsible for traditional medicine in 10 countries (Angola, Congo, Ethiopia, Guinea, Liberia, Mali, Senegal, Togo, the United Republic of Tanzania, and Zaire). In Benin, the Gambia, and the United Republic of Cameroon the responsibility rests with other ministries. A special agency assumes this responsibility in 3 countries (Burundi, Mozambique and Nigeria).

Three countries have passed legislation on the subject (Benin, Mali and Niger).

Healers' associations are operating under official auspices in 8 countries (Benin, Congo, Mali, Niger, Senegal, Togo, the United Republic of Cameroon, and Zaire).

Implementing institutes and their areas of interest. Traditional medicine appears on the syllabus of specialist institutes or university departments in 19 countries, Benin, Central African Republic, Congo, Guinea, Ivory Coast, Kenya, Liberia, Madagascar, Mali, Niger, Nigeria, Rwanda,

Senegal, the United Republic of Cameroon, the United Republic of Tanzania, Togo, Uganda, Upper Volta and Zaire.

The areas of interest are as follows:

Area of interest	Countries
Sociocultural aspects	Togo
Cancer	United Republic of Cameroon
Dermatology	Nigeria
Hepatology	Congo, Madagascar, Mali, Zaire
Parasitic diseases	Congo, Ghana, United Republic of Cameroon
General medicine	Benin, Congo, Ghana, Guinea, Madagascar, Mali, Niger, United Republic of Tanzania
Neurology/psychiatry	Benin, Congo, Ghana, Guinea, Mali, Niger, Nigeria, Rwanda, Senegal, United Republic of Cameroon, United Republic of Tanzania
Obstetrics	Benin, Ghana, Guinea, Mali, Nigeria, Rwanda, Senegal, United Republic of Cameroon, United Republic of Tanzania
Ophthalmology	Benin
Paediatrics	United Republic of Cameroon
Pharmacological research (Medicinal plants)	Ghana, Ivory Coast, Kenya, Madagascar, Nigeria, Rwanda, Senegal, Togo, Uganda, Zaire
Dental care	Benin, Nigeria, Rwanda, Senegal, United Republic of Tanzania
Sexology	United Republic of Cameroon
Traumatology	Guinea, Mali, Senegal

Meetings. Without asking to be prompted by international and regional organizations, a number of countries have organized meetings on traditional medicine. As shown in Table 2, among the 25 countries for which information is available action has been taken as follows:

—12 countries have held a meeting on traditional medicine; of these Benin has held 3 meetings and Zaire 2

—5 countries have paid special attention to the pharmacopoeia (Benin, Guinea, Kenya, Mauritius, Seychelles)

—2 countries have linked traditional medicine with primary health care (Kenya and Zaire).

International cooperation

Research

The priority assigned to research in traditional medicine calls for substantial efforts. Unfortunately budgetary constraints on WHO permit only modest activities:

—A Zambian investigator was able to receive 4 months' additional training in traditional medicine (study of active principles, isolation of chemicals, study of substances used and pharmacological trials on animals)

—Between 1980 and 1982, the University of Swaziland has received a grant of US $43 000 for research on the chemical isolation of active principles from certain medicinal plants, and a consultant in Ethiopia will undertake preparatory studies for a programme of traditional medicine.

Education and training

Students have visited Brazzaville to prepare their doctoral theses before defending them at the National School of Medicine and Pharmacy in Bamako (Mali). Two examples are:

—1976: Thesis by Dr Adama Koné on "Contribution of traditional medicine to the improvement of health services in Mali",
—1978: Thesis by Dr Lalla Haidara on "Prevention and control of the major endemic diseases by traditional practitioners".

WHO/UNDP collaboration

In collaboration with UNDP, the Regional Office helped to arrange training in China for Africans:

—to learn the techniques of Chinese traditional medicine which are suitable for application in the African countries (acupuncture, moxibustion): 69 trainees between 1977 and 1979;
—to observe how the Chinese health system has solved the problems of coverage and drugs through the use of traditional medicine: 25 trainees.

Organization of African Unity

The permanent presence in Addis Ababa of a WHO official bears witness to the cooperation with the Health Division of the Science, Technology and Research Commission (OAU/CSTR) and the Association of African Medical Schools. The Regional Office sends observers to the major meetings and finances the participation of some country delegates. For example, it enabled 5 people from the Region to attend the Third Inter-African Symposium is Abidjan in September 1979.

African and Malagasy Committee for Further Education (CAMES)

The work of this body is in line with the decisions on traditional medicine taken by the countries regarding the use of medicinal plants, refinement of traditional methods and techniques for increased utility, and the revision of training programmes for different types of personnel. The Regional Office sent observers and granted subsidies to 4 successive symposiums held by this body (Lomé, November 1974; Niamey, June 1976; Kigali, October 1977; and Libreville, April 1979).

Environment and Development in the Third World (ENDA)

This agency periodically sends the Regional Office its technical information in the form of leaflets on traditional medicine. These leaflets are practical and well prepared, and are an excellent means of encouraging the use of medicinal plants.

Collaboration with other organizations

At the request of Member States the Regional Office has financed the attendance by some participants at meetings likely to advance the work of the programme:

—Seminar on traditional practices affecting the health of women, Khartoum, 10–15 February 1979 (6 participants);
—WHO/Istituto Italo-Africano Meeting on Medicinal Plants, Rome, 2–6 April 1979 (2 participants);
—Consultation on acupuncture and moxibustion, China, 31 May–15 June 1979 (2 participants).

Development and future prospects of the regional programme

The development of regional activities will depend on requests received from Member States and the recommendations made by various international meetings.

The potential priority areas are as follows:

Pharmacopoeia for identifying all the medicinal plants and other substances used in drugs, giving therapeutic indications, methods of preparation, and dosage; this will contribute to the manufacture of simple and effective drugs.

Catalogue of techniques used by traditional practitioners and traditional birth attendants, with a view to preserving and improving them.

Collaboration between modern and traditional medicine. The factors which can influence this collaboration, whether favourably or unfavourably, are now known, as are the mechanisms for implementation. Each country will decide on the stages for introducing collaboration according to its specific requirements. A fruitful trial in the psychiatric field has been carried out in Mali.

Training. Some teaching in traditional medicine should be introduced into the curriculum for health personnel; conversely, traditional practitioners should be given practical training and orientation courses.

Implementation. The priority objectives can be achieved through:

—Assistance with the organization of seminars, workshops and study sessions, with the participation of health personnel, research workers, scientists from other disciplines and, above all, traditional practitioners. The participation of traditional practitioners in a seminar organized in Nigeria in April 1979 and in the Bamako and Accra consultations was highly encouraging, because it showed a trend towards the collaboration which everyone wanted;

—Strengthening of the documentation and information system. To achieve results more quickly, the exchange of scientific data on the research topics and the findings should be facilitated. Periodical bulletins, scientific journals, information sheets, and correspondence between the centres and individuals are all effective ways of giving encouragement and support, and of fostering technical cooperation;

—Contribution to the development of primary health care programmes which involve traditional practitioners and traditional birth attendants and make use of traditional drugs;

—Award of grants for research on traditional medicine in collaboration with other interested bodies and institutions;

—Technical logistic and financial collaboration in programmes for cottage or large-scale industries which aim to use the widely available raw materials of traditional medicine and to put the products within the reach of the rural population. This is fully in keeping with the policy on essential drugs and with the principle of technical cooperation among developing countries;

—The training of research workers so as to give health personnel access to better knowledge of the wider aspects of the problems of traditional medicine.

Finally, the time is ripe to consider conducting case studies to put the components of traditional medicine into better perspective; knowledge about the users, the practitioners, the techniques and the drugs, and the conversion of this knowledge into statistical data, would be beneficial from every point of view. The Regional Office is engaging short-term consultants for this purpose.

Table 1. Situation of traditional medicine in some countries of the African Region

Country	Bodies concerned			Area of interest	Professional association and legislation
	Responsible ministry	Public or private institutes	Universities		
Angola	Ministry of Health				
Benin	Ministry of Youth and People's Culture (Pharmacopoeia and Traditional Medicine Section)	Benin Applied Research Centre (CRAB)		General medicine Neurology Neuropsychiatry Ophthalmology Dental care Obstetrics	National Union of Healers Existence of legislation?
Burundi		National Commission for Research on Plants			
Central African Republic			Faculty of Health Sciences		
Congo	Traditional Medicine Unit, Ministry of Public Health	National Public Health Laboratory (ORSTOM)		Psychiatry Arterial hypertension Diabetes Rheumatology Snakebite Parasitic diseases	National Union of Congolese Healers
Ivory Coast		INADES (Abidjan)	Faculty of Sciences, Abidjan	Isolation of alkaloids from various medicinal plants	
Ethiopia	Ministry of Health	Coordinating Committee on Plant Medicine			
Gambia	Forest Department				
Guinea	National People's Medicine Service, Ministry of Health	Pharmaguinée	Faculty of Medicine	General medicine Obstetrics Traumatology Psychiatry	
Ghana	Department of Traditional Medicine, Ministry of Health; Administrative division of the regions (local government)	Centre for Scientific Research on Medicinal Plants	Universities of: —Legon —Cape Coast —Kumasi	Emergency care General medicine Mental diseases Parasitic diseases Obstetrics	Healers' Association
Upper Volta		Upper Volta Centre for Scientific Research			
Kenya			University of Nairobi: —Department of Botany —Department of Biochemistry	Pharmacology	

Table 1 (Contd.)

Country	Bodies concerned			Area of interest	Professional association and legislation
	Responsible ministry	Public or private institutes	Universities		
Liberia	Department of Traditional Medicine, Ministry of Health		Chair of Pharmacology, Dogliotti College		
Madagascar		Research Centre Itassy Applied Research Centre	Faculty of Medicine	Leprology Diabetes General medicine Pharmacology	
Mali	Traditional Medicine, Ministry of Health	National Institute for Pharmacological Research and Traditional Medicine		General medicine Obstetrics Psychiatry Snakebite Traumatology Hepatology	Malian Association for the Rehabilitation of Traditional Medicine Existence of rules on licence to practise
Mozambique		Study Group on Traditional Medicine			
Niger		Research at the Neuropsychiatry Department, Niamey Hospital		Group psychotherapy Study of the phenomenon of possession Differential psychology	Existence of legislation on traditional medicine
Nigeria	National Commission		University of Port Harcourt University of Lagos University of Ibadan University of Ife	Extraction of active principles from medicinal plants Communicable diseases Psychiatry Obstetrics Dermatology Dental care	Association of Traditional Healers
Uganda			Department of Pharmacology and Therapy, Makerere University, Kampala	Study and extraction of active principles from medicinal plants	
Rwanda		Institute for Research on Medicinal Plants	Butare University	Extraction of active principles from medicinal plants Mental disorders Obstetrics Dental care	
Senegal	Department of Research Planning and Training, Ministry of Health	ENDA Black Africa Institute ENFAD	Faculty of Medicine and Pharmacy Faculty of Science	Psychiatry Dental care Hepatology Traumatology Pneumology Obstetrics	Association of Traditional Healers
Togo	Department of Traditional Medicine, Ministry of Health	Institute for Research on Traditional Medicine in Togo	Benin University	Restriction of harmful practices of traditional medicine Social and Scientific aspects of traditional medicine Study of the major plants	Togolese Association for Scientific Research

Table 1 (Contd.)

Country	Bodies concerned			Area of interest		Professional association and legislation
	Responsible ministry	Public or private institutes	Universities			
United Republic of Cameroon	Ministry of Planning, Institute for Medical Research and Medicinal plants attached to the National Office for Scientific and Technical Research	National herbarium	Faculty of Science, University of Yaoundé	Neuropsychiatry Sexology Parasitic diseases Gynaecology Obstetrics ENT Cancerology Paediatrics		Association of Healers of Bamanda and Ntem
United Republic of Tanzania	Department of Traditional Medicine, Ministry of Health	Institute for Research on Traditional Medicine	Faculty of Medicine Dar-es-Salaam	General medicine Minor surgery Mental disorders Psychosomatic diseases Obstetrics Dental care		
Zaire	Department of Traditional Medicine, State Health Secretariat	Scientific Research Institute, (medical section) UNICOOP Mbuji-Mayi	National University of Zaire	Diabetes Botanical identification of plants Infectious diseases		Zaire Healers' Association

Table 2. Seminars, symposia and workshops on traditional medicine held in some countries of the African Region

Country	Year	Meetings on Traditional Medicine	Comments
Benin	1974	5–6 July: National Congress	
	1976	September: Seminar	
	1979	16–18 April: Seminar on the traditional medicine and pharmacopoeia of Africa	Participation of 8 other African countries and a WHO observer
Congo	1975	25–26 June: Seminar	With participation of the Regional Office
Guinea	1978	25–29 January: National Symposium on medicinal plants and people's medicine	Participation of the WHO National Coordinator
Kenya	1979	22–29 January: Symposium on the use of medicinal plants in primary health care	Organized by the Department of Pharmacy, University of Nairobi. The WHO National Coordinator took part
Madagascar	1974	4–7 September: Celebration meetings	
Mauritius	1978	6–12 November: Working group on the distribution of medicinal plants in the Indian Ocean area	Participation of ENDA and states of the Western Indian Ocean (Madagascar, Réunion, Seychelles)
Nigeria	1973	10–16 December: International Symposium	Organized by the Department of Chemistry, University of Lagos; sponsored by the Lagos State Government. 800 active participants and over 200 observers
	1979	30 April to 1 May: Seminar	Participation of almost 200 traditional practitioners
Seychelles	1979	12–18 November: Seminar on medicinal plants	Participation of ENDA Mauritius and Madagascar
Togo	1977	6–15 August: Congress	Organized by the Ministry of Health together with the Ministries of Education and Scientific Research
United Republic of Cameroon	1978	22–23 July: Symposium	
Zaire	1974	2–16 November: National Seminar	Organized by the national research and development organization (ONRD)
	1978	August: Seminar	Organized by the Institute for Healers' Medicine
Zambia	1977	9–13 May: National workshop on traditional medicine to promote primary health care	Participation of WHO and traditional practitioners

CHAPTER 21
Region of the Americas*

The role of the Pan American Health Organization[1]

When considering the role of the American Region in traditional medicine, it is necessary to keep in mind three facts:

First, medical anthropology as a discipline originated in Mexico and the United States of America and it is there that large numbers of publications appeared and university teaching on this subject continues to be offered.

Secondly, sporadic attempts to collaborate with traditional medicine men started in Latin America some two decades ago and much experience on this subject has been accumulated.

Thirdly, the concept and practice of primary health care, and the extension of health coverage to the entire population, presently the main policy of the whole WHO system, is often considered to have originated in the Pan American Health Organization (PAHO) although under another name, basic health services.

Almost 30 years ago, PAHO recognized the importance of collecting information on the customs and beliefs of the people regarding illness and traditional therapeutic methods. This is reflected in the relevant articles which have been published in the *Boletín de la Oficinia Sanitaria Panamericana*. The following examples may be cited:

In 1952 a paper on the influence of popular customs and beliefs on the services of a health centre (*1*) was published in the *Boletín*. This consisted

---

* Regional contribution compiled by Dr Boris Velimirovic, formerly Chief, Field Office of the Pan American Health Organization for the United States–Mexico Border, El Paso, TX, USA.

[1] The Pan American Health Organization (PAHO) comprises the Pan American Sanitary Conference, the Directing Council, the Executive Committee, and the Pan American Sanitary Bureau (PASB). PASB serves as WHO's Regional Office for the Americas.

of a summary made from a report *A cross-cultural anthropological analysis of a technical aid program* based on field work carried out by several American anthropologists. That report was edited by George M. Foster and was initially published in Washington by the Smithsonian Institution in 1951. After a discussion of popular opinions on various aspects relating to illness, recommendations are given on how this knowledge could be optimally applied in the establishment and operation of health centres in a number of Latin American countries.

In 1955, the *Boletín* published a paper on the food habits of the population of Guatemala (*2*) and in 1959 an article (*3*) which describes, *inter alia*, some of the dangerous traditional methods used in the treatment of diarrhoea in infants. It also evaluates research findings prepared for a PAHO-sponsored seminar which took place in Santiago, Chile, in 1956.

In June 1968 a special session was held during the Seventh Meeting of the PAHO Advisory Committee on Medical Research in Washington on the origin, present distribution and principal biological subdivisions of American Indians, including newly contacted Indian groups and groups in transition (*4*). The 14 papers presented at this special session were mainly focused on biomedical problems and, with the exception of one on food and nutrition of the Mayas from before the conquest to the present day, did not consider the cultural implications of health behaviour and beliefs. The session nevertheless represented a step towards an increasing appreciation of the health problems of traditional people.

Other articles have dealt with the application of social anthropology to public health programmes (*5*), with the use of hallucinogens in folk psychiatry (*6*), with traditional habits regarding sanitation (*7*) and with coca-leaf chewing (*8*). They all have the common aim of collecting information on the health behaviour of traditional population groups in the American hemisphere in order to better understand their attitude toward new health programmes and to develop strategies for strengthening "Community Participation in Health" (the theme chosen by PAHO for its 75th anniversary in 1977).

Traditional birth attendants (TBAs) attracted the attention of the health authorities much earlier than the new trend toward traditional medicine appeared. In Latin America, where the highest rate of population increase in the world occurs, up to 84% of deliveries are still today taking place at home without qualified supervision. In order to reduce or eliminate harmful practices, training courses were established where TBAs received instruction in fields such as basic hygiene, anatomy, germ theory, communicable diseases and, to a lesser degree, in first aid, family planning and health education. Such programmes were already under way in Guatemala in 1935 and in Brazil in the late 1940s.

In 1970 the Pan American Health Organization published a guide for training and supervising TBAs (*9*). This was specially designed for nurses and obstetricians responsible for training programmes.

Current practices and studies

With or without the assistance of PAHO, such training courses were carried out in many countries or territories of Latin America, including Belize, Bolivia, Colombia, Dominican Republic, Honduras, Mexico, Nicaragua, Suriname and Venezuela. Some countries formulated manuals for use by *parteras empíricas*; one example is the *Manual de Capacitación de Parteras Empíricas* which was prepared in 1976 by the Ecuadorian Health Ministry. A comparative analysis of the kind of obstetric attention sought after in Mexico City was undertaken in 1959 and then again in 1976 by the Mexican health authorities. In various parts of Mexico inquiries among TBAs were carried out in order to get an idea about their level of knowledge prior to training and before such training programmes were set up.

It is only recently that a general trend has appeared in WHO towards recognizing with interest and respect the values of the traditional systems and evaluating the resources, methods and procedures of which they make use. At present, in at least 8 countries of the Americas research is being conducted with a view to gaining a better understanding of the traditional system and assessing the advantages and benefits of its empirical knowledge as a community resource. In addition to the laboratory research being carried out, these studies embrace a wide range of subjects in the social field and in regard to real conditions in the communities. An increase in knowledge of the situation is being actively sought with a view to establishing the coordination machinery that will enable the two systems to work harmoniously together in meeting community health needs.

In the United States of America it is well known that traditional healers play an important role in the American Indian cultures, but little material has been available until recently on the importance of traditional medicine among other minority groups. More studies are now being made to explore the mechanism of self-help, especially in the area of mental health, among those groups.

One such study, begun in 1966 and continuing through 1975, was carried out as an integral part of the Tremont Residency Training Program of the Lincoln Hospital Mental Health Services (Department of Psychiatry, Albert Einstein College of Medicine, South Bronx, New York). Its purposes were to identify and examine instances where folk and professional systems of care for the mentally ill in the Bronx Puerto Rican community intersected, to discover the potential for collaboration and conflict, and, consequently, to help clinicians and planners develop models for a comprehensive system of mental health care (*10*).

Cooperation between medicine men and officials of the Indian Health Services and the existence of a training programme for traditional healers have been reported from the Navajo Reservation (*11, 12*).

In Latin America traditional medicine is practised mainly among Indian tribal groups, rural peoples, and lower-income urban groups. Folk healers such as herbalists, massagers, bonesetters, and spiritists coexist with, and in many cases take the place of, health professionals. The services of the traditional midwife (*partera empirica* or *comadrona*) are particularly used throughout the Latin American countries.

Studies on the evil eye, (*mal de ojo*), prolonged fright (*susto* or *espanto*), and the disturbances of the emotional or thermal (hot–cold) equilibrium have been carried out (*13*).

In Colombia folk medicine is widely practised, although the actual number of practitioners is not known. No official collaboration between health services and traditional healers exists, but a pilot project for the incorporation of previously trained traditional practitioners was scheduled to begin in 1977 in a particular area of the country.

In certain Andean regions of Peru more than 60% of the people—in some places as many as 80%—are treated exclusively by local healers (*curanderos*). The practice of folk medicine was officially prohibited in 1969, and no information is available on the current policy of the Peruvian Government towards it. One case of the utilization of folk practitioners in an unofficial capacity is particularly illuminating. In order to lead the population progressively toward modern medicine, the chief physician of a health centre in southern Peru decided to collaborate with the *curanderos* of his region by inviting them to his centre for instruction in the basic principles of hygiene and first aid. Each of the participants in his "courses" received a first-aid kit. These *curanderos* then returned to their communities and became local health educators. After some years under their influence, the change in the health behaviour of the people was reported as "visible" (*14*).

In Ecuador, 67% of births are reported to be attended by traditional midwives, but no information is available on the official policy toward traditional healers in general. Because of the high incidence of maternal and child morbidity and mortality in the country, the Ministry of Public Health established a project of training courses for traditional midwives in 1974, with the aim of incorporating them into the health services of rural areas. Still ongoing, these courses are meant to improve the midwives' performance as birth attendants and to instruct them in family planning methods. The midwives also act as intermediaries between the people and the local health services, and are expected to promote the use of maternal and child care services in the communities.

In the Dominican Republic, in an effort to extend maternal and child care, the Ministry of Health and Social Welfare maintains training programmes for traditional birth attendants in hospitals and health centres throughout the country. With the assistance of a PAHO/WHO nursing adviser, the programme was revised in 1973. Various working groups were set up to improve the norms for training and for supervision of *parteras empiricas*, offering them instruction in the basic concepts of hygiene and midwifery and in the practice of first aid.

Until the 1959 revolution, a considerable part of the Cuban population relied on the help of *curanderos*, spiritualists, and traditional birth attendants. After 1960, it was decided by the Cuban health authorities not to utilize practitioners of traditional medicine; *curanderos* were forbidden to practise, and the traditional midwives were slowly integrated into the system of health services as ancillary staff.

In Guatemala traditional healers are prohibited by law from practising; they are, nevertheless, active in both rural and urban areas. The Government has no plans at present to include folk healers in health services. Some 80% of all births in Guatemala are attended by traditional midwives who, since 1956, have been receiving some (not systematized) training. In 1974, these midwives held their first convention.

The work of Dr Berhorst at Chimaltenango in Guatemala in primary health care, training and utilization of auxiliary workers, disease prevention and community development (including a cooperative relationship with traditional healers) has led to his centre becoming a focus of international attention and its selection as a WHO demonstration centre.

At their Third Special Meeting, in 1972, the Ministers of Health of the Americas recommended to the Member countries that they "begin installing machinery during the decade to make it feasible to attain total coverage of the population by the health service systems in all the countries of the Region" (*15*). Since that meeting, the Member Governments have made laudable efforts to reach that goal.

The growing needs of the population make it necessary to consider new approaches and strategies for speeding up the process of extending the coverage of services to the entire population, and to give high priority to deprived and underserved rural and urban groups.

In its emphasis on primary health care and extension of coverage, PAHO is interested in the field of medical anthropology. There is no official policy statement as yet, but the following is indicative of the attitude taken (as stated at the Fourth Special Meeting of Ministers of Health of the Americas, Washington, DC, 26–27 September 1977).

> If the goal of universal coverage is to be attained, the services offered must not only be efficient, but must also meet the following conditions: they must effectively correct the situations or solve the problems that arise, be appropriate to, and consistent with the basic needs of the community and be accessible and acceptable to it (*16*, p. 23).

In any community there are two possible sources of services:

(*a*) *The traditional community system* set up by the community itself, and used by its members who resort to self-medication or to some members of the community recognized as an agent of the system;

(*b*) *The institutional health system*, consisting of public and private health institutions.

The traditional system frequently coexists with the institutional one, but sometimes it is the only source from which the health needs of the community are being met. In the former situation, whether more use is made of the traditional or the institutional system or whether they are equally popular depends on the educational or sociocultural status of the population and the characteristics of the institutional system.

One of the guiding principles for effective community participation is recognition of and respect for the knowledge the people possess, their human dignity, and their ability to contribute to their own development. Further community studies are needed to identify the inner dynamics of the role, organization and operation of the traditional system and its relations with other areas of community life.

PAHO participated in the WHO Interregional Consultation on Promotion and Development of the Traditional Medicine Programme (New Delhi, 4-8 October 1976). Regional experiences were presented on the status of traditional medicine in the Americas, stressing the training of certain types of lay personnel and traditional midwives and their inclusion in the official health services, rather than an integration with traditional medicine.

Aware of the need for more knowledge on the extent of, and the services operated within, the traditional health care systems, PAHO recognized that it was necessary to collect more data on traditional healers and indigenous systems of medicine, to analyse this information, to determine the relevance of traditional healing to primary health care and to the needs of the population, and to suggest guidelines for future action.

Bearing this in mind, the PAHO field office of El Paso, Texas, in collaboration with the Centre for Interamerican Studies of the University of Texas at El Paso, organized in January 1977, as a first step, a Workshop on Medical Anthropology in the Border Population. The aim was to provide an opportunity for a profitable exchange of ideas between medical anthropologists and health personnel and, at the same time, to gain insights through the comparison of the various experiences, both positive and negative, contributed by the participants.

The papers presented at this Workshop were subsequently published in English and Spanish (*17*). They deal with the particular border situation and with problems stemming from the clash of two cultures, from migrations within Mexico and from Mexico to the USA, from the existence of minority groups living in this area, all with regard to traditional (or parallel) medicine practised in some form or other in the border states. A follow-up workshop organized by the PAHO field office together with the Houston School of Public Health took place in Houston in November 1977. As a further step, a selective bibliography on medical anthropology was compiled by the PAHO field office of El Paso in 1978 for the use of health professionals working in national and PAHO projects.

Finally, an interesting and encouraging attempt to integrate modern and traditional medicine has been carried out in a study by the Institute of Nutrition of Central America and Panama (INCAP) in Guatemala. It should also be mentioned that at the Twentieth Pan American Sanitary Conference held in Grenada in September/October 1978 the technical discussions dealt in part with the utilization of medicinal plants and other natural products in view of their costs as compared to those of synthetic drugs. It was recommended that "research should be conducted to identify the active ingredients and specifications . . . their safety and efficacy should be confirmed clinically in scientifically conducted studies . . ." (*18*).

In this context, research in traditional medicinal plants has been carried out by the Botanical Institute for Therapeutic Plant Resources in San Marcos University in Peru, and in Mexico by the Medical Institute for the Study of Medicinal Plants (IMEPLAM) founded in 1975 under the sponsorship of the Mexican Government.

The lack of a declared policy statement requires explanation. PAHO has concentrated on primary health care and on aggressive action in pursuance of the strategy for health for all by the year 2000. The attitude in respect to traditional medicine is, as seen from the above, a positive one. It is similar to that of the large body of medical anthropologists, including Foster, that there must be much good in traditional systems that can be highly useful in primary health care, and that traditional systems have avoided many of the pitfalls into which modern medicine has fallen. Yet even with this bias, considerable scepticism has been expressed by a number of anthropologists as to how feasible this approach is.

In seeking an answer to this question, it is natural to consider the experience gained to date. Most of it is limited to two areas: the upgrading of indigenous midwives, and the use of traditional healers for mental illness. But success with midwives and mental illness treatment does not necessarily mean that other forms of care can as easily be incorporated into official health services.

In the case of pregnancy, both midwife and physician agree about the onset of the condition, its course and its duration, and its probable outcome. In the absence of complications, both do about the same things.

With respect to the treatment of mental illness, psychiatry is the least exact of all forms of medicine, the field in which it is most difficult to predict the outcome. The symbolic and supportive roles of traditional healers often seem to lead to successful outcomes, or at least to the alleviation of symptoms, to the extent that a patient can continue to live at home.

But beyond these two fields, the problems become more difficult. "When the physician diagnoses a malignant tumour requiring surgery, and the medicine man an intruded disease object that can be removed by sucking, are there real grounds for cooperation" (*17*, p. 7).

In the effort to extend the coverage to all people, PAHO relies more on the creation of new types of health manpower, which could involve the community, which could fit into the political and social culture and which could be harmonized with the effort for increased economic development. For this a thorough transformation of the traditional social structure is a precondition, and in that process traditional medicine could prove to be marginal or even sometimes outright antagonistic.

"Acculturation to the modern medical model would doubtless entail a denial of their own basic concepts and practices. It would even reduce the effectiveness of spiritual healing for the culturally patterned psychological and psychophysiological conditions for which it is best suited" (Kearney, reported by Foster, *17*, p. 7).

Another reason why incorporation of traditional healers into official health systems probably would not work well is the fact that removing *curanderos* from their neighbourhood environments and including them within a clinical organization and setting would destroy the therapeutic advantages provided by the intimate magicoreligious ambience of their home consultation rooms. Some health authorities even doubt that there is much role for indigenous midwives. Some of the reasons advanced, however, stem from political and professional reality, i.e., opposition of established health personnel. None the less, hospital births are supplanting *partera*-delivered births whenever there is a hospital.

Further doubts regarding the practicality of incorporating traditional healers into official medicine have been raised in a study of the Navajo. There are not as many healers as in the past, and those remaining appear to be less knowledgeable and less competent than their forbears. Reliance upon "official medicine" probably explains this decline. This observation is true of much, perhaps most, of the developing world. Serious consideration of incorporating traditional personnel into contemporary health systems is based on a false assumption—that traditional healers continue to be produced at the same rate as in the past. Abundant evidence indicates that this is not the case. Wherever the matter has been investigated the same situation recurs: many healers a generation ago; few, and less well-prepared healers today.

As Foster puts it:

> Do doubts as to the advisability of incorporating traditional curers into official health services mean that anthropologists feel traditional medicine can be ignored? The answer, clearly, is "no". Probably all anthropologists agree that health personnel should know more about, and understand, and appreciate, the contributions traditional (and "alternative") medicine makes, and can continue to make, to health care (*17*, p. 8).

REFERENCES

(*1*) GRANT, M. Influencia de las costumbres y creencias populares en los servicios de un centro de salud. *Boletín de la Oficina Sanitaria Panamericana*, **33**:283–298 (1952).

(*2*) FLORES, M. & REH, E. Estudios de hábitos dietéticos en poblaciones de Guatemala—I. Magdalena Milpas Altas. *Boletín de la Oficina Sanitaria Panamericana*, sup. **2**:90–128 (1955) (INCAP Scientific Publication).

(*3*) CUELLO, P. E., GOMEZ, T. V. & MUÑOZ, M. Estudio antropológico de las diarreas infantiles en la Comuna de Renca, Santiago, Chile. *Boletín de la Oficina Sanitaria Panamericana*, **47**:323–329 (1959).

(*4*) *Biomedical challenges presented by the American Indian: Proceedings of the special session held during the Seventh Meeting of the PAHO Advisory Committee on Medical Research, 25 June 1968*, Washington, DC, Pan American Health Organization, 1968 (PAHO Scientific Publication No. 165).

(5) SOLER, E. ET AL. Aplicación de la antropología social a nuestros programas de salud pública. *Boletín de la Oficina Sanitaria Panamericana*, **49**:350–354 (1960).
(6) CHIAPPE COSTA, M. El empleo de alucinógenos en la psiquiatría folklórica. *Boletín de la Oficina Sanitaria Panamericana*, **81**:176–186 (1976).
(7) BELCHER, J. C. Sanitation norms in rural areas: a cross-cultural comparison. *Bulletin of the Pan American Health Organization*, **12**:34–44 (1978).
(8) NEGRETE, J. C. Coca-leaf chewing: a public health assessment. *Bulletin of the Pan American Health Organization*, **12**:211–218 (1978).
(9) OFICINA SANITARIA PANAMERICANA. *Guía de orientación y supervisión de parteras empíricas*, Washington, DC, 1970 (Revision) (Informes de Enfermería No. 12).
(10) FIELDS, S. Folk healing for the wounded spirit—I. Storefront psychotherapy through science. In: American Institutes for Research, Palo Alto, CA. *Innovations: highlights of evolving mental health services*, **3**(1):3–11 (1976).
(11) FIELDS, S. Folk healing for the wounded spirit—II. Medicine men: purveyors of an ancient art. In: American Institutes for Research, Palo Alto, CA. *Innovations: highlights of evolving mental health services*, **3**(1):12–18 (1976).
(12) LEIGHTON, D. C. Cultural determinants of behaviour: a neglected area. *American journal of psychiatry*, **128**:1003–1004 (1972).
(13) RUBEL, A. J. The epidemiology of a folk illness: *susto* in Hispanic America. *Ethnology*, **3**:268 (1964).
(14) BRAUN, P. La médecine des Indiens de la Cordillière des Andes. *La presse médicale*, **77**: 2119–2121 (1969).
(15) *Ten year health plan for the Americas: Final report of the III Special Meeting of Ministers of Health of the Americas*, Washington, DC, Pan American Health Organization, 1973 (PAHO Official Document No. 118) p. 73.
(16) Extension of health service coverage based on primary health care and community participation strategies. In: *IV Special Meeting of Ministers of Health of the Americas. Final report and background document*, Washington, DC, Pan American Health Organization, 1978 (PAHO Official Document No. 155) pp. 19–42.
(17) VELIMIROVIC, B., ed. *Modern medicine and medical anthropology in the United States–Mexico border population*, Washington, DC, Pan American Health Organization, 1978 (PAHO Scientific Publication No. 359).
(18) The impact of drugs on health costs: national and international problems. In: *XX Pan American Sanitary Conference, XXX Meeting of the WHO Regional Committee for the Americas: final report*, Washington, DC, 1978 (Technical Discussions, document CSP20/DT/1).

CHAPTER 22
The South-East Asia Region*

The role of the WHO Regional Office

The Twenty-ninth World Health Assembly recommended action to encourage the development of health teams trained to meet the health needs of the population, including health workers for primary health care, taking into account, where appropriate, the manpower reserve constituted by those practising traditional medicine (resolution WHA29.72). In pursuance of this recommendation the Regional Committee for South-East Asia requested the Regional Director to organize seminars on traditional medicine to enable Member countries to exchange information and experience about their respective systems of medicine and discuss approaches for the best utilization of these systems in the provision of medical care to the population in this region (resolution SEA/RC29/R11).

An Intercountry Seminar held in Colombo in April 1977, made the following recommendations:

(1) Governments should make a policy declaration at the top national level to recognize, promote and rehabilitate the traditional systems of medicine prevalent in their respective countries and to maximize their utilization in health teams, particularly in providing primary health care to the rural population.

(2) Governments should conduct national surveys to collect information about the number of traditional medical practitioners (including traditional birth attendants), their methods of treatment, the nature of their training and such other information as may be necessary for their utilization in extending health care to large numbers of people.

(3) (a) Based on the information collected, steps should be taken to identify the most appropriate manner of participation by traditional medical practitioners in the health team with a view to promoting their activities in the provision of basic health care, particularly to the vulnerable sections of the rural population.

(b) After identification of the manner of their participation at various levels of the

---

* Regional contribution compiled by Dr Habibuz Zaman, Medical Officer, WHO Regional Office for South-East Asia, New Delhi, India.

nation's health care system, orientation/training programmes should be organized for these traditional practitioners in community surroundings in keeping with the needs of the people.

(4) Governments should design and supply standard medical kits to trained health workers which should contain traditional medicines for common ailments; wherever traditional medicines for such ailments are not available the kit may include certain specified allopathic drugs for the delivery of primary health care.

(5) Governments should intensify their efforts at:

(a) interdisciplinary research into the practice of traditional medicine;

(b) the proper training of personnel;

(c) documentation; and,

(d) the conservation and cultivation of medicinal plants.

(6) Governments should make freely available to other governments and relevant agencies information regarding traditional medicine practices, research findings, flora, fauna and minerals used in the preparation of traditional medicines.

(7) Governments should include in the curriculum of all health workers (medical and paramedical) an orientation course in the principles and practice of traditional/indigenous systems of medicine.

(8) WHO should:

(a) collaborate in the implementation of the above recommendations;

(b) assist Member countries in organizing group educational and research activities and award fellowships for training in research techniques, studies of health care systems and other technological procedures related to traditional/indigenous systems of medicine.

In May 1977, the Thirtieth World Health Assembly adopted resolution WHA30.49, on the promotion and development of training and research in traditional medicine, thus including traditional medicine as an activity in the overall programme of the Organization.

The WHO Regional Committee for South-East Asia, by its resolution SEA/RC30/R13 on traditional systems of medicine, also requested the Regional Director:

(1) to take steps for the implementation of the resolutions relating to the promotion and development of training and research in traditional medicine, and further

(2) to provide facilities for the necessary training in traditional systems of medicine to health workers and to prepare protocols specifying the training, role and utilization of the manpower available in the traditional systems of medicine in the basic health care programme.

The International Conference on Primary Health Care held in Alma-Ata in September 1978 discussed the role of traditional medicine in primary health care and made recommendations for the promotion and development of traditional medicine where appropriate (*1*).

In resolution SEA/RC33/R5 on drug policies, including traditional medicine, the Regional Committee requested the Regional Director, *inter alia*, to continue assistance and technical cooperation with the countries in the evaluation, utilization, and standardization of traditional medicines used in primary health care, in training programmes and in the dissemination of relevant information in the field of traditional medicine.

A WHO intercountry project was started in 1978 to collaborate with countries in the South-East Asia Region in:

(a) promoting and developing traditional systems of medicine;

(b) making maximum use of practitioners of traditional medicine for increasing the health coverage with particular reference to primary health care;

(c) providing training for trainers of prospective traditional practitioners.

In addition to providing a number of fellowships to teachers of institutions of traditional medicine in Bangladesh, Nepal, Sri Lanka and Thailand, a significant number of institutions in these and some other countries in the Region have received sets of books on traditional medicine.

Another important activity was the holding of an intercountry consultative meeting in New Delhi in April 1979. The meeting listed the following as constraints in the use of traditional medicine in primary health care:

(i) Inadequate knowledge of modern methods of preventive and promotive health care among traditional practitioners.
(ii) Lack of homogeneity between traditional and modern methods in this field.
(iii) Insufficient knowledge on the part of traditional healers and even trained and qualified practitioners in different aspects of curative and preventive health care.
(iv) Absence of standardization of traditional drugs.
(v) Lack of active involvement of traditional practitioners in primary health care programmes supported by adequate referral systems.
(vi) Lack of an organization for the procurement and supply of raw drugs and compound formulations.
(vii) Non-availability of basic guide books and manuals on common ailments.
(viii) Lack of adequate information and mutual exchange of information between practitioners of modern medicine and those of traditional medicine.

Taking note of the inherent advantages of the traditional systems of medicine, the meeting made a number of detailed and specific recommendations in regard to: (1) the use of practitioners of traditional medicine in primary health care, (2) their training including that of traditional birth attendants, (3) directions of research in traditional medicine, (4) exchange of information, and (5) collaboration between countries and various international agencies.

In the implementation of the various resolutions adopted by the Regional Committee, a number of short-term consultants were assigned for various periods to study the situation in respect of traditional medicine in nine countries of the Region—Bangladesh, Bhutan, Burma, India, Indonesia, Maldives, Nepal, Sir Lanka and Thailand. In general the tasks assigned to them were:

(i) to investigate the place that traditional medical preparations have in on-going or planned primary health care programmes and activities;
(ii) to report on the training of primary health care workers in the use of traditional medicines and suggest improvements as necessary;

(iii) to study the factors that determine the availability of traditional medicines at the primary health care level and recommend measures to improve the situation as necessary;

(iv) to compile a list of medicinal herbs (traditional medicines) in different countries of the Region so that each country's experience could be of mutual benefit; and

(v) to identify individuals and institutions which may be capable of carrying out research in traditional medicine and to stimulate nationals to submit protocols for research in the areas of priority already indicated by the Regional Advisory Committee on Medical Research.

The reports of these consultants have been compiled and circulated to the countries for appropriate action. They have not been published, but some of the data from them are presented in a subsequent section of this chapter.

Since the ongoing intercountry project became operational, several countries in the Region have taken active steps in developing a national programme in traditional medicine, Burma and Sri Lanka being most prominent in this respect. In Indonesia and Thailand some traditional medicines are being studied; and Nepal is continuing to integrate traditional medicine in the basic rural health service structure at the health post level.

In the meantime, another intercountry project (medicinal herbs and ayurvedic drugs), funded by the United Nations Development Programme and meant for the least developed countries, became operational during 1980. This project has limited objectives to be achieved by 1982 in 3 countries—Bangladesh, Bhutan and Nepal. These consist of organizing study/observation tours in neighbouring countries for senior health administrators in charge of traditional medicine programmes in these 3 countries; developing a small number of rural dispensaries in each country; developing medicinal kits; and training a small number of practitioners of traditional medicine through short-term fellowships; and a national workshop in each country to review the progress in integrating traditional medicine in the primary health care system.

Continuing support for the ongoing intercountry project will be required to sustain these collaborative activities in the other countries of the Region such as Burma, Indonesia, Maldives, Sri Lanka and Thailand, and to provide further incentive to the WHO/UNDP programme in traditional medicine in Bangladesh and Nepal mentioned above. The major emphasis of the project in the future will be integration of the practitioners of traditional medicine into the basic health services.

Research in traditional medicine

The Regional Advisory Committee on Medical Research at its third session, held in Colombo, Sri Lanka, in April 1977, drew attention to the need for enhanced research efforts in traditional medicine. The Committee, having considered the report of its Research Study Group, recommended that the following avenues of research in traditional medicine be accorded priority:

(i) listing those remedies that fall within the context of primary health care;
(ii) carrying out studies on the utilization of traditional healers in primary health care;
(iii) undertaking studies on the alternative strategies for training traditional healers for their contemplated participation as members of the health team delivering primary health care.

It was suggested that early consideration be given to:

(iv) assessing the efficacy, side effects and toxic effects of traditional remedies that could be used in primary health care, with their standardization and cost effectiveness, using scientific parameters, in order that they could be recommended for widespread usage.

Besides collaborating with the Indian Council of Medical Research since 1977 in a four-year research project on the efficacy of ayurvedic treatment of rheumatoid arthritis (*amavata* in Ayurveda) at Coimbatore, the Regional Office has provided support to enable a limited number of research scientists to visit research institutes in the Region and also to study research methodology.

A meeting on research in traditional medicine was held in Varanasi, India, in November 1980. A few research protocols emerged from this meeting and these will no doubt facilitate the further development of research in traditional medicine in countries of the Region.

In view of the large number of practitioners of traditional medicine in some of the countries of this Region, and the large masses of people who receive their services, it is important that various aspects of the practice of traditional medicine should be subjected to scrutiny through scientific research.

One of the important aims of research in the regional programme on traditional medicine is to explore all possible alternative approaches to meeting the basic health needs of the maximum number of people in the shortest possible time by the utilization of practitioners of traditional medicine in the health care system. Specifically, studies need to be carried out on the utilization of traditional healers in primary health care. Studies may also be undertaken on the alternative strategies for training traditional healers for their contemplated participation as members of the health team delivering primary health care.

The status and functioning of the major systems of traditional medicine in the Region

The major systems of traditional medicine being practised in the Region can be classified as (a) formalized systems of indigenous medicine which include Ayurveda, Siddha, Unani-Tibbi, the Chinese system of medicine, the *amchi* (Tibetan) system of medicine and Burmese medicine, and (b) non-formalized, traditional systems of medicine practised by herbalists, bonesetters, practitioners of *thaad* (element system), home remedies and spiritualists. In addition, yoga, nature cure and homoeopathy are being practised in some countries including Bangladesh and India. Almost all the countries have recognized the traditional systems of medicine and are making efforts to utilize the practitioners in their health care delivery programmes. There are at present 750 000 practitioners of traditional systems of medicine in the Region. The status and functioning of these systems of medicine in each of the countries are briefly indicated below.

Bangladesh

There are mainly two systems practised in the country, Unani and Ayurveda. A board has been set up for issuing registration, for maintaining the standard of the teaching institutions and for encouraging research. There are over 5000 registered practitioners in addition to about 3000 unregistered practitioners. Only 540 practitioners are institutionally qualified; there are four institutions which impart training in Unani and ayurvedic systems of medicine.

These institutes offer a four-year diploma course with an intake of 50 students per year in each institute. There is a research institute for conducting research on drug action and on common diseases such as asthma. There are no government dispensaries; there are only two ayurvedic dispensaries run by the *Zilla* (district) Boards.

About 14 pharmacies manufacture ayurvedic medicines worth over one crore Takas (one crore Takas = US $1 250 000) each annually. Two Unani pharmacies manufacture medicine worth slightly less than one crore Takas each. These pharmacies produce about 500 items of ayurvedic and 250 items of Unani medicines.

Burma

Nearly 30 000 traditional medical practitioners provide medical care to about 85% of the country's population. An indigenous medical institute and hospital is run by the Government as well as 34 dispensaries devoted to indigenous medicine which operate in different parts of the country.

There are 11 227 trained and about 22 000 non-institutionally trained practitioners in the country in addition to about 43 000 birth attendants. The Government believes that the development of indigenous medicine will gain momentum through its proper utilization in community medicine activities along with modern medicine.

India

The traditional systems practised in India include Ayurveda, Siddha, Unani, yoga, and the naturopathy and Tibetan systems of medicine. These systems have been recognized by the Government for the purpose of the national health services. There are 108 undergraduate teaching institutions in traditional systems of medicine awarding a degree following training for 4½ years in Ayurveda/Unani/Siddha. There are also two postgraduate institutes and 21 postgraduate departments awarding postgraduate degrees and doctorates. There is an exclusive Ayurveda University at Jamnagar in Gujarat—the only one in the world. A statutory Council has been established to regulate the practice of these systems of medicine. The Council has already prepared the syllabus and minimum standards of education for these systems, which are being followed by all the undergraduate colleges throughout the country. Currently there are 460 000 practitioners of traditional medicine in the country. Of this number, over 271 000 (223 000 Ayurveda, 30 456 Unani, and 18 128 Siddha) practitioners are registered under the state boards. Some 186 000 practitioners are not registered with any of the boards or councils. Of the registered practitioners, 117 774 Ayurveda, 10 268 Unani and 1559 Siddha practitioners are institutionally qualified. There are also about 145 000 practitioners of homoeopathy. In order to encourage research in traditional systems of medicine the Government has also established four independent Central Research Councils, one each for Ayurveda and Siddha, Unani, homoeopathy and yoga, and naturopathy.

Under these Councils about 50 research institutes and 200 units are carrying out clinical and drug research with a multidisciplinary approach, standardization, literary research, survey and surveillance, rural developmental programmes etc.

The Government of India has listed the traditional remedies for purposes of providing primary health care. The practitioners of traditional medicine are actively involved in the health care delivery programme. A composite kit containing simple and effective traditional remedies and those from other systems of medicine have been given to community health workers along with a printed manual about the administration of drugs, etc. A WHO collaborating centre for traditional systems of medicine has been established in Gujarat Ayurveda University, Jamnagar. In addition to a number of private pharmacies almost all the State Governments have their own pharmacies for the production of standard medicines. There also exist separate directorates for traditional systems of medicine in all the states; there is an adviser at the central level. There are, in all, 215 hospitals and 14 000 dispensaries in the country.

Indonesia

The traditional practitioners in Indonesia are the *sukun bayi* and traditional healers who mostly use herbal medicines in their treatment. A school of traditional medicine is run by the Government. A directorate for the control of traditional drugs has been established and research into the use of these drugs is also being conducted in the pharmacology departments of medical schools and in the schools of pharmacy functioning in the country. The Ministry of Health has registered 25 pharmaceutical companies producing traditional drugs. The Government recognizes that there is a great body of knowledge available among traditional healers on the treatment of various diseases and also for promoting health.

Maldives

The system of traditional medicine prevalent in the Maldives is a mixture of Arab medicine and other systems practised in the neighbouring countries of India and Sri Lanka. Most of these practitioners are located in the rural areas. Herbal medicine is much in use. There are 151 practitioners of traditional medicine; only two practise Unani medicine. There are no Government hospitals or dispensaries and no formal training programme available.

Nepal

Ayurveda is practised in this country. There are 82 ayurvedic clinics and a 50-bed ayurvedic hospital. About 75% of the population resort to ayurvedic treatment. Facilities are available for intensive education in this system; there is a three-year certificate course. There are 200 institutionally qualified practitioners and about 1000 traditionally trained persons. Drug research and survey activities have been taken up.

Sri Lanka

There are three traditional systems of medicine—Ayurveda, Siddha and Unani—being practised by 3500 institutionally trained and 14 700 non-institutionally trained physicians. There is a Government Ayurvedic College, which provides five years of systematic education to about 150 students every year. Research activities have been conducted at the Bandaranaike Ayurvedic Research Institute since 1962. There are four Government ayurvedic hospitals, four dispensaries and 240 ayurvedic dispensaries run by the local government institutions. The practice of traditional medicine is controlled by an Act. Drugs are being produced by several establishments on a commercial scale.

Thailand

In Thailand all the 35 000 traditional practitioners are registered. There are no recognized training institutions. Traditional practitioners are, however, trained by a few professional associations. These practitioners are not utilized by the Government for delivering health services at any level in the country. The Government is pursuing several research projects to study the action of various medicinal plants available in the country.

Trends for the future

Future efforts of WHO in the Region will be related to two distinct and broad areas for action to meet the goals of health for all by the year 2000. First, to effect the reorientation of the traditional healers, practitioners and physicians to meet the needs of primary health care. In this context, research will be stimulated on the utilization of practitioners of traditional medicine, as well as on the factors which enhance or retard their use by the community. Secondly, to support research on the treatment by traditional medicines of certain diseases for which modern medicine has no sure cure to offer, such as peptic ulcer, bronchial asthma, rheumatoid arthritis, urolithiasis, viral hepatitis and diabetes mellitus—conditions which have reportedly been successfully treated with traditional medicines.

REFERENCE

(*1*) WORLD HEALTH ORGANIZATION. *Alma-Ata 1978. Primary health care: report of the International Conference on Primary Health Care, Alma-Ata, USSR, 6–12 September 1978*, Geneva, 1978 ("Health for All" series, No. 1).

CHAPTER 23

The European Region*

A review of the health care systems in the European Region shows a rather complex situation and a vast number of both official and unofficial healing methods in use. There are, however, several similarities with health care systems in other parts of the world, and behind the facade of modern allopathic medicine, a considerable proportion of self-care and primary health care employs traditional medicine and alternative health care systems.

Many health therapeutic practices in Europe are not really traditional, as the traditional elements have been diluted over the centuries by what used to be official medicine. The term "folk medicine" is therefore more appropriate in this context (1).

Many of the little home remedies and practices of ancient or more recent origin, cherished and practised by many people in industrial societies, are neither truly folk medical practices nor are they essentially scientific. They can be regarded as manifestations of "popular medicine". Folk medicine, popular medicine and alternative medicine in Europe are classified as unofficial medicine, as opposed to scientific (Western) medicine.

In the framework of ethnology, traditional medicine is taught in university institutes in the Federal Republic of Germany, Switzerland, the United Kingdom, and in some other countries soon to include Austria. Research in medical anthropology is carried out at these institutes, and also by scholars of other disciplines such as sociology, history of medicine, pharmacology and botany. Research in folk medicine is going on in institutes for folklore, particularly in some East European countries. The Federal Republic of Germany has two working groups for ethnomedicine with members from German-speaking and other European countries. Both of these groups publish a scientific journal. The societies for medical

---

* Regional contribution compiled by Dr H. Velimirovic and Dr B. Velimirovic.

anthropology in Austria and in the United Kingdom, and several institutes of tropical medicine in a number of European countries are interested in the subject of traditional medicine, but the emphasis of the latter is on the situation in non-European countries.

Unofficial medicine in Europe

Traditional medicine

The survivals of true folk medicine in Europe which, according to Foster (2), are part of the culture of a pre-industrialized society, no longer belong to a genuine medical system. Independent manifestations can be found in individual households all over Europe, mostly in rural areas. The more popular traditional therapeutic practices include herbalism, balneotherapy, the use of mud and clay, cupping and bleeding. Hydrotherapy is widely applied in alternative medicine and, at the same time, it is a complementary part of official medicine in some countries.

Magic and religion

Popular medicine in Europe does not specifically include esoteric thoughts, but in folk medicine the spiritual aspect is still strong. Magic can be involved occasionally in therapeutic practices. In southern Italy, for example, a magic ritual is performed for the diagnosis and later for the treatment of headache caused by evil eye (3). In general, magic has been replaced in Europe by mysticism or religion although faith has always played an important part in the healing process. Christianity brought, for example, faith in saints with special healing powers.

Imported traditional medicine

Not all of the traditional therapeutic methods practised in Europe are of European origin.

Acupuncture. Acupuncture as practised in China has been known to the West for centuries. From the 19th century onwards, it has been at some time popular in France, in other European countries such as Austria and Germany, and in Scandinavia. The interest in acupuncture has diminished somewhat in the present century. For many years it was considered in Western countries as "superstition". Following intensified contacts with China in the late 1960s and early 1970s, the use of various forms of acupuncture analgesia in surgery received wide publicity by the mass media. Acupuncture is now more tolerated and partly accepted by official medicine. It is claimed that there are over 5000 acupuncturists in Europe (4), practising in Austria, Denmark, Finland, France the Federal Republic of Germany, Italy, Romania, the USSR and the United Kingdom. In East European and some West European countries they are always physicians. In the Soviet Union acupuncture is practised at the Institute for

Reflexology in Moscow. In the republics of the USSR it is taught at institutes of postgraduate training. Finland has 200 local health centres which provide acupuncture treatment (9). It is taught in two medical schools, and limited to physicians in order to avoid malpractice; however, it is not covered by the National Health Insurance of Finland. Acupuncture and conventional Western analgesia have been jointly used in a few hospitals for surgery in Austria (5), where there is a State-sponsored research institute for acupuncture. Teaching facilities are available in France, where it is also practised in some hospitals. Institutes for acupuncture are established in the Federal Republic of Germany, where the subject is also included in the curriculum of the college for practitioners of healing, and in many other European countries. In the Federal Republic of Germany health insurances cover the costs of acupuncture treatment. In the United Kingdom there are two colleges of acupuncture besides the British Acupuncture Association. In the latter the applicants for membership must be "registered medical practitioners, osteopaths, chiropractors, dental surgeons, physiotherapists or State Registered Nurses after a 1-year *ab initio* course". For a licentiate in acupuncture 2 years constitute minimum study time, 4 years for the Bachelor of Acupuncture, and 6 years for the Doctor of Acupuncture Award (6). The Nordic Acupuncture Society was formed in 1980. On the whole the teaching of acupuncture in Europe follows a variety of patterns. France and some other countries offer Westernized teaching, while in some the Chinese pattern is followed. Acupuncture analgesia courses are carried out in Austria, Greece, Italy, and Eastern Europe (7).

In most European countries the discussion is still going on whether the authorization to practise acupuncture should be limited to professional physicians.

Other forms of imported traditional medicine. In recent years Asian traditional medicine has gained ground in Britain. Due to the large numbers of immigrants from Bangladesh, Pakistan, and Moslem areas of India, traditional practitioners of the Unani system of medicine have established themselves in the country. It is estimated that there are about five resident hakims in every city of Britain with a large Asian immigrant community. Some hakims fly to Britain for temporary consultations. The clients of the hakims are from the Asian population who for reasons of language and cultural difficulties prefer to consult a practitioner of their own ethnic origin. However, one hakim reported that two-thirds of his patients were white, mainly young people dissatisfied with modern Western medicine or patients with chronic diseases. Although these practitioners are taking some of the burden from general practitioners, they present a number of problems to the health authorities, especially in connexion with the import of Asian drugs not licensed in Britain or with the traditional admixture of poisonous heavy metals in their remedies (8).

In some other countries of Europe, for instance in France, a similar situation arises when non-European immigrants in substantial numbers bring with them various forms of traditional medicine and practitioners.

Alternative medicine[1]

As a consequence of a multitude of factors, including the growing dissatisfaction with and unfulfilled expectations from bureaucratic medicine, alternative medicine in Europe is becoming increasingly popular. "One of the roots of the present (if latent) crisis of our scientific medicine seems to be that it has been busy developing its own scholarly codes which are no longer shared by the patients"(9).

Some 20 years ago it was possible to sort the alternative therapies into a few well-defined categories. Today their practitioners are increasingly being tempted to learn and practise a variety of methods. Old forms of therapies, too, are being imported, revived or adapted (14).

A list of the commoner and more established therapeutic practices and curing theories known and applied in the European countries, based with some alterations on *A Visual Encyclopedia of Unconventional Medicine* (11), is presented in Annex 1.

An idea can be given of the status of some of the more frequently met practitioners and therapies of alternative medicine in European countries:

Heilpraktiker. Under a variety of names *Heilpraktiker* (Healing practitioners, naturopaths) are working all over Europe. Some are applying a variety of therapeutic methods while others have a special technique which is used as standard treatment for any ailment.

In the Federal Republic of Germany the practice of the healing practitioner is authorized on condition that he has passed an examination conducted by a local public health officer. There is no legal obligation to attend a school in preparation for the examination, as long as the student fulfils the requirements. The Bundesverband Deutscher Heilpraktiker (Federal Association of German Healing Practitioners) organizes training courses of 20 months in 29 cities of West Germany, as well as special courses and practical training. Among other things the curriculum offers subjects such as neuraltherapy (an injection therapy applied in the treatment of pain), iris diagnosis, acupuncture, homoeopathy, acupressure, chiropractic, phytotherapy, psychotherapy, and ozone therapy. Most healing practitioners, however, concentrate on only a few of these methods. The courses are open to German nationals, and lately also to citizens of the member states of the EEC. *Heilpraktiker* in the Federal Republic of Germany are not authorized to attend a birth, to give medicines needing a prescription, to recommend opiates, to vaccinate, to treat venereal disease, or to issue death certificates. The medium income of a practising health practitioner was given in 1974 as between US $3000 and US $10 000 per month (12). The legal recognition of the *Heilpraktiker*'s activities is based on the law of 1939 which stipulates, however, that he cannot call himself a physician (*Arzt*). On the other hand, some academically trained physicians are using the methods of the *Heilpraktiker*.

---

[1] See also Chapter 16, "Selected individual therapies".

Only a few private health insurance agencies cover the costs of the treatment by a healing practitioner.

In Switzerland, only the Canton of Appenzell gives healing practitioners (*Naturaerzte*) the permission to practise, although with a number of restrictions. In Austria, no such permission is granted, although it is known that a number of *Heilpraktiker* practise illegally, sometimes under the cover of a legal occupation. They are prosecuted only in cases where their treatment leads to complications.

Heilpraktiker have organized a number of associations, aiming *inter alia* to establish teaching institutions, inform the public, issue journals or give courses in various techniques.

Herbalism. The use of herbs, presumably for therapeutic purposes, is reported in Europe from archaeological findings from a number of neolithic sites. Herbs have been used for centuries by the people themselves and by lay practitioners as an important part of the official medical system. Herbalism persisted in all parts of Europe with more or less intensity and even today there is hardly any household without some knowledge of at least a few plants used for teas, compresses, inhalations, etc. In fact, it became a consistent part of alternative medicine.

In industrialized countries medicinal plants have become industrial products through methodical cultivation, import and export, industrial processing, packaging, and marketing. Various companies for the cultivation and distribution of plants have representatives in many countries. A number of producers of medicinal plant drugs are listed for Austria, France, the Federal Republic of Germany, Italy, Switzerland and USSR. Plant remedies were formerly produced mainly for the official medical systems, but are now sold in pharmacies or drugstores and, according to the regulations in each country, in supermarkets and newly established health-food stores (*13*). More than 200 species of herbs are used in the USSR for production of "elixirs of health".

In the United Kingdom herbalism was the main system of healing until the 20th century. It gradually declined in popularity when chemical drugs were introduced, but some people still prefer this kind of treatment (*14*). An act of Parliament to protect herbalists continued in force until 1968, when the Medicines Act regulated the practice of herbalists and the use of plant medicines. The National Association of Medical Herbalists was started in 1964 and the Faculty of Herbal Medicine in the 1940s. They are the two main training centres for herbalists today besides the Tutorial School of Herbal Medicine in Kent. At the present time the United Kingdom has around 12 000 practising herbalists who received their training in one of these schools. A Herb Society is active in London, with a publication entitled *The Herbal Review*. It provides a list of over 600 health food stores in the United Kingdom (*10*). Various therapies based on flowers have emerged recently and there are 3 institutes responsible for "flower healing" in Britain, and an Aromatherapy Training Centre in London.

In some European countries, herbalists are not officially authorized to practise but are tolerated; in others they have the approval of the health administration and some have legal recognition. The *Heilpraktiker* in the Federal Republic of Germany, for example, includes herbalism in his repertoire. In the less industrialized countries of Europe with larger rural populations and more individual knowledge in the field of medicinal plants, their use is more evident, as has been reported for instance from Bulgaria (*17*), Greece, Poland (*15*, *16*) and Romania (*18*). In Romania herbal remedies are sold in special State stores *Plafar* (plant pharmacies).

Balneotherapy. The healing temples of Greek antiquity, dedicated to Aesculapius, were usually built in the vicinity of springs believed to have healing powers. Many of the spas in a number of European countries were already in use in Roman times and are still popular today. In European practice balneotherapy has always been integrated into official medicine. It is not considered as an alternative but as a complementary curative method.

In countries where medicinal springs occur, for example in Austria, France, Federal Republic of Germany, Italy, Switzerland, Yugoslavia and USSR, health authorities have a more favourable attitude to their assumed therapeutic value than in other countries. Physicians will recommend water therapy for a number of ailments according to the chemical content of the water, and health insurances will cover the costs. On the other hand, in countries without their own medicinal springs, the medical profession remains sceptical.

Consumers of the traditional water therapies are mostly people with chronic diseases (traumatic or degenerative conditions of the joints, rheumatism, heart and circulation diseases, gynaecological and intestinal complaints, diseases of the mouth and respiratory tract, skin diseases, obesity, etc.) and rehabilitation patients.

In addition to treatment with water, underwater massage, whirlpools, cold and hot jets, and underwater exercise, some modern establishments of water therapy offer electrical treatment, chiropractic and osteopathic manipulation, and official medical therapy.

The drinking of mineral water is so common today that nobody thinks about the age of this custom. Mineral water is taken for preventive or therapeutic purposes, whether recommended by a physician or not, or simply because some mineral waters are pleasant beverages.

The traditional element of hydrotherapy has been rationalized and accepted by official medicine. Treatment and rehabilitation in spas with water rich in substances claimed to be favourable for all kinds of conditions have been incorporated into the official systems. The curative value, however, as opposed to the social or recreational value, is regarded with scepticism by many physicians.

Of minor importance, yet traditionally known, is the application of hot clay or mud in baths or as packs, compresses and poultices for chronic or rheumatic diseases. This therapy is used in some of the European spas, individually or by alternative healers. Medicinal mud or clay is available in the pharmacies of some European countries, and mud extracts are exported from Romania. From Poland it is reported that in rural areas potters are still today using clay internally or externally to treat a number of ailments including skin conditions, burns, or rheumatism. This practice was very widespread in the past but is now limited to the treatment of friends and relatives (*19*).

Cupping and bleeding. In Europe as in many other parts of the world cupping and bleeding are very old therapeutic methods. In the Middle Ages these techniques became standard practice in official medicine, together with purging and the application of complicated medicinal compounds combined according to the theories of Galen. They remained in use also during the Renaissance. In some European countries bleeding (with the use of leeches, *Hirudo medicinalis*) and cupping were still part of official medicine well into the present century, and cupping is still used today in official medicine in some East European countries. The last vestiges of this practice in a rural area of central Finland were reported as curiosities (*20*). Both cupping and bleeding have been taken over today as therapeutic methods by alternative healers in Austria, France, the Federal Republic of Germany, Switzerland, and elsewhere.

Osteopathy and chiropractic. The difference between osteopathy and chiropractic appears minimal. Osteopaths tend to use leverage, rotating and lifting of the patient, whereas chiropractors prefer well-directed thrusts at particular vertebrae. Techniques overlap considerably, however, and some manipulators prefer to use the term "osteopractic" (*12*).

Osteopathy was brought to Europe from the United States of America, where it originated around 1870. In 1918 the British School of Osteopathy was founded, but osteopathy did not spread much on the European continent where a well-established scientific orthopaedic specialization and physical treatment had existed for several decades.

Chiropractic, too, had its origin in the USA (1895). It was introduced into Europe through a plebiscite in Switzerland, when in 1939 the Canton of Zurich decided that chiropractors should be authorized to treat sick people, in opposition to the recommendations of a number of scientific advisers. So far Switzerland and the Federal Republic of Germany are the only countries in Europe where chiropractors are recognized by the State. Recognition has been requested in Denmark, where osteopathic treatment is covered by the health services if referral is made by a physician, in Norway, and it seems also in the United Kingdom (*21*) where considerable pressure exists from some physicians and occasionally also from politicians to bring osteopaths and chiropractors into the National Health Service, and to make registrations and proper training compulsory for manipulation therapists in order to protect patients from unqualified practitioners and charlatans. If they are not recognized, the problem is that anybody may call himself an osteopath without breaking the law. There are said to be between 500 and 3000 unqualified people practising in the United Kingdom under the title of osteopath, chiropractor, physiologist, reflexotherapist and others; the president of the British Association for Manipulative Medicine has stated that at least a million manipulations are performed every week and only a tiny proportion of these are done by medically qualified manipulators.

It seems that the resistance to recognition among physicians and authorities is slowly giving way. More and more doctors are referring patients for osteopathic treatment, measures unthinkable some years ago when, for example, in Britain a physician was struck off the register by the General Medical Council for making referrals to "unorthodox" practitioners.

There are several institutions for training in osteopathy and chiropractic in the United Kingdom. The Anglo-European College of Chiropractic, for example, provides four-year courses, a minimum requirement for practitioners of chiropractic. The British Chiropractors Association has a register of all qualified practitioners in the United Kingdom, limited to graduates from approved chiropractic colleges (21). The British Association of Manipulative Medicine gives short courses for practising physicians on osteopathic techniques of manipulation. In the Federal Republic of Germany the Bundesverband Deutscher Heilpraktiker (Federal Association of German Healing Practitioners) includes chiropractic among other healing methods in its curriculum of training courses. In 1976 the number of practitioners of chiropractic was: 1 practitioner for 46 875 population in Denmark, 1 for 74 324 in Switzerland, 1 for 81 395 in Norway, 1 for 125 000 in Belgium, 1 for 336 957 in Sweden, 1 for 516 670 in France, and 1 for 635 542 in the United Kingdom (figures quoted by Breen, 22).

Homoeopathy.[1] Homoeopathy is not uniformly considered as a "system" of medicine, although it satisfies most of the criteria to be called so.

For some time homoeopathy was seen as competition for orthodox medicine. In the second half of the last century the United Kingdom had about 300 homoeopathic doctors with homoeopathic hospitals established in several cities, and the Royal Household had a homoeopath among its staff of physicians. By 1970, however, there were only 100 medically qualified homoeopaths. However, homoeopathy has gained ground lately, although most physicians are not very enthusiastic about it. The number of patients at the London Homoeopathic Hospital has increased by 10% over the last five years and lately the Society of Homoeopathy has declared that it will liberate homoeopathy from the "dominance of the medical profession" (10, p. 145), to the dismay of medically trained homoeopaths.

Because of the lack of medically qualified homoeopaths to meet the demand, patients turn to unqualified practitioners who have adopted homoeopathy as one of their therapeutic methods.

The United Kingdom has a Faculty of Homoeopathy, one college and several societies, six hospitals and one outpatient clinic. The British Homoeopathic Association provides addresses of about 100 chemists who

---

[1] See also Chapter 10.

supply homoeopathic remedies. In France homoeopathy is more popular than in Britain, and there are about ten times as many doctors practising homoeopathy. They receive training at the French homoeopathic faculty. Austria has a State-supported research institute for homoeopathy and a society for homoeopathy. Successful animal treatment and experiments are alleged to prove the claim that homoeopathy does not work through suggestion, and debate continues whether its practice should be restricted to physicians. There are outpatient departments for homoeopathy in the USSR, and homoeopathic pharmacies are allowed, sales being restricted to drugs without noxious substances. In the Federal Republic of Germany homoeopathy is taught at the training courses for healing practitioners and a Chair in homoeopathy is planned in Munich. Qualified physicians frequently take supplementary courses in order to incorporate homoeopathic methods. Homoeopathic remedies are prescribed by a wide range of alternative practitioners. Health insurance agencies reimburse homoeopathic treatment. The first official handbook for homoeopathic drugs appeared in 1901.

Anthroposophical medicine. Anthroposophical medicine dates back to the Austrian Rudolph Steiner (1861–1925). His philosophy was based on the notion that physical matter was formed and activated by cosmic forces, and that there is a dynamic equilibrium between man and the universe. The organs of the body are correlated with the parts of plants. Steiner's theories on three autonomous but interacting and interpenetrating systems of organs gave rise to the theories of anthroposophical medicine. He never practised medicine himself, but gave courses on therapeutics exclusively for physicians and medical students. A School of Spiritual Science (Goetheanum), at Dornach in Switzerland, includes a medical department. Eurhythmy, a form of dance therapy, was developed from his ideas about the art of movement (23).

After Steiner's death his philosophy spread in Europe, particularly in Austria, Germany and Switzerland. There are now more than 1000 physicians practising anthroposophical medicine, while about 2000 medical practitioners are prescribing remedies based on its theories. Physicians with an anthroposophical orientation, for example, believe in a cancer remedy made of mistletoe, developed by Steiner. The Federal Republic of Germany has 2 large anthroposophical hospitals and about 10 smaller hospitals, including a psychiatric clinic (23). The spread of anthroposophical medicine was slower in the United Kingdom, and more centred on the treatment of handicapped and emotionally disturbed children. Village communities for handicapped adults probably emanated from anthroposophical initiative.

Hand healing. In the United Kingdom there are many more healers than all other practitioners of alternative medicine and, according to Forbes, there are about 20 000 healers compared with probably fewer than 2000 practitioners of other health systems and 55 000 trained physicians (24). Healing is performed by lay persons, by practitioners of other alternative methods and by a few physicians, all of them believing that they have specific healing powers. Besides the National Federation of Spiritual Healers with more than 2000 members, there are a number of other associations extending membership to healers, such as the Aetherius Society, the Atlanteans and the White Eagle Lodge (*24*). Some groups are religiously oriented. The Healing Research Trust gives courses of three weeks in hand healing. Theoretically, British physicians are permitted to recommend a healing seance to their patients but such activities are difficult in hospital practice. As healers understand their healing powers to emanate from God, many do not take payment except in the form of donations (*25*). The teaching of healing practices is not included in the curriculum of the "Münchner Heilpraktiker Kolleg", the School of the Federal Association of German Healing practitioners.

All over Europe healing is a widespread therapeutic method, usually performed without the specific approval of health authorities. It is not accepted by health insurance agencies for reimbursement.

Special cases of unorthodox therapies

A number of unorthodox therapies relating mainly to certain specific drugs gained popularity for varying periods in Europe but were later abandoned when their effectiveness or safety could not be demonstrated.

Examples of these drugs which figured mainly in cancer therapy are vitamin B5 (pangamate), Krebiozen, Calcaron and Amygdaline-Laetril (*26*), and in therapy for arteriosclerosis vasolastine (in Holland), fresh-cell therapy, placenta extracts, rejuvenating drugs, etc. Efforts to ban their use usually meet with organized resistance from vested interests.

Self-care in Europe

The role of lay persons, mothers, grandmothers, and other family members, neighbours, colleagues, etc. as the first providers of health care in preference to professional health workers, has recently gained considerable popularity.

"Self-care" is applied to various self observations, examinations or procedures such as urine testing, breast self-examination, insulin injections, blood pressure measurement, home kidney dialysis, self-medication for asthmatics and physical therapy. It is usually not medically initiated, e.g., in symptom-induced self-care when a patient treats himself or is treated by family members before the physician has been consulted. Some trends put more emphasis on meditation, Eastern philosophies and religion, diet, exercise, etc.

Health authorities are beginning to recognize self-help as a means to relieve official medicine of some of the unnecessary demands on health care, and as a tool for health education that could enable people to help themselves where professional care is not essential any more. Self-care based on algorithms prepared by the official medical services is encouraged for isolated populations, e.g., in Arctic areas of the USSR. Proponents of self-care are the providers of official medical care and also the practitioners of popular medicine. The people learn from each other, from family, friends and neighbours and from the media and other popular sources.

* * *

Some of the practitioners of alternative medicine are constantly trying to obtain official recognition. The need for a careful scrutiny and appraisal of all medical methods and therapies, and for quality control of drugs is likewise increasing. European health and research institutes are particularly well placed to apply modern science and technology to traditional methods of practice and therapy in order to evaluate herbal medicaments in particular. Health authorities would also wish to satisfy themselves regarding the cost-effectiveness of traditional health care in relation to official health care.

Appendix

Some Therapeutic Practices and Curing Theories

Homoeopathy
Anthroposophical medicine
Astrological diagnosis
Iris diagnosis
Tongue diagnosis
Applied kinesiology
Psychic diagnosis
The aura
Kirlian photography
Biorythmus
The Luscher colour test
Acupuncture
Reflexology
Shiatsu
Moxibustion
Osteopathy
Chiropractic
Impact therapy
Rolfing
Manipulative therapy
Touch for health
Skin brushing
The Bates method of eyesight training
Mesmerism
Radiant heat
Wax baths

Breathing
Sun baths
Ultra-violet radiation
Mono diets
Fasting
Gerson therapy
Urine therapy
Cymatics
Psionic medicine
Medical radiesthesia
Radionics
Lakhovsky oscillatory coils
Orgone therapy
Pyramid energy
Naturopathy (*Heilpraktiker*)
Metaphysical healing
Human cybernetics
Psychosynthesis
Dianetics
Autosuggestion
Hypnosis
Autogenic training
Neurophysiological psychology
Galvanism
Cupping
Bleeding

Faradism
Sinusoidal current
Interferential therapy
High Frequency therapy
Diathermy and microwave therapies
Ultrasonics
Pulsed high frequency therapy
Endogenous endocrinotherapy
Gems and copper therapy
Clay and mud
Balneotherapy
Herbalism
Vita florum
Exaltation of flowers
Aromatherapy
Wholefood diet
Vegetarianism
Veganism
Macrobiotics
The Bircher-Benner method
Raw food
The Hay diet
High protein diet
High fibre diet

Biochemic remedies
Orthomolecular medicine
Biofeedback
Meditation
Arica
Somatography
Bioenergetics
Biodynamic psychology
Psychodrama
The new primal therapies
Gestalt
Co-counselling
Encounter
Sensitivity training
Enlightenment intensive
Transactional analysis
Colour therapy
Music therapy
Yoga
The Alexander technique
Dance therapy
Curative eurythmy
T'ai chi ch'uan
Faith healing

REFERENCES

(1) REDFIELD, R. The folk society and culture. In: Wirth, L., ed. *Eleven twenty-six, a decade of social science research*. New York, Arno Press, 1974.
(2) FOSTER, G. M. What is folk culture? *American anthropologist*, **55**:159–173 (1953).
(3) HAUSCHILD, T. Sind Heilrituale dasselbe wie Psychotherapien? Kritik einer ethnomedizinischen Denkgewohnheit am Beispiel des sünitalienischen Heilrituals gegen des bösen Blick. *Curare*, **2**:241–256 (1979).
(4) NEWTON, J. Acupuncture. In: Hulke, M., ed. *The encyclopaedia of alternative medicine and self-help*. London, Rider & Co., 1978, pp. 21–22.
(5) Use of acupuncture in modern health care. *WHO Chronicle*, **34**:294–301 (1980).
(6) Associations and societies. In: Hulke, M., ed. *The encyclopaedia of alternative medicine and self-help*. London, Rider & Co., 1978, p. 212.
(7) SCHATZ, J. A common purpose. *World Health*, December 1979, pp. 21–23.
(8) EAGLE, R. Your friendly neighbourhood hakim. *World medicine*, July 26 1980, pp. 19–22.
(9) HONKO, L. The ethnological aspect in health research. In: Heikkinen, et al., ed. *Research on health research*, Helsinki, Suomen Akatemia, 1980 (Publications of the Academy of Finland, No. 11), pp. 87–90.
(10) INGLIS, B. *Natural medicine*. London, Collins, 1979.
(11) HILL, A., ed. *A visual encyclopaedia of unconventional medicine*. New York, Crown Publishing, 1979, & London, New English Library, 1979.
(12) *Studienprogrammen*. München, Müncher Heilpratiker Kolleg, Schule des Bundesverbandes Deutscher Heilpratiker, 1980.
(13) VELIMIROVIC, H. & VELIMIROVIC, B. Do traditional plant medicines have a future in third world countries? *Curare*, **3**:173–191 (1980).
(14) DIDCOTT, E. F. Herbalism. In: Hulke, M., ed. *The encyclopaedia of alternative medicine and self-help*. London, Rider & Co., 1978, pp. 98–101.

(15) TYLKOWA, D. *Die Volkspharmakologie der Dorfbewohner in den polnischen Karpathen*, Freiburg/Br., 1980 (Paper presented at the 5th International Conference on Ethnomedicine, Ethnobotany and Ethnopharmacology).
(16) KOWALSKA-LEWICKA, A. *Der Knoblauch in der polnichen Volkskultur*, Freiburg/Br., 1980 (Paper presented at the 5th International Conference on Ethnomedicine, Ethnobotany and Ethnopharmacology).
(17) PETKOV, V. Bulgaria's folk remedies stand the test of time. *The UNESCO Courier*, July 1979, pp. 39-41.
(18) DUNARE, N. *Les recherches roumaines sur l'ethnobotanique pharmacologique*, 1980 (unpublished document).
(19) CZUBALA, D. Lehm-ein Heilmittel der Töpferzunft. *Curare* 3:107-112 (1980).
(20) DANNER, R. Bericht über die letzten Zeugnisse eines volkstümlichen Behandlungsverfahrens in Finnland. *Curare*, 3:67-69 (1980).
(21) COOPER, R. G. Chiropractic. In: Hulke, M., ed. *The encyclopaedia of alternative medicine and self-help*. London, Rider & Co., 1978, pp. 58-61.
(22) BREEN, A. C. Chiropractic. In: Hill, A., ed. *A visual encyclopaedia of unconventional medicine*. New York, Crown Publishing, 1979 & London, New English Library, 1979, pp. 73-77.
(23) DYSON, J. A. & HOLLMAN, C. Anthroposophical medicine. In: Hill, A., ed. *A visual encyclopaedia of unconventional medicine*. New York Crown Publishing, 1979 & London, New English Library, 1979, pp. 29-33.
(24) FORBES, A. Healing. In: Hill, A., ed. *A visual encyclopaedia of unconventional medicine*. New York, Crown Publishing, 1979 & London, New English Library, 1979, pp. 176-179.
(25) BAERLEIN, E. Hand healing. In: Hulke, M., ed. *The encyclopaedia of alternative medicine and self-help*. London, Rider & Co., 1978, pp. 88-91.
(26) VELIMIROVIC, B. Laetrile-the case of a disputed drug. In: Soda, T., ed. *Drug-induced suffering, medical, pharmaceutical and legal aspects*, Amsterdam, Excerpta Medica, 1980 (International Congress Series, No. 513) pp. 236-248.

CHAPTER 24

The Eastern Mediterranean Region*

Traditional medicine in countries of the WHO Eastern Mediterranean Region enjoys a rich cultural heritage from several ancient civilizations. In historical perspective, various African, Babylonian, ancient Egyptian, Persian and Arabian concepts of health and approaches to disease have left their marks on traditional medicine. Other influences from outside the Region, notably the Chinese, Indian, Greek and Roman beliefs and medical practices, have also had their effect. The works of Hippocrates, Galen, Dioscorides and other physicians were introduced to the Region in the pre-Islamic era through the Nestorian monks who established the medical school at Jondisapur (Iran) towards the end of the 5th century (*1*). The blend of these important sources of knowledge and wealth of experience resulted in the development of various healing arts. For more than ten centuries, however, the mainstream of medical practice continued to flow along the general lines of Graeco-Arab medicine. Because of this historical background, traditional medicine in some countries, particularly Pakistan, is known as Unani (Greek) medicine, thus denoting one of its main sources.

More recently, historical events have changed the course of traditional medicine. Towards the end of the 19th century, the majority of countries in the Region came under foreign domination and new approaches in medicine were introduced. Initially, the use of the newly introduced medical system was generally limited but, under the growing impact of Western-style medicine, traditional medical care receded from a central position to a peripheral one and a new medical era began. Within the past two decades, however, and especially following political independence and self-rule, many of the developing countries have become increasingly aware

---

* Regional contribution compiled by Dr Taha Baasher, Regional Adviser on Mental Health, WHO Regional Office for the Eastern Mediterranean, Alexandria, Egypt.

of the importance of the long-neglected traditional and indigenous systems of medicine, their potentialities and manpower resources.

Unfortunately, despite the great advance in modern medicine, a striking disparity in health care between countries and within countries, as well as between urban and rural populations, has been generally apparent. It has become more and more evident that the existing pattern of health care in developing countries does not resolve the critical issue of the inadequacy and inequalities of health care. Indeed, if the system of health care continues as it exists today, the cherished social goal of the attainment of an acceptable level of health for all people by the year 2000 will remain a dream (2).

Naturally, this goal has become a growing challenge for many countries and alternative systems have to be sought. The question is what will be the role of traditional medicine in the attainment of this goal? An attempt will be made here to describe the present state of traditional medicine in the Region and its future prospects, with special reference to WHO's efforts to promote and develop research activities in this connexion.

Attitude and policy

The general attitude and the official policy towards traditional medicine vary greatly from country to country, depending on the historical background of the development of health care, the political system, socioeconomic conditions and cultural background. In practically all the countries two systems of health care are in operation—allopathic or modern medicine, which comes under official regulations by the State, and traditional medicine, which is community-related and generally self-developed. It therefore seems appropriate to consider the views of the practitioners of allopathic medicine, the official policy, and the community attitude towards traditional medicine.

Professional attitude

With the development of modern health sciences, attempts to study and understand traditional medicine have been rather scanty and generally scarce. In practically all medical faculties of the Region, for example, there is hardly any reference in undergraduate medical teaching to organized training programmes on traditional health care. Similarly, seldom is any attention given to traditional medicine in postgraduate training, nor has any systematic research been organized.

In the absence of an operational framework linking the conventional and traditional systems of medicine, a wide gap exists between workers in modern health services and traditional practitioners in the community. This has resulted in lack of communication, inadequacy of information, suspicion, mistrust and sometimes open antagonism. In the great majority of countries, graduates of Western-type medical schools regard traditional medicine as an outmoded, unscientific and inappropriate practice. Even in medical specialties such as psychiatry, where interest in traditional psychotherapeutic practices has been generally shown, some of the leading psychiatrists, for no convincing reasons, show strong aversion to folk practices and traditional practitioners. In contrast with this latter attitude, the traditional midwife has been accepted in some countries and valuable efforts have been made by health administrators in her training and effective incorporation in the general health care system.

Official policy

Official attitudes and policy regarding traditional medicine vary greatly. In the majority of countries in the Region, though traditional healing practices are not officially recognized, they are not legally prohibited. There are several countries where traditional medicine suffers from benign neglect and from a policy of isolation.

Exceptionally, in a few countries, attempts have been made to regulate and promote traditional medicine. In this respect, the developments which have taken place in recent years in Pakistan are worth recording here.

In 1965, the Government of Pakistan established an Autonomous Board for Tibb (medicine) and Homoeopathy with a view to enabling the traditional medical practitioners to train and practise their systems independently by supplementing them with such modern advances as the Board may from time to time determine. Relevant to the growing needs, it has rightly been recognized that the cost of using modern medicine to provide proper health care for the entire population of Pakistan would be rather prohibitive, and that other options have to be duly considered. Consequently, and in view of the results obtained in neighbouring China, the issue of integrating inexpensive traditional practices into the general health services was raised. In 1974 an Indigenous Medicine Commission was formed to explore such a possibility. Though no practical measures have been adopted to enforce this policy, major decisions have been taken at the All Pakistan Tibbi Conference which was recently held under the chairmanship of the President of Pakistan. A special Advisory Board was appointed to: (*a*) review the Unani, Ayurvedic and Homoeopathic Practitioners Act, 1965, and recommend suitable amendments; (*b*) re-examine the report of the Indigenous Medicine Commission, 1975, and formulate necessary recommendations as seems appropriate; and (*c*) study the medical, legal and other aspects which empower *tabibs* (traditional practitioners) to issue medical certificates.

Another Board has been set up to review the working of existing Tibbi colleges and to make recommendations for improvements and provincial extension. Other important recommendations included the development of Tibbi hospitals and dispensaries especially in rural areas; utilization of the services of appropriately selected *tabibs* and the establishment of a Tibbi

Research Institute to organize and supervise relevant studies in this field.

From this it is clear that increasing official support has been given in Pakistan to the promotion and enhancement of traditional medicine which is regulated under an established system of registration and licensure.

The situation is different, however, in the majority of the countries. In Afghanistan, Iran, Oman, Somalia and the Sudan, for example, there is no registration, licensure or certification for traditional practitioners. The *attar* (herbalist) in these countries, however, needs to obtain a licence and it is not uncommon to find herbal medicine dispensed at a traditional drug store adjacent to a modern pharmacy.

Community attitude

Traditional medicine in these countries, as in other parts of the world, is firmly based within the local sociocultural context and is therefore readily accepted by the community.

The traditional healer is usually an active member of the community; he speaks the native language and is easily available to his clientele. This obviously facilitates the practitioner–patient relationship and helps in the therapeutic situation. The healing process is often carried out in an atmosphere of mutual confidence and shared expectations. It is therefore not surprising that the failures of traditional practitioners are often rationalized and calmly accepted.

In the assessment and analysis of diseases, traditional practitioners in some countries such as the Sudan divide the medical problems into two major categories—those which are treatable in hospitals and those which are manageable by community healers. The former are often referred for treatment by medical professionals. However, due to the lack of an organizational framework, there is hardly any feedback of information to the traditional practitioner. Clearly this constitutes a major defect in the functional unity of health care.

Manpower resources in traditional medicine

Categories of traditional practitioners

There are a variety of names by which traditional practitioners are designated. Popular names include the *hakim* (medical practitioner), the *attar* (herbal seller), the *mullah*, the *fekki*, the *sheikh* (religious healer), the *kujur* (medicine man), the *mutawae* (volunteer), the *daya* or *dai* (midwife), the *mujabirati* (bonesetter), and, under various names, the barber.

In present-day terminology, traditional practitioners can be briefly categorized as follows:

—the *hakim* as the medical practitioner
—the *attar* as the pharmacist

—the religious and medicine man as the psychotherapist
—the bonesetter as the orthopaedic surgeon.

The designated names are generally interesting and culturally meaningful. In the United Arab Emirates, for example, the *mutawae* is usually a religious teacher or leader. Etymologically, it is interesting to note that this name seems to be derived from the Arabic word *mutatawae* which means to volunteer for action (*3*) and this corresponds to the state of early Arab physicians as well as the majority of traditional practitioners who practice the art of healing as volunteers and serve the community on a self-elected basis.

Traditional techniques

The traditional practitioner generally relies on what he sees and observes or what he hears from the patient and his family. The diagnosis is essentially based on general observations and history taking. Usually no resort is had to medical instruments or to laboratory tests to establish a diagnosis.

The techniques used in treatment can be broadly grouped under physical remedies, social and psychotherapeutic practices. The physical remedies are mainly the prescription of certain diets, the use of drugs and chemicals, cautery, simple surgical operations, bonesetting, massage, hydrotherapy, cupping, blood-letting, etc.

There are also a variety of social and psychotherapeutic practices. Apart from community support, traditional techniques may involve an elaborate process of social analysis to establish the underlying causal factors, prior to the prescription of the course of action to be taken (*4*). The psychotherapeutic practices may be simple devices for protection or may entail a complex group interaction and abreactive measures. The ancient cultural *Zar* cult, for example, is a psychodramatic technique based on musical therapy and group activity (*1*).

Number of traditional practitioners

The only available statistical data are for the traditional birth attendants (TBA) (*5*), and even these are limited. They nevertheless indicate the important role TBAs play in maternal and child care services. It has been found, for example, that in rural areas TBAs attend to approximately 99% of mothers in Pakistan, 80% in Iraq, 60% in Iran and 50% in Egypt.

At country level, with the exception of a few countries such as Pakistan, only rough estimates of the number of traditional practitioners are available. On the whole there is an extremely wide variation between countries. For example, while it is reported that the role of traditional practitioners in medical care in Cyprus is negligible, it is estimated that in Somalia about two-thirds of the population are served by them.

In Pakistan, where there is regular registration, a clear picture is obtainable of the traditional manpower resources. Traditional practitioners are classified in three categories, namely hakims, ayurvedic practitioners and homoeopaths. Under the 1965 Act, all these have been granted registration and the records in 1979 show that there were 34 258 hakims, 19 903 homoeopaths and 439 vaids engaged in the practice of traditional medicine. It is important to note that there are approximately 14 000 conventional doctors in the country providing health care to a population of more than 70 millions. These figures indicate a sharp difference in manpower resources between the traditional and the conventional systems of medicine. Furthermore, the great majority of the medical professionals are located in urban centres and their services cover approximately one-fifth of the population. On the other hand, the traditional practitioners work independently from the official health system, mostly in rural areas and mainly as primary health workers.

Training in traditional medicine

In recent years serious concern has been shown for the development of traditional manpower resources and the improvement of practitioners' knowledge and skill through training. Naturally, questions are raised regarding the objectives of training, the type of workers to be trained, how to select them, who should select them, what should be the content and duration of the training programme, what are the most appropriate methods and media of training, and who should be responsible for the training.

Obviously, however, as the experience and conditions of countries differ, so does the training programme. Models of other countries must be appropriately modified and adapted to local conditions for, as has been rightly pointed out, they may not be "transportable". Even in countries well known for their vast experience in training traditional health workers, such as China, it is advocated that training programmes should be different for different parts of the country to suit local needs and conditions (6, 7).

Although there are no organized training programmes for traditional practitioners in a number of countries, others have a long and rich historical background in the field of training. In the training of TBAs, for example, several countries have developed practical and relevant programmes. Indeed, in some of them innovative approaches have been introduced.

The experience of the Sudan and the model developed there seem extremely interesting. In 1921, training of TBAs was initiated in the Sudan and two village midwives were selected for this purpose. The number was gradually increased and the method applied in training was simple, practical and pragmatic. It was based on the systematic learning process of "demonstration and repetition". The illiterate TBAs were taught to recognize drugs, for example, by sight, smell or taste, and their equipment consisted of simple, readily available household items. Very soon the training programme became popular and the centre was developed into a recognized school of midwifery. During the period 1950 to 1975, 3889 village midwives were successfully trained, officially registered and regularly provided with special field kits containing the appropriate equipment and the necessary drugs. It was through this practical and proper approach that it was possible to extend maternal and child care to rural areas and effectively penetrate into remote areas of the country.

Another example of training of TBAs can be seen in Afghanistan, where the *dais* are trained for three weeks in the care of pregnant mothers and safe delivery techniques. They are also trained for two weeks in child care. The training is provided by mobile training teams and in district towns close to the *dai*'s home. Some 600 TBAs have undergone this training and it is planned to train about 1000 *dais* every year for the next five years.

Formal training of traditional practitioners has been exceptionally well developed in Pakistan. At present, there are 17 recognized teaching schools in the country. Ten of these are for teaching the Tibbi system and 7 for the homoeopathic system of medicine. The duration of the course is 4 years during which, in addition to training in traditional medicine, the students are oriented in basic sciences, particularly anatomy, physiology and modern materia medica. From each of these teaching institutions 20-60 students graduate annually and the number will increase when these colleges, as recently recommended, have been extended to other provinces.

Apart from formal training, traditional medicine in several countries is learnt by apprenticeship and association with leading practitioners. There are several reference books, such as *The Canon of Medicine* by Avicenna, which provide resourceful knowledge and practical example in the field.

Of special interest are the reference books on herbal medicines and drugs. Historically, much effort has gone into the collection, identification, production and use of herbal medicines. The number of medicinal plants, mineral substances and animal products is inexhaustible and a variety of classical works provide useful background as learning material and for consultation. Valuable contributions have been made to traditional pharmacopoeia by pioneer workers such as Al Biruni (*8*), Al Bitar, Al Attar, Al Antaki and others. All these reference books include useful compilations on medicinal plants and still form rich sources of information.

Research activities

General

Research activities in the field of traditional medicine have been neglected to a great extent. In recent years, however, more interest has been shown and a number of individuals and various university centres have been actively involved in research studies on traditional medicine, including its history, philosophical background, chemistry and pharmacology, and on traditional pharmacopoeias.

Medicinal plants

The growing literature on medicinal plants in several countries clearly indicates the potential resources and the growing movement in this direction (*9, 10*). The list of medicinal plants used in eastern medicine (*11*) is highly impressive and forms a useful basis for future studies.

As a result of the evolving activities in phytochemical studies on medicinal plants, new therapeutic agents have been isolated, identified and usefully produced. Workers in Egypt, for example, have successfully investigated pharmacological substances in a number of traditionally known medicinal plants. *Khellin*, for example was isolated from *Ammi visnaga* and has been effectively used in the treatment of angina pectoris and renal colic.

Investigations of other medicinal plants such as *Nigella sativa* (Habbat El Baraka) and *Cymbopogon proximus* have yielded useful therapeutic agents which are now commercially processed.

Several research centres in Iran, Pakistan, Somalia, the Sudan and other countries have been involved in systematic studies of medicinal plants and encouraging results have been obtained.

A promising model for intercountry cooperation in this respect is the collaborative programme between Egypt and the Sudan. Steps which have been recently taken have strengthened the evolving programme and opened up new possibilities for future research activities.

The role of WHO in the promotion and development of research

At its second meeting held in Alexandria in 1977, the WHO Regional Advisory Committee on Biomedical Research approved a statement by the Regional Director, Dr A. H. Taba, that "one of the resources of the Region which had received scant attention until now was the area of traditional medicine". It was recommended that possibilities of research into means of associating traditional healers with the network of health services delivery should be explored.

As a follow-up to this recommendation, a research programme in traditional medicine was initiated with the following objectives:

(1) Promotion of collection of baseline information on traditional practitioners, diseases known and successfully treated by traditional healers, traditional herbal medicine and pharmacopoeia, literary and bibliographical sources, etc.

(2) Promotion of traditional medicine in health care services, with special emphasis on primary health care. There are several possibilities such as selection of essential medicinal plants and development of proven and useful techniques, such as acupuncture.

(3) Development of special programmes:

(*a*) Educational programme. This aims at general community orientation, dissemination of appropriate information and promotion of favourable positive attitudes towards traditional medicine.

(*b*) Manpower development. This implies the development of relevant training programmes for traditional medicine workers with a view to promoting their knowledge and skill and maximizing their contribution in health care.

As an initial step, a structured questionnaire for the collection of baseline information on traditional medicine was developed and distributed to potential research workers and to the authorities concerned in 20 countries of the Region.

The responses from the countries are being analysed at the time of writing, and the findings processed. Subsequently, micro-case studies on specific areas and on practical issues, along the lines which have already been indicated, will be undertaken.

One of the challenging issues, and one which has often been raised, is the possibility of effective integration of traditional medicine into primary health care. Though this is highly desirable, it will depend on finding a proper solution to a number of problems. Some of these are:

(*a*) The nature of the organizational relation between the conventional and traditional system of medicine.

(*b*) To whom are traditional practitioners to be responsible and accountable; how to assess their credibility and acceptability in the community; and who should supervise their work.

(*c*) The extent to which community development mobilizes and supports the integration between the two systems.

(*d*) The establishment of priorities in health care which can be provided by traditional practitioners, and its economic aspects.

(*e*) The transfer of appropriate health technology to improve the quality and extend the scope of traditional health practice.

The research programme sponsored by the WHO Regional Office for the Eastern Mediterranean aims at determining the right approaches to these problems in order that traditional medicine may be optimally utilized. It is envisaged that a realistic and practical programme, based on the findings and recommendations emanating from country studies and regional meetings, will be developed for the effective use of the potential resources in traditional medicine and for the better extension and appropriate promotion of health care.

REFERENCES

(*1*) HOWELLS, J. G., ed. *World history of psychiatry.* New York, Bruner/Mazel, 1975.
(*2*) WORLD HEALTH ORGANIZATION. *Global Strategy for health for all by the year 2000.* Geneva, 1981 ("Health for All" Series No. 3).

(3) IBN MANZOUR, A. G. M. *Lisan el Arab* [The tongue of the Arab]. Beirut, Dar Sadir, 1956.
(4) BAASHER, T. A. Traditional treatment of psychiatric disorders in Africa. *African journal of psychiatry*, 1:77–85 (1975).
(5) VERDERESE, M. DE L. & TURNBULL, L. M. *The traditional birth attendant in maternal and child health and family planning*, Geneva, World Health Organization, 1975 (WHO Offset Publications No. 18).
(6) RONAGHY, H. A. & SOLTER, S. Is the Chinese barefoot doctor exportable to rural Iran? *Lancet*, June 29 1974: 1331–1333.
(7) HUANG YU-HSIANG The training of barefoot doctors. In: Hetzel, B. S., ed. *Basic health care in developing countries: an epidemiological perspective*. Oxford University Press, 1978, pp. 128–136.
(8) SAID, H. M., ed. *Al Biruni's book on pharmacy and materia medica (Kitab el Saydanah fi al Tibb)*. Karachi, Hamdard National Foundation, 1973.
(9) RIAD, A. & MACKSAD, A. *Medicinal plants in Kuwait*. Kuwait, Assriya Printing Press, 1974.
(10) KHAN, A. H. ET AL. *A note on the plants of medicinal value found in Pakistan*. Karachi, Government of Pakistan Press, 1957.
(11) SAID, H. M., ed. *Hamdard pharmacopoeia of eastern medicine*. Karachi, Institute of Health and Tibbi Research, 1969.

CHAPTER 25

The Western Pacific Region*

This review does not pretend to be exhaustive with respect either to the countries of the Western Pacific Region or to the many variations of traditional medicine which are currently in use. Nevertheless, it remains apparent that traditional medicine is respected and extensively used by the people of the Region, who often prefer it in particular types of sickness on account of deep-rooted beliefs or family experience, and in view of the relatively high cost of modern medicine and its limited accessibility. Governments, which are now showing appreciation for the value and contribution of some forms of traditional medicine in primary health care, are taking steps to identify and train its practitioners as well as to verify the pharmacological effectiveness of cheap and easily obtained local herbal remedies. The tools of modern scientific research are also being used to explore the nature of the psychophysiological mechanisms underlying traditional healing procedures and to attempt to explain their known therapeutic value.

The various systems of traditional medicine in the countries of the Region share several characteristics, including a long history usually dating back many centuries. The resources in medical plants are rich, especially in the subtropical and tropical zones, although their development in different countries is unequal. However, while accepted by the general population and particularly popular among the rural inhabitants, traditional medicine is often rejected or ignored by modern medical practitioners and by the more affluent and educated classes in some countries.

Practices observed in countries of the Region follow one of two patterns. One model is highly institutionalized, with formal academic training in a variety of disciplines in recognized schools, professional associations and official recognition. The Chinese system follows this pattern, and has been

---

* Regional contribution compiled by Dr Kuang An Kun, Consultant, WHO Regional Office for the Western Pacific, Manila, Philippines.

widely practised for many centuries. Some of its methods, notably acupuncture, are being increasingly used by practitioners trained in Western medicine. Chinese medicine has been characterized by a strong adaptive tendency and a growing concern for research to identify and validate the physiological bases of its practices.

Hindu medicine follows a similar pattern, involving the rational use of naturalistic theory to organize and interpret systematic empirical observations. It is widely practised in only a few countries of the Region. Ayurveda is the leading branch of Hindu medicine, practised to a significant degree in those countries to which substantial numbers of people from the Indian subcontinent have migrated—Malaysia, Singapore, Fiji and to a small extent Australia.

The second pattern is less well-defined and institutionalized but nevertheless deeply rooted in the culture of the particular community in which it is practised. In these forms of traditional medicine, common among South Pacific peoples and rural populations in the Philippines and Malaysia, formal training does not exist. Procedures usually consist of secret herbal remedies, ceremonial rites, incantations, sorcery, bone manipulation and massage. Official recognition is seldom accorded to its practitioners but there is a growing interest by governments in studying the contribution which they make to health care delivery and their possible integration into primary health care.

Traditional healers in the Region

Many kinds of practitioners are found in the Region. Their role in primary health care is most obvious in the underserved rural communities and among the poor in the larger cities, but very little documented information is available regarding their methods or effectiveness. It is true that the shortage of health manpower is most acute in these localities but there is also an important element of cultural choice in the selection of a traditional healer in preference to a modern Western trained physician or nurse. Often the healer is an important, respected and perhaps admired or feared personality having the same ethnic and sociocultural characteristics as the patient. His fees are relatively low and his methods are socially approved and well regarded. He does not ask difficult or embarrassing questions and does not resort to hospitalization of his patients in most cases.

Healers exert their skills in a number of specialist areas. They may be herbalists, acupuncturists, bonesetters, midwives, psychic or ritualistic practitioners or magicians. Some are highly trained, others claim special powers, while some derive their skills from family inheritance or apprenticeship to acknowledged masters.

Their integration into governmental health care programmes has been close and effective in China and in countries where Chinese medicine is widely used. Traditional birth attendants have been officially recognized in many countries and modern training provided, and they have been incorporated into the primary health care approach of governments. Often, however, official recognition of the traditional healer is hampered by inadequate communication, educational problems, and professional and community attitudes, which tend to be negative toward the traditional practitioner.

There is a growing awareness that many traditional healers exhibit considerable skill in diagnosis, minor surgery, drug therapy, psychosocial management and perinatal care. The need to utilize the prestige, skill and close community contact of the healer in the prevention of disease and impairment is being increasingly recognized, and has been encouraged by the success in training traditional birth attendants, who are now well accepted as members of the primary health care team.

The Chinese system of traditional medicine[1]

Traditional Chinese medicine is a great treasure-house with profound experience and knowledge accumulated through thousands of years. It has a theoretical system of its own. The human body is considered as a single entity, all the organs being interrelated functionally and pathologically in the case of disturbances. The traditional Chinese concept of the universe conceives of the elemental forces yin-yang and *wuxing* as being in harmonious balance. Yin and yang are seen as opposing and interlocking dynamic forces which complement each other and remain in a state of permanent change. Excesses create imbalance and consequently disease. All branches of traditional Chinese philosophy, including medicine, are dominated by this concept of the harmonious balance of elements. The doctrine of yin-yang, together with the influence of *wuxing*, the five elements—wood, fire, earth, metal and water—are factors in this balance.

The concept of *zang fu* (internal organs) and *jing luo* (channels and collaterals) is another factor. The twelve meridians bear the names of twelve organs associated with the flow of *qi*, a vital force that circulates in the human body through the meridians. It is believed that the continuous and undisturbed flow of *qi* promotes health and that, should the flow be broken at any point, one organ will have an excess of *qi* while another will be deficient. Acupuncture at particular points along the twelve meridians aims to restore the flow of *qi*. Further, it is believed that, by stimulating the appropriate meridian, yin or yang can be stimulated. Numerous herbs are thought to be imbued with special properties which help to restore the balance when disturbance, manifested as illness, occurs. For example, herbs may be prescribed to make up a deficiency of yang or to aid the fire element against the water element. An inspection of any traditional Chinese

---

[1] See also Chapter 6.

pharmacy reveals the vast number of drugs derived from plants, animals and minerals, which are selected for use under various conditions.

Chinese medicine has been much concerned with prevention as well as treatment. Therapy often resorts to modification of the patient's diet, surroundings and associations. In clinical practice, the principle of *bianzheng shizhi* or the determination of treatment according to different conditions, is stressed. Early diagnosis and management of organic disease are also accorded considerable importance. Hygienic principles proscribing unwholesome or uncooked food and unboiled water and encouraging regular bathing have from the earliest times sought to deal with environmental health problems. Besides herbal medicine and acupuncture, many other types of treatment are also widely used, e.g. bonesetting, breathing exercises, cupping, massage and manipulations.

It is generally recognized in China that some of the most important modern medical developments can be credited to early traditional practitioners. For example, the relationship of endemic goitre to drinking-water was known and described in China well over 2000 years ago and there are records of the administration of seaweed rich in iodine to cure goitre. Diabetes was also a recognized and clearly described disease at that time. Herbal anaesthesia was first used in performing abdominal operations by Dr Hua To in the 2nd century of the present era by mixing herbal powder with wine.

Traditional medicine in China today

The integration of traditional medicine with Western medicine is one of the major policies in China's national health development. Great efforts have been made towards the development of an integrated system of new medicine.

Doctors of Western medicine are encouraged to learn traditional medicine, while doctors of traditional medicine learn the strong points of Western medicine. Young and middle-aged doctors are assigned to assist and learn from veteran traditional physicians. All of them aim to inherit and systematize the rich experience of traditional medicine and to explore and raise it to a higher level. Most health workers at various levels have been trained to use both systems for the prevention and treatment of diseases, particularly in the rural areas.

China recognizes that the scientific achievements of modern medicine, like those of traditional medicine, began with very simple methods of treatment, and developed through empirical experience. In both systems, herbs, minerals or insects were commonly used for their observed pharmacological properties. As time went on, early medicine was gradually replaced by a more scientific discipline, based on new theories and following new methods of investigation. The invention of microscopy opened a new era in physiology, pathology and related sciences. Advances in biochemistry led to the development of endocrinology, synthesis of hormones and other drugs of great potency, and modern laboratory methods made possible the detection of minute quantities of hormones, drugs or other substances in blood, tissue and body fluids. A similar development pattern is now being used in the scientific study and development of Chinese traditional medicine, and links are being forged between the two systems. Much progress has already been achieved in theoretical studies of traditional medicine, applying modern scientific research.

The concept of yin and yang has been, for many, difficult to accept, just as humoral theories of health and disease have been largely abandoned by modern medicine. However, some work has been performed in China in an attempt to find a scientific basis for yin and yang by animal experimentation. In one study, groups of mice were given cortisone in high dosage, with severe effects on protein metabolism and general health. Other groups of mice received similar dosage of cortisone plus decoctions of yang-stimulating drugs and were found to remain in good health. Control groups to which both cortisone and modern anabolic drugs were administered presented a better picture than the first-mentioned experimental group but were more adversely affected than the groups given the yang-stimulating drugs.

Chinese endocrinological research in humans has also suggested that hormones and enzymes with mutually antagonistic characteristics may play a part in physiological imbalance and disease.

Good results have also been noted in clinical and laboratory studies of some principles of treatment in traditional medicine. For example, by using the principle *huolitueh huahu* (invigoration of circulation to relieve blood stasis), remarkable improvements have been observed in the treatment of coronary heart disease, scleroderma, rheumatoid arthritis, etc.

Acupuncture.[1] From ancient times, acupuncture treatment has been widely used in China. More than 300 diseases can be treated by acupuncture and moxibustion, of which about 100 show marked therapeutic results. The mechanisms of its functioning have been systematically studied and are now better understood. Acupuncture anaesthesia is estimated to have been used in about 2 million surgical operations. Effective surgical anaesthesia is achieved in 20–30 kinds of operative procedures.

Standardization of technique and terminology is being actively promoted in the practice of acupuncture and moxibustion. Variations in nomenclature and in anatomical description of meridians and acupuncture points have been common both within China and in countries where Chinese traditional medicine is extensively practised. Research projects are now being pursued with WHO technical collaboration to establish an internationally agreed nomenclature.

Herbal drugs. Major research programmes are also being directed

---

[1] See also Chapter 7.

towards the study of traditional herbal drugs, particularly by evaluation of therapeutic effects and scientific promotion of the production of known pharmacologically active preparations.

Continuous study of medicinal plants and research into traditional Chinese and folk medicine have been carried out in China so that the resources of herbal medicine and other traditional therapeutic procedures can be better documented and more fully utilized. Studies are also being undertaken on the cultivation of medicinal plants. Crude extracts are first made to test clinical effects as it has often been shown that the therapeutic effect of a total extract is more pronounced than, and quite different from, that of a single constituent.

Besides the traditional medical practices using Chinese medicines which are recorded in ancient pharmacopoeias and other classics, there is also a great deal of scattered knowledge in folk medicine which utilizes unrecorded medicinal plants of different localities. Certain findings arising from clinical practice have given rise to investigations with a view to generating an understanding of new drugs which may be used clinically in the future. Research institutes also seek to isolate active principles and elucidate their structure and biochemistry so that active constituents present in small amounts in a herb can be synthesized.

A notable development in recent years has been the development in China of training programmes in the English and French languages for foreign students. Many physicians and other health workers from all over the world have attended these courses in China with the assistance of the United Nations Development Programme and WHO. Study tours within China demonstrating traditional medicine at work in all its forms have also been provided for senior health officials from many countries.

Traditional Chinese medicine in other countries of the Region

The theory and practice of traditional Chinese medicine have been adopted and extended to include local variants and herbal pharmacopoeias in many countries of the Region, including the Lao People's Democratic Republic, Japan, Malaysia, Republic of Korea, Singapore, and Viet Nam. China, however, remains the greatest single resource of expertise and has retained its historical approach which favours constant exploration and revision of traditional methods.

Viet Nam. The system of traditional healing which is extensively practised in Viet Nam was derived from Chinese medicine but has been modified over the years to include a large local herbal formulary and Vietnamese methods of diagnosis and physical therapy. A special form of gymnastics is also in use.

Government policy is to integrate traditional and modern medicine and an intensive research programme has been mounted to identify and test useful traditional healing methods in the national health care delivery programme. About 20 000 traditional healers are recognized by the health services and many clinics and hospitals have been established both in urban and rural areas. A proportion of beds in modern hospitals has been reserved for traditional therapy. Traditional medicine is taught in all six faculties of medicine in Viet Nam and, in addition, there are a number of national and provincial institutions providing lengthy courses in traditional medicine. In the provision of traditional health services, priority has been assigned to the common acute diseases, but extensive use is also being made of traditional methods in treating chronic diseases, such as collagen diseases and asthma, which are often resistant to modern medical treatment. Wide use is also being made of acupuncture for surgical anaesthesia.

More than 1000 indigenous plants are known to be pharmacologically active. Studies of their geographical distribution, cultivation and active constituents, and of therapeutic experience concerning them are being carried out. To promote the production of useful medicinal plants identified by these studies 5000 gardens have been established. Many pharmacies prepare and distribute plant preparations, although standaridization of products is not yet established. Much of this research work is being carried out by the National Institute of Vietnamese Traditional Medicine, which has been functioning since 1961. It has a large staff and a considerable budget, which enables it to undertake large-scale research in clinical application, pharmacology and production methods. A second research institution was opened in Ho Chi-Minh City in 1975.

Malaysia. Traditional Chinese medicine in Malaysia follows the classical concepts and therapeutic practices, including acupuncture, moxibustion and the therapeutic use of numerous herbs and some products of animal origin. Modernization of drugs and other research developments are closely followed by Chinese physicians in Malaysia. Medicinal teas are very popular for sickness prevention. The dispensing of drugs is carried out by a variety of people, including street "tea sellers", herbalists and trained Chinese physicians. Patients usually view the various medical systems available in Malaysia, including modern medicine, as complementary rather than antagonistic, and move freely from one system to another in their search for relief and cure. This is particularly so for those suffering from severe or chronic illness, regardless of ethnic background.

Four-year training courses for Chinese medicine practitioners are freely available in Malaysia and four schools of traditional medicine are available for this purpose.

Republic of Korea. Three universities provide formal training in traditional medicine and more than 3000 practitioners are licensed. Their practice is widely recognized although they do not form part of the governmental health care services. Very great reliance is placed on herbal medicine for the prevention of many degenerative diseases such as gastrointestinal disorders and hypertension. A regionwide revival of interest in Korean traditional drugs has led to modernization of the production of many of the older preparations. Manufacturing enterprises now produce pills and other convenient forms of traditional medicines for both the home and export markets.

Japan. Traditional Chinese medicine has been practised in Japan for over 1000 years and has, like Vietnamese medicine, developed its own national variation (*kampo*). It has gained strength in recent times parallel with the development of modern medicine. Reasons for this increased popularity seem to include a widespread feeling that *kampo* drugs are free from the adverse side effects which are known sometimes to follow modern drug therapy. Also the very personal approach of the *kampo* practitioner is attractive to patients, whereas the increasing specialization of modern medicine and its advanced technology are less supportive to Japanese psychological needs in health and disease. In *kampo* medicine, great importance is attached to the patient's complaints and concerns and not so much to precision of diagnosis.

In recent years, traditional drugs have been extensively studied in Japan using the methods of the natural sciences. Japanese scientists have also been interested in the electrophysiological relationships between the meridian system of acupuncture and the pathophysiology of internal organs. As in China, significant findings are emerging from these studies, some of which tend to support the practical everyday experience that therapeutic results follow the use of traditional methods in a number of conditions.

Practitioners of *kampo* medicine in Japan must first be licensed in modern medicine. Acupuncturists are however permitted to practise without medical licensure and are viewed as allied health professionals. A proportion of them are blind as acupuncture has been viewed as a suitable occupation for the blind.

Folk and tribal medicine in the Philippines and rural Malaysia

Extensive though the spread of Chinese traditional medicine has been, it has not penetrated every country, nor has it displaced ancient and socially accepted folk medicine in a number of countries. The Philippines and rural Malaysia possess particularly rich and varied traditions of herbal medicine as well as numerous healers, who receive no recognizable formal training but are respected for their powers of physical and psychological therapy.

The Philippines

The value of medicinal plants (herbal medicines) is acknowledged by the Government and the use of bioassayed local medicinal herbs is being promoted nationally as part of the effort to reduce dependence on expensive imported drugs and thereby reduce the cost of medicines to the State. To ensure that sufficient emphasis is placed on this, the Ministry of Health is planning a Bureau of Herbal Medicines. In the meantime, rural health units and *barangay* health stations have begun to establish small medicinal plant gardens.

The National Science Development Board of the Ministry of Science, has funded a five-year research programme, the Integrated Medicinal Plants Programme, now in its fourth year of operation. Part of its official contribution has been to set aside two 200-hectare sites in Mindoro and Zamboanga for the cultivation of medicinal and pesticidal plants.

Over 10 000 species of higher plants are to be found in the Philippines. Of these over 1000 have been used as herbal medicines by *herbolarios*. The most authoritative work on potential medicinal plants lists nearly 1000 species of medicinal plants, 63 of which are listed in various pharmacopoeias.

Healers in the Philippines practise a number of skills; they include *hilots* (traditional birth attendants), *herbolarios* (general healers), faith and other quasi-religious healers, acupuncturists and acupressure practitioners, and *medicos* (healers who combine the traditional system of healing with modern medicine).

Hilots. It is estimated that there are some 40 000 *hilots* (traditional birth attendants) in the Philippines. The Government has been active in providing training of *hilots* to augment the present health manpower of the country by attaching them to the health team. This has also helped to wean them from harmful or potentially dangerous practices. Gradually, the Government aims to replace *hilots* with trained midwives but this will not be possible for some considerable time. The broad objectives of *hilot* training are: recognition by the *hilots* of the importance of their role in the care of the child-bearing woman and her newborn infant; discontinuance of beliefs and practices that directly or indirectly endanger the health of the mother and child; and recognition of high-risk cases for timely referral. The Government hopes that acquisition of knowledge and skills will lead to the safer handling of maternity cases, and better care for the newborn and young infant. Nutrition and family planning are also taught as integral components of maternal and child care, with special emphasis on the prevention of neonatal tetanus.

Herbolarios. The *herbolario* is the Philippine "general practitioner" of traditional medicine and is well versed in the use of medicinal plants. He performs procedures for diagnosis and treatment and deals with both natural and supernatural illnesses. Unlike the *hilots*, *herbolarios* have never been nationally surveyed or trained under government auspices, and much less is known about their training, backgrounds or practice. Nevertheless, it is estimated that there are about 100 000 *herbolarios* in the Philippines. About 50% of the population is thought to utilize the *herbolario* before consulting a modern physician. *Herbolarios* are known to refer patients to one another as well as to modern physicians. They do not usually keep consultation hours and are on call throughout the day and night. They do not charge fees but accept token gifts and cash according to the means of the patient and family. They may diagnose and treat patients at a distance, on the basis of the history supplied by a relative. Some *herbolarios* rarely use herbs but tend to rely on special oils used for anointment, accompanied by prayers and the laying on of hands. There are no official plans to register or train *herbolarios* and attach them to existing health teams.

Faith healers and other quasi-religious healers. Many faith healers practise in the Philippines. A small elitist group is located in the mountains in and around Baguio catering largely for foreign tourists. The majority of faith healers cater for the local population; they are estimated to number about 1000. They vary in their styles of practice, some performing psychic surgery and psychic anaesthesia for dental extraction. Nearly all claim supernatural powers. The majority are full-time practitioners and will attend to all illnesses, particularly the chronic and "incurable".

Another type of quasi-religious healer is the *magluluop* (diviner), who specializes in diagnosing illness through rituals using the smoke of burning alum or incense. Finally there is the *manggagaway* (magician), who reputedly possesses supernatural powers to cause harm. Naturally, few will admit that they are *manggagaways*, nevertheless, they are also reputed to heal.

There is no official recognition of faith healers and other quasi-religious healers, nor are there plans to utilize them.

Acupuncturists. The Professional Regulation Commission of the Philippines has ruled that acupuncture may be performed only by trained physicians and then only for research. A number of physicians, both private and governmental, have received training in acupuncture. However, ethnic Chinese in Manila and elsewhere have always practised acupuncture and continue to do so although their practice is restricted to other ethnic Chinese. In accordance with the ruling of the Professional Regulation Commission, they may not legally practise acupuncture for other patients.

Medicos. In certain places, the people use this Spanish word to describe healers who combine traditional and modern medicine. Many were peasants who started as *herbolarios* and subsequently received some basic training in modern medicine, perhaps while they were medical orderlies in the army. There are no clear estimates but they are thought to number several thousands in certain parts of the Philippines. About half of their prescriptions comprise solely modern medicines, the remainder being either traditional medicines or a combination of the two. Officially, the use of modern medicines, particularly antibiotics, by *medicos* is not permitted.

Rural Malaysia

While the majority of the population are Malay (46.8%) or Chinese (34.1%), the nation is characterized by wide ethnic diversity. A similar diversity of traditional medical systems also exists, including Malay, Indian and Chinese folk medicine.

All Malay traditional healing variants are based on a concept of soul substance or *semangat*. Disease is thought to be the result of one or more of three factors—predisposing factors, supernatural causes and physical causes. Predisposing factors include the loss of the vital soul substance, *semangat*, which may lead to possession by evil forces or diminished capacity to handle otherwise normal nutritional or environmental problems. Some foods as well as socially incorrect behaviour are also thought to predispose individuals and their families to sickness. Supernatural causes include *hantu* (malevolent spirits), witchcraft, and "the will of God". In this group, the Malay includes the *badi*, some supernatural aura that emanates from slain animals and men. The *badi* is reputedly able to cause illness when it enters a person's body. Physical causes include certain poisonous foods, perhaps fish which is reputed to cause worms, heat and cold, "wind" which may cause swellings, vegetable poisons, physical trauma, *kuman* (a distorted notion of the germ theory), and organic impairment as in the case of epileptics and senile persons.

Traditional Malay healers (*bomoh*) and traditional birth attendants use a variety of therapies, which can be classified in four groups. The first group includes simple rituals such as incantations and spells to identify the cause of sickness, most often of a supernatural nature, and to exorcise it. In the second group are more elaborate rituals or psychodramas in which the healer, the patient and assistants as well as musicians perform a play, helping the sick person to organize his chaotic symptoms into an orderly pattern. The third category includes the use of herbs, of which there are many, and the last group includes physical therapies such as bonesetting, cupping, labour management and postpartum care. Epidemic illnesses are dealt with by elaborate community ceremonies, sacrifices and special offerings to the spirits.

Among the Indian community in Malaysia, extensive use is made of the various systems of Indian traditional medicine, Ayurveda, Unani, Siddha and homoeopathy, but Ayurveda is perhaps the most common. Like Chinese medicine, Ayurveda postulates that the organism, human and animal, exists in a balance of elements, imbalance causing disease. Poor nutrition, excess of wastes, or disturbance of the circulating fluids and vital organs are the primary causes to which therapy must be applied, both in prevention and cure.

The *vade mecum* of ayurvedic drugs which are used in these systems is very extensive and some may only be used by certain healers. Indian traditional medicines are imported into Malaysia from the many manufacturing pharmacies in India.

Unlike the numerous and varied healers practising folk medicine in the Philippines and Malaysia, practitioners of Ayurveda and the other Hindu healing systems receive lengthy formal training in colleges in India, most of which are affiliated to universities. Qualifications for admission are similar to those required of medical students. In addition to lengthy basic training, postbasic institutions also exist, particularly for Ayurveda.

Malaysia is thus of special interest as it possesses two of the three great systems of traditional medicine (Arabic, Hindu and Chinese) as well as an extensive network of folk medicine and village healers.

Folk and tribal medicine in the South Pacific

All island countries of the South Pacific have considerable numbers of healers who employ methods similar to those used in the Philippines and Malaysia, although each country has individual variants of both healing practices and drugs.

Papua New Guinea

The National Health Plan (1974–1978) in Papua New Guinea categorized traditional beliefs and practices affecting health and disease into those which are of value in maintaining and promoting health and which need to be preserved, those which lead neither to ill health nor to improved health and need only to be noted, and those which lead to ill health and need to be changed. It also recognizes that many valuable beliefs and practices are being displaced by acceptance of Western ideas and practices.

Some fundamental research has been carried out in Papua New Guinea on traditional beliefs affecting health and disease but, in spite of considerable efforts, only a relatively small amount of information has been collected. The fact that there are at least 717 language groups in Papua New Guinea, each with its own customs and beliefs on almost every aspect of the cycle of life from birth to death including health and disease, indicates the vast quantity of information that remains to be catalogued. Further to complicate the issue, Papua New Guinea is perhaps one of the most rapidly changing areas in the world. The influence of different groups on one another, now made possible by the development of a lingua franca (chiefly, pidgin, English and Motu) and the effects of European contact, Christianity, the Second World War and independence, have brought major sociocultural changes that make beliefs and practices affecting health and disease an ever-changing scene.

Of the several components of traditional medicine considered important in Papua New Guinea, the promotion of beneficial traditional health practices in nutrition, and in particular concerning breast-feeding, has received the most official attention.

The majority of traditional medicaments in Papua New Guinea are of plant origin but medicines are sometimes brewed together with animal tissues, particularly pork, which are believed to be valuable adjuncts to treatment. A considerable amount of work to collect and identify the medicinal plants of Papua New Guinea has been carried out and, so far, 245 different species of plants used by traditional healers of Papua New Guinea have been botanically described.

Official policy recognizes that some traditional healers may be defective in their concepts of the causation of diseases and harmful in their practices, even sometimes deliberately endeavouring to cause as well as to cure disease. Consequently, there are no plans to arrange for the licensure or registration of traditional medicine men, but there are no moves to suppress traditional health care, the emphasis being on studies to evaluate the remedies used.

In Papua New Guinea, while common ailments and fevers are usually attributed to natural causes, most illnesses that afflict people in their prime are attributed to supernatural causes. The processes by which these causes can produce illnesses can be classified into three groups:

(*a*) those by which some morbific object or substance, for example a mixture of herbs, the exudate of a corpse, or the dead man's bones, has been projected into the victim's body;

(*b*) those by which something, such as the soul substance, has been abstracted from the victim's body;

(*c*) those by which the sorcerer acts on some part of the body of the victim or on some object which has had contact with the body of the victim, such as his hair, sweat, excrement, semen, remains of food or a piece of wood touched by the victim.

Social misbehaviour is also considered to be important in the causation of disease, which may be a consequence either of the sufferer's violation of a social or moral norm or of his having provoked someone into attacking him, usually through sorcery. Diagnosis is not based on physical symptoms and signs, but is related to social events at the time of sickness. Prognosis also is not related to signs and symptoms but to the likelihood of involvement of any sorcery.

Traditional healing methods are of two main types; one is concerned with counteracting the alien or evil power, while the other seeks to strengthen the sufferer's personal power. Techniques include consumption of therapeutic substances such as herbs or foods, application of herbs and sometimes tobacco smoke to the injured or painful part, purification or elimination of harmful substances by venesection or scarification, and catching the soul substance and enticing it to return into the victim's body.

The response to illness and death, which can hardly be called healing but is nevertheless associated with it, is revenge or "pay back". Relatives of the deceased may resort to sorcery to avenge the death. Consequently, traditional medicine in Papua New Guinea is associated not only with healing but with preventing attempts that cause illness and death.

A great deal of variation exists among healers in Papua New Guinea. In some smaller communities, traditional medicine cannot be distinguished from magic. In such circumstances, medicine men as such cannot be found; at the other extreme, particularly in more densely populated communities, traditional medicine is distinguishable as a special area of expertise. There may be specialists in sorcery, in divination and in healing. In some communities there are healers that specialize in malaria and fevers, or in contraception and abortion, or in bonesetting and wounds.

Many sick individuals will use modern drugs to relieve their pains, fever and other symptoms, and simultaneously seek the traditional medicine man to counteract the alien or evil powers and to augment their own personal power. Consequently, it is fairly common to find that patients admitted to hospitals will also use traditional medicine. It is also common to find a sick individual being guarded by one or two relatives in order to protect him from possible sorcery or harm from any adversary.

Even in hospital, it has been repeatedly observed that some individuals under proper treatment remain in poor condition and are unable to eat or drink as they sincerely believe that they are the victims of sorcery and as such cannot be adequately cured until the alien or evil power has been appropriately neutralized. Consequently, some physicians have permitted and even encouraged selected patients to seek the aid of traditional medicine men for their psychological support.

It can be assumed that the 3 out of 4 births that are not professionally supervised in Papua New Guinea are assisted by "untrained" birth attendants or are self-managed by the mother herself. Such births may proceed unassisted or the mother may receive the help of an older woman, often of her own family, or a traditional midwife.

Kiribati

In Kiribati, there is no clear distinction between laymen and professionals. All mature adults are supposed to have some knowledge of medicine. When some slides of plants are shown to people in appears that certain plant remedies are known to most of them. Moreover, the great majority of people have secret family remedies. A person who is regarded as an expert healer (*bakuaku*) would be one having an unusually good reputation as a healer and with a large number of secret remedies. However, with the drift from the outer islands to the urban centres, healers are emerging who depend for their livelihood mainly or even entirely on their therapeutic skills.

Most types of traditional art and technology are secret, including médicine. Knowledge of these techniques is considered private property and a high value is attached to them. They may, however, be exchanged, e.g., medical knowledge for fishing technique.

Two forms of physical therapy are used in Kiribati, one dealing with trauma to bones and joints and the other involving the use of massage in the diagnosis and treatment of conditions of general medical nature. Bonesetting tends to be practised as a specialty by certain healers, some with a considerable reputation, and people believe strongly in the superiority of traditional medicine for the treatment of fractures. Examination of some hospital records covering many years of both inpatients and outpatients showed few fracture cases, but the end results of poorly united fractures were not visible in the community.

For certain conditions, e.g., *te pabobo* (fever which may lead to jaundice), the healer massages the abdomen for diagnostic purposes. Parts of the body are also thought to be prone to malalignment; here massage, generally along the axis of the limbs, is both diagnostic and curative, and seeks to detect and realign any malalignment. *Te kaikeike* (asthma) is also treated by massage.

Knowledge of psychological medicine is possessed by only a small minority, perhaps by one or two people in each village. Most psychological illness is perceived as being basically different from physical disease, and is usually ascribed to the effect of *te ans* (ghosts or demons). Alternatively, they may be induced to exert their effect by a magician of evil intent. This is called *manibuog* and its signs include loss of appetite, sleepiness and timidity. The best magician supposedly can cure all magically induced mental disease, which may also present as an ordinary physical disease which fails to respond to other means.

Some preliminary work on the preparation of a catalogue of medicinal plants has already been carried out. However, secrecy about the preparation of medicinal plants is closely guarded. The use of plant preparations is usually accompanied by religious or other rituals to combat the ill effects of evil spirits.

The revival of traditional medicine, with Government support for activities integrated into primary health care, will be assisted by further government-sponsored studies on indigenous medicinal plants. As an initial step, it is intended to collect information on traditional healers and their mode of practice. It is thought that they number about 2000, for whom a programme of education consistent with the Government's health plans will be needed.

Fiji

As in Malaysia, Hindu, Chinese and folk medicine all flourish in Fiji, serving the corresponding ethnic groups which maintain their own traditions. There is little to be said of the formalized Hindu and Chinese medicine, which are not peculiar to Fiji. However, folk medicine among the Fijian ethnic population is worthy of some attention.

Traditional healers are active and numerous in all parts of the country and they attract many patients. As in the other South Pacific countries, healing is associated with the use of herbs, rituals, mysticism and various physical procedures. In their practice healers use either psychic and spiritual methods or solely physical and pharmacological methods. All use the drug *yaqona*. Massage is also frequently used to divine the cause of illness and to strengthen the organ's response to sickness. About 300 native plants are used as medicines, and are prepared as infusions or decoctions for oral administration.

Some of the estimated 500–1000 healers specialize in particular ailments but most deal with any medical or psychological condition that is presented. The majority are part-time healers and no formal training exists other than apprenticeship to a recognized healer.

The Government has taken the view that traditional healers must be taken seriously as one means of improving the health of the people. Meantime, it feels that much more research is needed into the practice of popular forms of healing, including the scientific study of the plants which are used.

WHO regional policies in the Western Pacific on traditional medicine

The Region is committed to collaborating with governments in increasing the utilization of those practitioners of traditional medicine whose practice can be validated in support of the goal of health for all by the year 2000. Efforts are being made to identify and study the pharmacologically active components of herbal remedies, to collaborate with countries in the compilation of schedules of effective drugs, and to encourage the standardization and production of those deemed valuable in the treatment of common disorders.

An important policy of the Region is to stimulate research and development in traditional medicine, and research institutes in China and Viet Nam are currently being supported. Finally, the training of traditional practitioners to increase their effectiveness, safety and integration in health care delivery systems is being actively encouraged.

The WHO Regional Office for the Western Pacific will continue to collaborate with Member States in the further development of traditional medicine, including programmes to share research findings, field experience and managerial studies. It may be expected that group educational experiences supported by WHO will increase during the next two decades as governments intensify their interest in making full use of the more effective healers and healing practices in their respective countries. A particular goal will be to strengthen existing training and research institutions for traditional medicine and, where these do not exist, to stimulate the interest of institutions of modern medicine in the study of appropriate traditional practices. The continuing study and classification of medicinal plants and their pharmacological properties must also be fostered. Finally, the Regional Office will encourage highly regarded and experienced traditional healers to participate in information-sharing publications and activities.

Part Four

Organizational and legal aspects of traditional medicine

CHAPTER 26
Organizational aspects

G. S. Mutalik[1]

In the preceding chapters, the role of traditional medicine in providing health care to the community and the various systems which survived the vicissitudes of history and are flourishing in different countries have been described. It is now widely recognized that there is a great potential in traditional medicine to contribute to primary health care, especially in developing countries. Such a potential is clearly due not only to the wide acceptance of these systems at the community level but also to their simple, inexpensive, non-toxic and time-tested remedies for the alleviation of disease and disability. Furthermore, the fact that vast numbers of formally and non-formally trained practitioners of traditional medicine live and work in remote rural communities underlines the need to consider seriously in what way they could be associated with primary health care for the attainment of the universal goal of health for all by the year 2000.

Aspects of organization

Efforts to organize traditional systems and to mobilize their vast untapped resources of healing practices for primary health care must take into account the following considerations.

These systems, in order to contribute usefully to primary health care, must be functionally integrated into the country's health system.

A thorough study should therefore be made of the prevailing traditional systems in their entirety—the type of system, the available manpower, the existing training programmes, including any linkage to the official health services, and the budgetary requirements. The identification of the areas of health care to which these systems can contribute effectively and problems

---

[1] Chief, Coordination with Other Organizations, Division of Coordination, World Health Organization, Geneva, Switzerland.

relating to their further development also require careful scrutiny. Such studies will entail a systematic, coordinated and broad-based national effort with appropriate international support, and should take account of the socioeconomic, cultural and developmental situations in the country concerned. Evidently, such an undertaking will require firm policy support at the highest national level.

Policy support

In most countries where traditional systems of medicine are prevalent, and particularly in those of Asia and Africa, national governments have supported and encouraged these systems as a part of their national heritage. At the political level, therefore, these systems certainly do have firm support. However, there are several gaps between policy support and its actual translation into practice resulting from the lack of an organized approach to ensure an optimum contribution to the national health systems. First and foremost, barring exceptions such as Ayurveda in India, Unani in Bangladesh and Pakistan and traditional healers in China, most practitioners of these systems of medicine are in the non-official sector. This fact alone contributes to the prevalent isolation of these systems and their subsequent non-utilization in the national health services. Further, in most countries, the health care models as well as the health service system are largely based on modern medical and health sciences, and the manpower employed generally does not have any knowledge or understanding of the traditional systems. The result is that the latter tend to be dismissed as unscientific or ineffective. This is also the basis of the resistance of professional groups to accepting traditional medicine as a part of the country's health system. Thus, despite the growing political support at the implementational level, little if any headway has been made in recent years in resolving this complex issue and recognizing the merits of traditional systems for application at the community level. Any organizational effort, therefore, must be directed towards an integrative plan, starting with appropriate manpower planning and the development of training programmes, and including appropriate utilization of the trained manpower. The recognition by the Twenty-eighth World Health Assembly in 1975 (resolution WHA 28.88) of the importance of training health personnel possessing appropriate levels of skill within an organizational structure which ensures their effective support and guidance, in this context, was an extremely useful step in consolidating the existing policy support at the national level for further organizational efforts in several regions. This important development was followed by regional initiatives for active promotion of traditional systems of medicine in several parts of the world. These actions at the international level, such as WHO Regional Committees, have included the designation of WHO collaborating centres in traditional medicine for research, development and training, consultative meetings and conferences with national and international personnel, regional programmes aimed at securing information for exchange among countries, and so on. More recently, with support from WHO and the United Nations Development Programme, groups of nationals have been visiting countries such as China and India where traditional medicine is well organized as a part of the national health systems. Subsequent World Health Assemblies have also emphasized the importance of recognizing the role of practitioners of traditional medicine in meeting the health needs of the population including their utilization in primary health care programmes (see, for example, resolution WHA 30.49).

Main areas for action

In April 1979, under the auspices of WHO, a Regional Consultation on the Development of Programmes in Traditional Medicine in the South-East Asia Region deliberated upon the organizational aspects of traditional medicine (see document SEA/Trad.Med./7, 4 October 1979) and recognized the following as areas for urgent action.

(i) Utilization of traditional medicine in primary health care including its application in nutrition, maternal and child health, family planning, immunization programmes, control of communicable diseases, and treatment of common diseases and chronic illnesses.

(ii) Utilization of practitioners of traditional medicine in the referral services of the comprehensive health care delivery systems.

(iii) Training of vast numbers of personnel practising traditional medicine with or without formal training as primary health care workers, with particular emphasis on continued use of disease-preventive and health-promotive practices in their work.

(iv) Training of traditional healers as motivated health educators for the betterment of the health of the community.

(v) Collection of information on traditional birth attendants and programmes for their appropriate training.

(vi) Utilization of these traditional birth attendants as family health workers for maternal and child health programmes at the community level.

This meeting also made recommendations on

(a) Identification of the commonly used drugs and formulations for the treatment of common ailments in defining an essential list of drugs for use in primary health care.

(b) Establishment of a suitable mechanism for study of locally available herbs together with steps for standardization of indigenous drugs and medicines.

(c) The organization of an appropriate pharmaceutical supply system for traditional drugs.

(d) Direction of skills, through training programmes, towards surveying the existing botanical wealth in traditional medicine and its conservation for optimum utilization.

As regards training, the important areas recognized in addition to those mentioned above, were:

(a) Full exposure of the trainees of existing undergraduate and postgraduate traditional medicine courses to all aspects of primary health care and particularly the preventive and promotive aspects.

(b) The desirability of introducing short courses in traditional medicine to fulfil the pressing manpower needs for primary health care and higher studies in traditional medicine for those already trained at the basic level.

These recommendations cover some of the most crucial areas for the organization of these systems for primary health care. In recent years, most countries where these systems are prevalent have made increasing efforts to develop national plans for tackling these issues successfully.

Manpower planning

The mere fact that an enormous number of practitioners of traditional medicine are in the field and largely working outside the national health service system (with the notable exceptions of China, India and a few other countries) underlines the importance of health manpower planning if the potential of this system is to be utilized for primary health care. For example, Table 1 shows the number of traditional practitioners in eight countries of the WHO South-East Asia Region.

Likewise, China has an even greater number of traditional practitioners who have been integrated with its closely-knit national health care system.

The important requirements for organized health manpower planning in this area are:

(a) Preparation of an accurate inventory of the available manpower together with categorization of their levels of training, expertise and location.
(b) Assessment of specific manpower needs at different echelons of the health care systems including the community level.
(c) Identification of the availability of the manpower so defined for specific tasks in health care systems along with a definition of their roles in the health teams.
(d) Consideration of active steps for manpower management to incorporate such available

Table 1. Numbers of traditional practitioners in some countries of the South-East Asia Region[a]

Country	Traditionally-trained manpower	Institutionally-trained traditional practitioners	Total
Bangladesh	6 850	600	7 450
Burma	22 000	11 277	33 277
India	341 408	108 592	450 000
Indonesia	200 000	—	200 000
Maldives	151	—	151
Nepal	1 000	200	1 200
Sri Lanka	14 860	3 030	17 890
Thailand	34 025	—	34 025

[a] Data from: GUNARATNE, V. T. H. *Voyage towards health*. New Delhi, McGraw-Hill, 1980, pp. 98–99.

manpower into the health systems through appropriate service provisions, career structures, employment conditions, incentives etc.

(e) Translation of health manpower needs into health manpower production efforts through the organization of appropriate training programmes in regard to both the qualitative and quantitative aspects of manpower development.

(f) Continued effective manpower planning, production and utilization as well as development of appropriate educational and training technologies.

One of the organizational aspects for manpower planning is that of official recognition through the registration of traditional practitioners. In most countries, with the notable exception of China, there are considerable difficulties in this area. These can be attributed to the variety of such practitioners as well as the prevalence of a vast number of untrained or non-formally trained practitioners. The absence of a rational way to classify and accord appropriate registration categories has often resulted in a conflict of interest between different categories of traditional manpower. Here, the national policies have to address themselves to the rationalization and simplification of the existing classes and the establishment of precise qualification requirements for registration of the various categories. Opportunities for career prospects and the requisite training courses for advancement would be equally important for preserving the dynamics of manpower development efforts.

Traditional medicine at the community level

One of the basic issues that demands careful study relates to the use of traditional practitioners as community health workers.[1] While programmes to promote the use of traditional medicine emphasize the vast potential that exists in this area, many difficulties have hindered actual implementation in most parts of the world. The difficulties in training these types of persons to work in health care programmes include the fact that most traditional practitioners are elderly persons, while their attitudes and their pecuniary interests in private practice can also be cited as negative factors. On the other hand, in view of their wide acceptance by the community and their familiarity with traditional systems that have many health-promoting and disease-preventing practices, it would seem logical to stress the importance of providing an effective package of day-to-day medical care rather than pursuing organizational efforts to use traditional practitioners in primary health care. Perhaps greater selectivity in choosing traditional practitioners for primary health care may prove necessary.

One of the aspects mentioned above, namely, articulation of private traditional practitioners with primary health care programmes at the community level with the attendant linkage between official public health services and the private sector, would underline the importance primary

---

[1] See also Chapter 28.

health care attaches to the larger issue of cooperation between governmental and non-governmental sectors. Even in those countries where primary health care has emerged as a major programme with varying degrees of success, such linkages between official and non-official sectors tend to be tenuous, *ad hoc* and uncertain. The essence of primary health care is to be a community-oriented developmental activity; this requires that all sectors work closely and harmoniously for the common purpose. In Thailand, for example, certain non-official programmes, such as the community-based family planning programme, are working with commendable harmony and cooperation with official health services. An analysis of the factors which have contributed to the success of such programmes underlines the importance of purposeful initiatives on the part of both official health services and non-governmental agencies and organizations to bring about such harmony. The success of the integration of traditional systems of medicine and primary health care demands such initiatives.

The utilization of traditional systems of medicine in primary health care, including the deployment of traditional practitioners in health care programmes, involves certain expenditure for which the necessary resources will have to be provided to ensure success. As the traditional practitioners depend for their subsistence on private practice, the assignment of new health care tasks to them would certainly raise the question of appropriate remuneration or incentives. Costs are also involved in the design and implementation of carefully planned training programmes for them. Ensuring a steady supply of medicines, drugs and herbal preparations derived from the traditional systems would also entail financial outlays. Experience in some countries in Asia and Africa shows that while such resources are well within the limits of conventional primary health care programme budgets, careful attention in planning these details is most important.

Other problems that could arise are connected with the referral services. The health teams which provide back-up services to primary health care today are, as a rule, trained in the modern health care systems irrespective of the category of the health workers. Their functional linkage to the traditional practitioners for technical support and supervision would again be an area which would pose some problems that can only be solved by specific policies for development of integrated health teams and supported by appropriate training programmes.

Research

For the promotion of research in traditional medicine, the facts that these systems which took root a long time ago were primarily derived from empirical experience and that their growth and their introduction into organized "scientific" disciplines were interrupted by historical events such as foreign invasions need to be emphasized. While in most countries where these systems are in use the availability of many effective and proven remedies has been sufficiently demonstrated, few, if any, scientific studies furnish systematic evidence of the efficacy of those remedies, their active principles, modes of action, or short-term and long-term toxicity, or deal with the great problem of their standardization. A number of priority areas have been recognized for research in traditional medicine with emphasis on primary health care. These are:

(a) Investigation into the effectiveness of traditional drugs and methods in the treatment of common diseases.
(b) Multidisciplinary drug research programmes for identification of new drugs or herbs and for studying the existing ones in terms of safety, efficacy, easier preparation, cost, preservation, modes of administration, etc.
(c) Clinical research and standardization of drugs and active principles.

Other areas which fall into health service research but which are even more pertinent to primary health care are those related to:

(a) Current utilization of traditional healers by the community.
(b) Features of traditional medicine which influence community acceptance.
(c) The cost-effectiveness of traditional remedies and practices.
(d) Surveys of background, education and training currently received by different categories of traditional practitioners.
(e) Determination of the body of knowledge and skills that should be imparted to traditional practitioners in order that they may function effectively in primary health care programmes.
(f) Determination of the best "mix" of traditional and Western healers in the team approach to primary health care at the village level with the determination of the role of each member of the team and their training needs as individuals and as a team.
(g) Evaluation of the performance of traditional healers in relation to the performance of modern health practitioners operating in the same locality.

Other areas for research

While carrying on research programmes, the specific known "strengths" of each traditional system of medicine should be reinforced. Thus, the wide and diverse use of acupuncture for various ailments and basic research into its neurophysiological and possible biomedical aspects, the health promotive practices of Ayurveda, particularly the practices of yoga, the practices and procedures of African traditional medicine and its known application in psychiatric and psychosocial conditions, and the critical evaluation of many remedies claimed by these and other systems to be effective against specific chronic diseases for which there are no fully satisfactory treatments in modern medicine, are all matters that should receive appropriate attention. Some of the diseases that could be included in such investigations are diabetes mellitus, peptic ulcer, bronchial asthma, hypertension, anxiety neuroses, mental health and drug abuse, ischaemic heart disease, rheumatoid arthritis, thyrotoxicosis, urinary infections and ulcerative colitis.

In our quest towards health for all by the year 2000, there is every need for the imaginative promotion, development and utilization of traditional medicine as a part of primary health care all over the world. The primary health care approach is based on integrated community development. It would be only logical that these systems, which were born at an early stage of civilization and which have nurtured and sustained communities through the vast expanse of time, should fit well into such a community development endeavour of which health and health care are essential components.

WHO's role in promoting traditional medicine

In keeping with the policy mandate derived from resolutions of the World Health Assembly and regional committees, WHO has been actively promoting traditional medicine as an integral part of primary health care through its technical cooperation programmes with Member States. Such cooperation is aimed at promoting and strengthening various systems of traditional medicine in different parts of the world as well as in providing active support for the exchange of information and experience among Member States. In the last few years, a useful programme to encourage visits of teams from different countries to China has been carried out in collaboration with the United Nations Development Programme. Several centres have been designated WHO collaborating centres in traditional medicine in different parts of the world. WHO was a cosponsor of the International Conference on Asian Medicine held in Canberra, Australia, in 1979. Several seminars, workshops, consultative meetings and other group educational activities have been held under WHO auspices for the promotion of various aspects of traditional medicine, both at headquarters and at the regional level. Some of the WHO regional offices have initiated action on research in traditional medicine by establishing research panels and by developing research protocols on various problems. The focus in the entire programme is on coordinated and integrated efforts to foster these systems and to maximize their usefulness towards the attainment of health for all.

* *
*

For the effective use of traditional systems of medicine in primary health care, organizational efforts need to be directed principally towards:

(1) Utilizing the existing manpower of traditional systems in primary health care programmes after appropriate orientation, training and motivation.
(2) Developing a realistic approach to traditional medicine to ensure that it

acts not only as a complement to existing modern systems but is functionally integrated into the larger health system.

(3) Studying and evaluating traditional medicine in the light of scientific methodology with a view to enhancing its value and usefulness in primary health care.

(4) Promoting the integration of proven knowledge, skills, practice and procedures of traditional medicine into the health care system.

Such an organization would call for a stupendous effort in which various communities, national governments and international agencies can work in close harmony and partnership to ensure better health for vast populations.

FURTHER READING

DJUKANOVIC, V. & MACH, E. P., ed. *Alternative approaches to meeting basic health needs in developing countries: A joint UNICEF/WHO study.* Geneva, World Health Organization, 1975.

Traditional medicine: views from the South-East Asia Region. *WHO Chronicle*, 31:47–52 (1977).

WHO Technical Report Series, No. 622, 1978 (*The promotion and development of traditional medicine*: report of a WHO meeting).

CHAPTER 27

Legal aspects

I. Patterns of legislation concerning traditional medicine
Jan Stepan[1]

Since the advances in modern scientific medicine began, the legal regulation of health care has followed a similar if not uniform pattern, first developed throughout continental Europe. Legislation was designed to regulate the delivery of health care as a monopoly of formally educated physicians and a few other professions. Subsequently, even the practice of the allied and auxiliary health professions was limited to licensed persons. The organization of health care as a medical and paramedical monopoly spread from Europe to both North and South America. As almost all the rest of the world, with the exception of China and Japan, was under the colonial domination of a few European countries, the concept of health care regulated by law as a monopoly or prerogative of licensed professions was introduced by colonial legislation throughout what we now call the developing world. The type of health care so provided was based exclusively on modern scientific medicine. Thus, throughout the present century, it was, in theory, illegal for anyone not a physician with university education to practise medicine in the villages of French-speaking Africa or in the forests of South America, just as in Paris or Los Angeles.

The motive underlying such laws was partly concern for the health of the population, perceived as requiring protection against unqualified healers and charlatans, and partly a geniune belief of the medical profession that every attempt at healing outside the framework of recognized medicine was ineffectual, damaging and equivalent to quackery. Such concerns were combined with the hope that the technical progress of mankind would in the not too distant future make it possible for qualified health care to be delivered to all in need of it. There was, in addition, a secondary motive underlying monopolistic or preferential legislation, namely protectionism in favour of those already established in their occupations. Attempts to relax

---

[1] Harvard Law School Library, Cambridge, MA, USA, and Swiss Institute of Comparative Law, Lausanne, Switzerland.

the monopoly in some fields of health care met with strong resistance from organized professions which, under the existing laws, enjoyed monopolistic positions.

At the same time, however, people of most nations and of many cultures relied, and still rely, on various forms of what we have now come to call traditional medicine—from applications of herbal medicine to faith-healing and other practices based on the supernatural. In advanced and affluent societies these forms of healing are sought in addition to the system of scientific health care; in vast areas of the poor world, where access to formal medical institutions is minimal or totally lacking, traditional medicine still is, and will no doubt continue to be, the only form of health care delivered to hundreds of millions of people.

Thus, since approximately the middle of the 20th century, exclusive reliance on the formal Western system has been recognized as an inadequate solution to problems of health care delivery. The governments of the developing world were obliged to recognize that an exclusive system of formalized medicine was both impracticable and indeed harmful to public health in those areas where existing health care resources were unable to assure even the most basic needs of primary health care. The legislatures of many of the countries that had recently become independent were faced with the task of relaxing the legal prohibitions against practitioners of indigenous traditional medicine and of incorporating these practitioners in a looser and more flexible system of health care delivery. To a lesser degree, a surprisingly broad current of public opinion even in the developed countries appeared to support legal liberalization of some forms of "non-scientific" medicine.

Looking at the current legal trend in its broadest outlines, it may be affirmed that most of the countries in South and East Asia have introduced more or less substantial changes in their health laws for the purpose of either tolerating or recognizing some formerly prohibited systems of health care. In the independent states of most of the African continent, the colonial concept of health care systems based on professional physicians, pharmacists, and dentists still persists in theory, although the policies of many governments reflect their recognition that changes are needed. One political aspect of the problem is becoming visible in the sub-Saharan region; there one often encounters policies emphasizing that the indigenous forms of traditional medicine are part of older national cultures that should be revived. A certain lack of legislative reaction to the issue of traditional medicine can be discerned in most "transitional" countries of South and Central America. Except for occasional provisions dealing with medicinal plants, traditional birth attendants or specific disciplines such as chiropractic, little has been done to regularize traditional medicine even in the vast rural areas of the continent. In various developed countries of the Western world, legislation permits and regulates the practice of some specific non-orthodox fields of health such as chiropractic and osteopathy: more recently acupuncture has come under legal regulation. In the socialist countries of Eastern Europe, where the health professions have as a rule become integrated into the public services, health care is provided exclusively on the basis of modern medicine.

This chapter attempts to describe the various forms and patterns of laws now in force in the developing, and to some extent also in the developed, countries in so far as they affirmatively or negatively regulate the practice of traditional medicine in various regions and countries of the world. In view of the manifold variety of the relevant legal texts, sometimes accessible only with difficulty, and on account of the lack of substantial prior research in this field, such an attempt must naturally be modest in scope. Its purpose is to provide interested health administrators and legislators with examples of possible legislative approaches and solutions to the various problems involved in regulating traditional medicine.

For the purposes of this chapter, the term "traditional medicine" is interpreted in a broad sense. It includes, *inter alia*:

(*a*) "formalized" traditional systems of medicine, such as Ayurveda, Unani, and traditional Chinese medicine;

(*b*) the practice of traditional healers as defined by an African Expert Group in 1976 in the following terms:

> A traditional healer is a person who is recognized by the community in which he lives as competent to provide health care by using vegetable, animal and mineral substances and certain other methods based on the social, cultural, and religious background as well as on the knowledge, attitude and beliefs that are prevalent in the community regarding physical, mental, and social well-being and the causation of disease and disability (*1*).

(*c*) the practice of chiropractic, naturopathy, osteopathy, homoeopathy, and even Christian Science.

For the purpose of presenting the manifold legislative approaches to traditional medicine, the following broad categories of policies for the legal regulation of health care in individual countries will be examined:

—*The exclusive (monopolistic) systems*, where only the practice of modern, scientific medicine is recognized as lawful, with the exclusion of and sanctions against all other forms of healing. The actual enforcement of such strict legislation varies from one country to another.

—*The tolerant systems*, where only the system based on scientific medicine is recognized, although, at least to some extent, the practice of various forms of traditional medicine is tolerated by law.

—*The inclusive systems*, in which systems other than scientific medicine are recognized as legal; their practitioners may practise their form of healing legally, provided they conform to certain standards.

—*The integrated systems*, in which there is official promotion of the integration of two or more systems within a single recognized service; integrated training of health practitioners is the official policy.

The exclusive (monopolistic) systems

During the 19th and the first half of the 20th century, the health laws of most of the countries of the European continent and of the Americas (as well as those of many of the then colonies) were formulated as diverse modifications of the monopolistic system under which health care was dispensed by university-educated physicians and a few other professions with formal training, such as dentists, pharmacists and nurses. Several patterns can be distinguished within this system.

(a) *A strict, total, and enforced monopoly*, as in France or Belgium. Under French law (sec. 356 ff., 372 ff. of the Public Health Code), any person other than a licensed physician who pursues activities broadly described as "medical acts" is guilty of committing the contravention of illegally practising medicine. Over a period of several decades, dozens of reported judicial decisions, indicative of the strict enforcement of these legal provisions in actual practice, have applied the restrictive provisions in a far-reaching manner. The French High Court has repeatedly held that the penalization of illegal "practice of medicine" is not limited to scientific treatment. Even during the 20th century, the courts have punished as being contraventions chiropractic, hypnosis, psychoanalysis, treatment of baldness by a pharmacist, and even such activities as advice as to the positioning of a bed. Supernatural and religious healing practices have been tolerated by the courts, but it has been held that such acts lose their religious character and become "curative" when they include a physical intervention on the person being treated, or the prescription of drugs. Several decrees were issued in the 1960s and 1970s establishing lists of "medical acts" which may be performed only by physicians or by members of specific allied health professions.

In Belgium and Luxembourg, a similar legal regime has established a professional monopoly on the diagnosis, treatment, and prevention of illness.

During the first half of the 20th century, such legislation spread to most of the French and Belgian colonies in Africa, where it remained in force, at least in theory, even after those countries became independent. Not until the 1970s did some governments begin proclaiming policies intended to liberalize the system and legalize the hitherto formally illegal practice of traditional medicine.

In the United States of America there are at the present time statutes in all the states which provide that any person practising medicine or surgery must possess a licence or a certificate of qualification.

(b) Austrian law defines medical acts in a narrower, less universal manner: under sec. 1 (2) of the Federal Medical Law (as amended in 1964), the practice of medicine "includes all *activities based on medico-scientific knowledge*" used for the purposes of diagnosis, treatment, prophylaxis, etc.

(c) The system of health care in the USSR and in the European socialist countries is characterized by the exclusiveness of health care provided by the State. Except for a few remnants of private practice, health care in these countries has become a public service. The Fundamental Principles of the Health Legislation of the USSR and of the Union Republics, which came into force on 1 July 1970, declare that the population is to be provided with "free, qualified medical care, provided by State health institutions and accessible to everyone" (sec. 4); the practice of medical and pharmaceutical activities is limited to persons who have undergone appropriate training in medical or pharmaceutical educational establishments, and the practice of such activities by unauthorized persons is unlawful and punishable (sec. 12); physicians are required to use diagnostic, prophylactic, and therapeutic methods and the pharmaceutical products authorized by the USSR Ministry of Health (sec. 34).

In their efforts to cover the needs of the entire population with an organized network of medical establishments, the socialist countries continue to employ systems based on the exclusivity of modern scientific medicine.

> [Even] the injunction to reexamine the clinical merits of (folk medicine and folk remedies) was usually coupled with the admonition to separate what was scientifically valid from what was useless. The development of two parallel systems was never encouraged ... charlatans, quacks, faith healers, and native practitioners ... are stigmatized in official publications as the last remnants of superstition and ignorance to be rooted out by an enlightened and scientific approach, and not as the valuable heritage of a national culture (2).

Characteristically, when in 1976 and 1981 Ministerial Instructions regulating the use of acupuncture were issued in Czechoslovakia, not only was the use of this method restricted to physicians, but even then only to physicians with special training; no department may specialize exclusively in acupuncture. A guarded, if not negative, attitude towards at least some branches of traditional medicine can also be witnessed in some of those developing countries that have chosen the socialist system. Thus, the Public Health Code of Algeria promulgated on 23 October 1976, in part influenced by the French model, introduces a monopoly in favour of the licensed medical professions, the illegal practice of medicine being made an offence. There is no exception in favour of practitioners of traditional medicine, and sec. 47 (3) expressly prohibits medical auxiliaries from using "secret or occult procedures". It has been reported that healers are prohibited from practising in Democratic Yemen, while in Mongolia the Government "does not wish to encourage" traditional medical practitioners. Indeed, in this country sec. 13 of the Health Law approved on 27 June 1977 specifically lays down that "the practice of medicine and pharmacy other than under the prescribed conditions" is prohibited. However, the opposite seems to be the case in the Democratic People's Republic of Korea (see, p. 308).

(d) As has already been mentioned, in the case of the former French and Belgian colonies, Western European laws, generally based on a monopoly of modern scientific medicine administered by licensed professionals, were reproduced in the then colonial countries prior to the

Second World War and also embodied in the legislation of most of the Latin American countries. The usual legislative pattern was that the law authorized the practice of medicine, midwifery, dentistry, or pharmacy only by persons who had been duly trained and registered. This implied a prohibition on healing activities by persons who were not members of the "medical professions". Such prohibitions were sometimes declared expressly, and penal sanctions were laid down in the case of violations. Sometimes, the prohibitions are specific in nature, such as those prohibiting some forms of healing by supernatural forces (see the section on witchcraft below), whereas elsewhere the prohibition may be formulated in broader terms, as is the case in the Health Code of Honduras, the relevant provisions of which read as follows:

> 130. The practice of naturopathy (*naturalistas*) homoeopathy, empiricism and other professions considered to be harmful or useless by the Secretariat for Public Health and Social Welfare shall be prohibited.

It is self-evident that in regions where the expensive and complicated structure of modern scientific medicine is unable to satisfy even the most basic health needs of the population, and where people have since time immemorial been used to native forms of healing, legal prohibitions on traditional medicine are unrealistic. The dead letter of the law does not interfere with the daily practices of all sorts of traditional healers. Unless "something goes wrong"—mostly where a conspicuous death results from evident malpractice—such healers are unmolested, informally tolerated, although they have no official recognition; this is true even in cities, although to a lesser degree than in rural areas. However, the system of the written law, the "law in books", still remains rigidly in force.

The governments of such developing countries accept this situation, and thus *de facto* toleration of indigenous systems of healing is the usual pattern of health care at present in many countries in the Middle East, in both North and Sub-Saharan Africa, and in South and Central America. The effect of prohibitive legislation is minimal or non-existent. This may be one of the reasons why, during the period of several years after becoming independent, many developing countries did not repeal or amend their monopolistic laws and did not pass legislation supportive of traditional medicine. Another factor is the resistance of a high proportion of the indigenous professionals, who were trained and grew up in modern medicine and inherited the traditional feelings of mistrust towards any alternative systems of health care.

The tolerant systems

In contrast to the "exclusive" systems described above, some developed countries with particularly advanced health care systems do not prohibit healing by individuals not possessing a formal degree or healing by non-scientific methods. Such is the case in the Federal Republic of Germany and the United Kingdom. In both of these countries, medical care is, of course, based on scientific medicine and provided by professionals having formal degrees and qualifications. This is best demonstrated by the fact that only registered professionals are included in the National Health Service in the United Kingdom, or can provide treatment under the health insurance systems in the Federal Republic of Germany. However, neither of those countries prevents non-physicians from providing non-orthodox health care, although a monopoly does exist in the field of dentistry.

In pre-war Germany there existed a "freedom to treat" (*Kurierfreiheit*), that was limited neither by a monopoly extended to formally educated physicians nor to treatment according to the *lex artis* of the established medical sciences. Healing could be practised by anyone, without a licence or official authorization. Although a non-physician was obliged to recommend medical treatment in a situation where life might be endangered, he could legally use methods in which he sincerely believed. In a well-known 1930 case, the German High Court (*Reichsgericht*) acquitted a healer "of low intelligence" who was self-taught in homoeopathy through reading and who used a homoeopathic method to treat a child suffering from diphtheria; the child subsequently died. In 1939, a law was promulgated regulating the occupation of "lay health practitioner" (*Heilpraktiker*). Under the provisions of this law, as amended in 1974, this profession can be practised by anyone (above the age of 25) who has received an authorization from the competent administrative agency. This situation legalizes treatment by various kinds of non-medical healers, although certain statutes prohibit such practitioners from performing medical activities such as obstetrics and gynaecology, dentistry, the treatment of communicable and venereal diseases, and the prescription of certain drugs. Lay health practitioners may not provide treatment under the health insurance systems.

The British system, too, does not establish a monopoly in favour either of licensed physicians or of modern medicine. What is protected by law is the status of registered physician, i.e., the title of "registered medical practitioner". Under the Medical Act of 1956, those who have fulfilled the statutory qualification requirements are entitled to registration as fully registered medical practitioners. The completion of formal medical qualification is one of the requirements for registration. Such registered practitioners enjoy exclusive privileges, such as:

—entitlement to recover in the courts fees for treatment and advice;

—employment by and dispensing of treatment under the National Health Service;

—holding appointments in public hospitals and other public establishments;

—issuing such medical certificates as are required by law;

—performing certain medical acts (for example, abortion, treatment for reward of venereal diseases, and removing tissues from cadavers);

—issuing prescriptions in respect of certain drugs as provided for by the Medicines Act 1968.

An offence is created by sec. 31 of the Medical Act 1956, as follows:

> ... any person who wilfully and falsely pretends to be or takes or uses the name or title of physician, doctor of medicine ... surgeon, general practitioner ... or any name, title, addition or description *implying that he is registered* ...

Subject to the above exceptions, it is lawful for anyone to practise any form of medicine. Thus, the communities made up of immigrants from Asia can be treated by practitioners of ayurvedic or Unani medicine. Homoeopathy is practised and homoeopathic treatment is provided by physicians in the National Health Service; the legality of this state of affairs was confirmed in July 1979 by the health minister. There exists a private Act referring to homoeopathy, viz. the Faculty of Homoeopathy Act 1950. Osteopaths, chiropractors, and acupuncturists may practise in the private sector.

On the other hand, registered dentists enjoy a monopoly in the United Kingdom. Under the Dentists Act 1957, the "practice of dentistry" is defined as the performance of any such operation and the giving of any such treatment, advice, or attendance as is usually performed by dentists. The practice of dentistry by a person who is not a registered dentist (or a registered medical practitioner) is an offence under sec. 34 of the Dentists Act.[1]

During the last two decades, both in the developed and developing world, a trend has become evident for more freedom for other forms of health care than those provided by modern scientific medicine.

In the Western world the basic idea is to allow individuals more freedom in choosing the sort of healing they want. The need for this seems to be felt especially in the countries with an "exclusive" system. A draft bill is being prepared in the Netherlands to introduce a new regulation of "occupations providing individual health care". The provisions of this draft would introduce a tolerant system, allowing to everyone the freedom to provide health care, with prerogatives for members of registered health professions somewhat similar to those in the United Kingdom (see above) or in Scandinavia. One of the basic ideas is to respect "the right of the individual's autonomy". A Commission for Alternatives in Health Care, appointed in 1977 by the Netherlands Ministry of Public Health and Environmental Hygiene, published an extensive report in 1981 (*3*). (An action committee "for the freedom of therapy", concerned with individual freedom of choice of health care, exists in Belgium).

---

[1] The section dealing with the legal situation in the United Kingdom has been substantially revised by the author on the basis of extensive comments kindly made by the late Mr A.R.P.P.K. Cameron, a lawyer in the Solicitor's Office of the Department of Health and Social Security, London. Mr Cameron's comments do not necessarily reflect the views of the Department of Health and Social Security.

In the United States of America, in addition to state legislative regulation of some branches of "non-Western" medicine such as acupuncture, the liberalizing approach was based on the "right to privacy" in a recent constitutional case. A Federal District Court in Texas held that the right to obtain medical treatment was within the fundamental right of privacy. The Court wrote, *inter alia*:[1]

> Health care decisions . . . are, to an extraordinary degree, intrinsically personal. It is the individual making the decision, and no one else, who lives with the pain and disease. It is the individual making the decision, and no one else, who must undergo or forego the treatment. And it is the individual making the decision, and no one else, who, if he or she survives, must live with the result of that decision.

In the developing world there has been growing interest in the value of traditional forms of healing. This recognition is stimulated by the desperate need to provide health care to populations; sometimes it is strengthened by the political motive of reviving the older cultural heritage of newly independent nations. A few countries have taken the first modest legislative steps towards the legalization of traditional medicine, either in general or in respect to specific branches.

The following are a few examples of this kind of "tolerant" legislation in countries where the established health care structure is, in theory, still firmly if not exclusively based on the concepts and organizational forms of modern scientific medicine.

In some Latin American republics there is a pattern of somewhat tolerant legislation and policies limited to only a few forms of traditional medicine, typically those of herbal medicine and traditional birth attendants (see below). In these countries, legislation tends rather to make certain special exemptions from the prohibition of unauthorized practice of the healing arts, as opposed to permitting the practice of indigenous methods of healing in general. As shown above, the actual practice seems not to enforce such prohibitions.

In those African countries that were under the preliberation influence of French legal traditions, the trend towards liberalization of traditional medicine has been cautious, not to say hesitant. For example, in Mali the first step was the establishment in 1973 of a National Institute for Research on the Traditional Pharmacopoeia and Traditional Medicine. On the basis of regulations dealing with the functioning of this Institute, some practice of traditional medicine was legalized. A further innovative measure was the establishment by an Order dated 16 May 1980, issued by the Minister of Public Health and Social Affairs, providing for the establishment of a Scientific and Technical Committee to work in conjunction with the Institute; it is clear that the Committee's tasks have been defined within the context of the overall health care needs of the country. This Committee has elaborated a first draft of a regulation of the practice of traditional medicine (*4*, *5*).

---

[1] *Andrews v. Ballard*, 498 F. Supp. 1038 (1980).

In Upper Volta, Title IV (Traditional Medicine) of the Public Health Code of 29 December 1970 includes the following provisions:

> 49. The practice of traditional medicine by persons of known repute shall be *provisionally tolerated* [emphasis added]; such persons shall remain responsible, under civil and penal law, for the act which they perform.
>
> Subsequent items of legislation shall define the practice of this form of medicine and the status of persons engaged therein.
>
> A medical and scientific commission appointed by the Minister responsible for public health shall conduct a study of the practice of traditional medicine and shall undertake investigations, notably in respect to traditional therapeutics, in order to identify the mode of action and nosology of the drugs involved.

The tendency in the Commonwealth countries, generally more liberal in recognizing indigenous practitioners, can be understood in the light of the former British colonial policies which were based on minimal interference with native customs. A typical legislative technique in these countries was to include in the basic medical law provisions which exempt all or some forms of traditional medicine from the general limitations on the practice of medicine by non-professionals.

Under the Medical Registration Ordinance of Hong Kong, the practice of traditional medicine is permitted subject to certain limitations.

In Sierra Leone, the Medical Practitioners and Dental Surgeons Act, 1966, provides that nothing in the Act is to be construed as prohibiting or preventing the practice of "customary systems of therapeutics", provided that such systems are not dangerous to life or health.

The Medical Practitioners and Dental Surgeons Act, 1968, of Uganda prohibits unlicensed persons from practising medicine, dentistry or surgery; however, sec. 36 allows the practice of any system of therapeutics by a person recognized by the community to which he belongs to be duly trained in such practice, provided that the latter is limited to that community only and to such persons.

In Malaysia, the Medical Act of 1971 contains a broad general exemption:

> 34. (1) Subject to the provision of subsection (2) and regulations made under this Act, nothing in this Act shall be deemed to affect the right of any person, not being a person taking or using any name, title, addition or description calculated to induce any person to believe that he is qualified to practise medicine or surgery according to modern scientific methods, to practise systems of therapeutics or surgery according to purely Malay, Chinese, Indian or other native methods, and to demand and recover reasonable charges in respect of such practice.

In Ghana, the Medical and Dental Decree 1972 and the Nurses and Midwives Decree 1972 authorize the practice of indigenous forms of therapeutics, provided that the practitioner is an indigenous inhabitant of Ghana, and provided further that no act is performed that is dangerous to life.

Subsection (2) limits the treatment of eye diseases to practitioners of modern medicine. Moreover, under the Poisons Ordinance 1952, substances listed in that Ordinance may be used only by practitioners of Western medicine, and not by traditional healers. Both Western and indigenous practitioners are prohibited from advertising their skills or services by the Medicines (Advertisement and Sale) Ordinance 1956.

An exemption, limited to licensed persons only, from the prohibition on the practice of medicine by unqualified persons has been accorded to some traditional healers in South Africa. The legislative technique used is rather remarkable, as the exemption authorizing the practice of general traditional medicine is included in the Homoeopaths, Naturopaths, Osteopaths and Herbalists Act, 1974. Sec. 8 (Bantu medicine men and herbalists) of the Act reads as follows:

> 8.(1) Notwithstanding anything to the contrary in any law contained a licence to practise as a Bantu medicine man or herbalist shall not be issued unless the authority of the Minister of Health for the issue thereof has first been obtained.
>
> (2) The provisions of this Act *and of the Medical, Dental and Supplementary Health Professions Act* [emphasis added], 1974, shall not be construed as derogating from the right which a Bantu medicine man or herbalist may have by virtue of any licence issued as contemplated in subsection (1).

In contrast to the above provisions exempting traditional healers from the general prohibition on medical practice, a statute exists in Lesotho (the Natural Therapeutic Practitioners Act 1976) which regulates the practice of traditional medicine and limits such practice to registered practitioners. Sec. 2 defines the term "natural therapeutics" to mean the provision of services for the purpose of preventing, healing or alleviating sickness or disease or alleviating or preventing or curing pain "by any means other than those normally recognized by the medical profession". Sec. 3 prohibits practice as a "natural therapeutic" by any person not registered as such. Applicants for registration must be at least 21 years of age, be citizens of Lesotho, and be recommended as qualified by the Natural Therapeutics Practitioners Association of Lesotho. Persons who were practising prior to the date of commencement of the Act are deemed to be qualified.

Authorized persons under the Act are prohibited from carrying out certain procedures (including: performing operations on or administering injections to any person; practising midwifery; withdrawing blood from any person; treating or offering to treat cancer; performing an internal examination on any person; and using designations such as "medical practitioner" or "doctor"). It is also prohibited to prevent or improperly influence any person from being treated by a medical practitioner.

In Swaziland, the Control of Natural Therapeutic Practitioners Regulations of 1978 limit the definition of "natural therapeutic practitioner" only to persons practising chiropractic, homoeopathy, naturopathy or electropathy. The prohibitions on professional practice are similar to those in force in Lesotho.

A recent act of the Republic of Kiribati—the Medical and Dental Practitioners (Amendment) Act 1981—authorized some aspects of the indigenous healing art as follows:

Nothing in the Medical and Dental Practitioners Ordinance shall affect the right of any I-Kiribati to practise in a responsible manner Kiribati traditional healing by means of herbal therapy, bonesetting and massage, and to demand and recover reasonable charges in respect of such practice;

Provided that a person so practising shall not take or use any name, title, addition or description likely to induce anyone to believe that he is qualified to practise medicine or surgery according to modern scientific methods.

The exclusion of non-physical methods of healing and the emphasis put on the "responsible manner" of the practice should evidently function as safeguards against unqualified quackery or against more dangerous or controversial methods.

It may be noted that even where a form or forms of traditional medicine have been exempted from the monopoly of modern medicine and thus legalized in particular countries, this does not necessarily signify the automatic removal of all legal obstacles to useful cooperation between physicians and other professionals administering modern medicine and persons practising traditional medicine. The usual prohibitions against cooperation with non-physicians included in codes of medical ethics and other laws regulating professional conduct have not been formally repealed. Should future legislation rephrase such provisions to demonstrate that cooperation between the practitioners of both systems is not only permitted but is desirable, it may help to weaken the old attitudes hostile to such contacts.

The inclusive systems

This category of legal regulation of health care covers laws of those countries where two (or possibly more) systems of general health and medical care coexist. This is the present state of both statutory law and its implementation in practice in large parts of South Asia. In several countries in this part of Asia, systems of traditional medicine are not merely tolerated (in addition to medical care based on modern scientific medicine), but they are in fact recognized as part of the State-regulated structure of health care, and are supported as such by the governments. Accordingly, the Medical Council Act 1973 of Bangladesh and the Medical Ordinance of Sri Lanka define the scope of the medical practice therein regulated as "modern scientific" medicine.

To be suitable for such organizational inclusion, it seems advantageous that the particular traditional system be, as a consequence of long historic development, formalized to a considerable degree, i.e., to have medical traditions, literature, and teaching systems that can be studied and continued. The Asian experience shows that such systems are particularly suitable for institutionalization within the structure of a State-regulated or State-supervised system of health care. It is characteristic of the professional level of, for example, the ayurvedic system that its old as well as recent literature and its leading organizers have placed and continue to place strong emphasis on the necessity to combat charlatans and quacks.

The traditional systems recognized in South Asia are those based on Ayurveda (including Siddha) and Unani, and their modifications in Burma and Thailand, as well as homoeopathy.

During the 19th century in South Asia, as elsewhere, Western medicine was considered by the colonial administrations to be the only acceptable system of enlightened health care, while the overwhelming majority of the population continued to be treated by practitioners of the domestic traditional systems and by various kinds of folk healers. Early in the 20th century in India (in territories including what are now Bangladesh and Pakistan) and in Ceylon (now Sri Lanka), attempts began on a broad basis to achieve recognition for the traditional systems. Revival of the domestic systems, growing numbers of traditional practitioners, and nationalistic feelings were important factors and the national and state governments reacted.[1] No less than 11 committees were set up in the Dominion of India between the 1920s and independence. The reports of these committees, the most famous among them being the Usman Report of 1923, recommended State recognition of and support for Ayurveda and Unani and regulation of professional practice and education. However, when the report of the first comprehensive health survey undertaken in British India was submitted by the Bhore Committee, it avoided the issue of traditional medicine. Another all-Indian committee, appointed as a result of a general feeling of disappointment with the Bhore report, namely the Chopra Committee, submitted a report in 1948 that strongly recommended full professionalism for Indian traditional medicine and a certain degree of synthesis of Indian medicine with Western medicine. The legal situation of traditional medicine in South Asia after the end of British rule can be summarized as follows:

India. The legislatures of the Indian states enacted laws to regulate the teaching and practice of and research in Ayurveda and other systems, examples being the Madras Registration of Practitioners of Integrated Medicine Act of 1956, the Mysore Ayurvedic and Unani Practitioners Registration Act of 1962 and the Mysore Homoeopathic Practitioners Act of 1961. The states are responsible for the strengthening of traditional colleges, hospitals, dispensaries and pharmacies. Almost all the states have established Directorates of Indian Medicine for the development of traditional systems.

At the national level, provision for the development of such systems has been included in the Indian Five Year Plans. The sums of money involved show the growing extent of recognition and support. The total sums allocated for the traditional systems of medicine were Rs 4 million in the first plan (1951–1956), Rs 160 million in the fourth plan, and Rs 257 million in the current (fifth) Five Year Plan (6).

---

[1] The material on which the information dealing with India and Sri Lanka is based was kindly supplied by Professor Charles Leslie of the University of Delaware.

There is a section in the Ministry of Health and Family Planning, headed by an Advisor, to deal with traditional systems of medicine.

A Central Council of Indian Medicine, established by an Act of Parliament, is responsible for regulating the teaching and controlling the practice of Ayurveda, Siddha and Unani. A Central Council of Homoeopathy was established by a 1973 Act. In 1976 there were in India approximately 200 traditional hospitals, 14 000 dispensaries, 460 000 practitioners (of whom 240 000 were registered) and over 100 educational institutions. In 1969, a Central Council for Research in Indian Medicine and Homoeopathy was established. In 1976 it was responsible for the supervision of 15 research institutions and 130 research units.

Provisions regulating ayurvedic and Unani drugs and homoeopathic medicine were introduced by the Drugs and Cosmetics Act, 1940, as amended in 1966, and the Drugs and Cosmetics Rules, 1945, as amended in 1964 and 1970. "Ayurvedic and Unani drugs" are defined as medicines intended for internal or external use for or in the diagnosis, treatment, mitigation or prevention of disease in human beings, mentioned in, and processed and manufactured exclusively in accordance with the formulae described in the authoritative books of the ayurvedic and Unani systems of medicine, as specified in further texts. "Homoeopathic medicines" include any drug which is recorded in homoeopathic provings or has known physiological effects as causing the syndromes which it is administered to alleviate, if it is used in a dose insufficient to cause active physiological effect, but shall not include a drug which is administered by the parenteral route.

As Professor Charles Leslie has stated, "indigenous and cosmopolitan medicine are not officially integrated in India as they are in China in a state-sponsored hierarchy of medical institutions", although substantial *de facto* integration between the different sections of the Indian medical system exists (7).

Pakistan. In 1962, an Ordinance was issued "to prevent the misuse of the allopathic system". It provided that only registered medical practitioners were entitled to use the title "doctor", to perform surgery, or to prescribe any specially listed antibiotics or dangerous drugs. These prohibitions were applicable to practitioners of traditional medicine. Medicines of the Unani, ayurvedic, homoeopathic or biochemical systems of medicine were authorized for sale only if the true formulas of such medicines were conspicuously displayed.

The Unani, Ayurvedic and Homoeopathic Practitioners Act, 1965, applied to *tabibs* (i.e., practitioners of the Unani system) and to *vaids* (i.e., practitioners of the ayurvedic system), both categories being prohibited from using the title "doctor"; homoeopaths were authorized to use the title "homoeopathic doctor". Under the Act, a Board of Unani and Ayurvedic Systems of Medicine and a Board of Homoeopathy were established in order to arrange for the registration of qualified persons, for adequate standards in recognized institutions, to conduct research and to perform other activities. Requirements for the registration of practitioners were laid down; the course of training in recognized institutions was to be four years.

The Government thereafter issued the Unani, Ayurvedic and Homoeopathic Systems of Medicine Rules, 1965, which included implementing provisions on the registration of practitioners, on elections to the Boards, and on the recognition of teaching institutions.

Bangladesh. During the period when the country constituted the eastern part of Pakistan, the Board of Unani and Ayurvedic Systems of Medicine referred to above was operative in Bangladesh. After independence was achieved in 1972, a Government Order restructured this body as the Board of Unani and Ayurvedic Systems of Medicine, Bangladesh. There are four teaching institutions under the Board's control, which offer diplomas after courses of four years' duration. The Registrar of the Board also functions as the Controller of Examinations. A Research Institute has been functioning under the Board since 1976. In that year, traditional practitioners in Bangladesh were not employed in general health services in the country.

Sri Lanka. The interest in traditional medicine and the activity of the profession even prior to independence led to the promulgation of the Indigenous Medicine Ordinance in 1941; this Ordinance provided for the incorporation as governmental institutions of the Board of Indigenous Medicine (whose duties included the registration of practitioners), the College of Indigenous Medicine and the Hospital of Indigenous Medicine.

With the establishment of a Department of Ayurveda within the Ministry of Health by the Ayurveda Act of 1961, a veritable landmark occurred in the modern history of Ayurveda (defined in the Act to include Siddha, Unani, and any other system indigenous to Asian countries). The Act also provided for the duties of the Ayurvedic Medical Council (responsible, *inter alia*, for the registration of ayurvedic physicians, pharmacists and nurses and for the regulation of their professional conduct), the Ayurvedic College and Hospital Board, and the Ayurvedic Research Committee.

Made under sec. 18 of the above-mentioned Act, the Ayurvedic Physicians Professional Conduct Rules, 1971, were issued by the Ayurvedic Medical Council and approved by the Ministry of Health.

The Homoeopathy Act of 1970 (which defines homoeopathy as "the system of medicine established by Dr Hahnemann") provided for the setting up of a Homoeopathic Council, responsible for the registration of homoeopathic practitioners. It exempted persons practising medicine, pharmacy or nursing according to homoeopathy from the provisions of the Medical Ordinance, and empowered the competent minister to make regulations as regards the control of professional conduct and other matters.

Detailed hygienic and other standards to be fulfilled by ayurvedic pharmacies were laid down in the Ayurvedic Pharmacies Regulations, 1973.

The importance attached by the Sri Lankan Government to Ayurveda was further expressed by the creation in early 1980 of a separate ministry known as the Ministry of Indigenous Medicine. The portfolio was assigned to a senior Parliamentarian, himself an ayurvedic practitioner by profession.

Burma. Burmese indigenous medicine is based on ayurvedic concepts and has been influenced by Buddhist philosophy. Prior to the Second World War, certain committees recommended that this system be recognized by the Government, but no action resulted. After independence (1948), the Burmese Indigenous Medical Committee was formed (in 1952). It drafted the Indigenous Burmese Medical Practitioners Board Act, which was passed in 1953. This Act was amended in 1955 and again in 1962. It established an Indigenous Burmese Medical Practitioners Board, whose functions are to advise the Government on, *inter alia*, the revival and development of indigenous Burmese medicine, related research, and the promotion of public health, another function being the "suppression of charlatans or quacks who are earning their living by means of indigenous Burmese medicine" (sec. 11). The Board is also empowered (subject to the prior sanction of the Head of State) to prescribe the subjects for examination in indigenous Burmese medicine, to register practitioners thereof, or to remove their names from the register if a defect in character or infamous conduct was proven.

Sec. 24 of the Act prescribes that, subject to the provisions of sec. 23 of the Burma Medical Act, only registered indigenous medical practitioners may sign certificates required by the law. Similarly, except with the prior sanction of the Head of State, no person other than a registered indigenous medical practitioner may hold certain appointments in publicly supported hospitals and other health facilities.

The Indigenous Burmese Medical Practitioners Board Rules, 1955, provide (sec. 7) for the registration of such practitioners in six classes. The system of classification is essentially based on the division of Burmese medicine into four branches (viz. *dhatu,* Ayurveda, astrology and witchcraft). Details are given in sec. 9 of the Rules of the knowledge required in order to be registered in the particular classes. Provision is also made, in sec. 10, for the registration of medical practitioners who are authors of publications in the field of indigenous medicine (such registration is made in one of three classes); it is indicated in this section that monks are debarred from registration as medical practitioners.

Under sec. 12 of the Rules, the Board is assigned the task of seeking ways and means of effecting as far as possible the consolidation of the four branches of medicine currently practised into one single system; the Board is likewise made responsible for undertaking studies and research and for advising the competent authorities with a view to bringing about uniformity in the methods of treatment being provided in dispensaries operated by the Government.

The Indigenous Burmese Medical Practitioners Board Amendment Act of 1962 introduced new secs. 22-A and 28-A empowering the Chairman of the Revolutionary Council to (*a*) cancel the registration of indigenous medical practitioners, (*b*) prescribe qualifications for registration, and (*c*) terminate the services of any or all of the members of the Board and appoint new members in their place. Under those powers a new Board was appointed with a view to initiating the reregistration of practitioners.

It has been reported that an educational institution known as the Institute of Indigenous Medicine was established in 1976.

Thailand. Traditional healing practices have been recognized in Thailand as a branch of the "art of healing". The original 1936 Act for the Control of the Practice of the Art of Healing was re-enacted under the same title as Act No. 7 of 30 December 1966 (it was subsequently amended by an Act dated 30 September 1968). Its provisions cover the practice of medicine, dentistry, pharmacy, nursing, and midwifery. In order to be registered and licensed as a practitioner in the "old-fashioned art of healing" the applicant is required to undergo a course of training and instruction with a registered and licensed practitioner for not less than three years, and must pass an examination set by the Commission for the Control of the Practice of the Art of Healing. Examinations are held once a year; according to a report submitted to a WHO regional seminar on traditional medicine held in Colombo in April 1977, very few applicants pass the examination. All types of traditional practitioners are registered with the Medical Registration Division of the Ministry of Public Health.

Under the Drugs Act 1967, as last amended by the Drugs Act (No. 3) 1979, a licence is required in order to engage in the manufacture, importation, and sale of drugs, both modern and "old-fashioned". The latter are defined in sec. 4 of the Act as "drugs intended for use in the practice of the old-fashioned art of healing or veterinary medicine, included in the old-fashioned pharmacopoeias notified by the Minister [of Health] or drugs declared by the Minister to be old-fashioned drugs or drugs whose formula has been granted registration as an old-fashioned drug".

The integrated systems

In the countries covered in what we have described as the "inclusive" category, practitioners of traditional systems of medicine are recognized and their work is fully legalized and regulated by law; they may be employed in public health institutions and perform some official medical functions. Nevertheless, they still form a system that is separated from the main structure of health care which, since the 19th century, has essentially been based on modern scientific medicine. The two systems in that category are not yet integrated in the sense that professionals trained in different systems of medicine work together as members of a single national health care network.

Under the policies endorsed by the World Health Organization, some form of integration of modern and traditional medicine needs to be attempted in order to achieve optimal coverage of health care needs. At present, it seems that only two countries have integrated traditional medicine in their health care system in the real sense of the word, namely China and Nepal. The difficulty that arises in endeavouring to summarize legal aspects of health care in these countries derives not only from the lack of accurate information but also from the absence of the normal legal, i.e., statutory, regulation of medicine. In another country, the Democratic People's Republic of Korea, there are indications of efforts to integrate the two systems in the new Public Health Law adopted on 3 April 1980.

China. In the first half of the 20th century, the health services in China were organized under the Western system of medicine. The revival of the old Chinese medicine that occurred after the Second World War in the People's Republic of China resulted in a unique, and it would seem truly integrated, system of health care.

The procedures and structure of the health care apparatus are determined by Party policies, and their implementation is undertaken by representative agencies in the field. Professor Milton I. Roemer has declared that one of the proclaimed political principles in China was to unite traditional and Western medicine. He states that:

> ... it was important to the new government to assure that everyone had access to health care. This meant that traditional doctors, with their herbals, acupuncture, and moxibustion, must be used to serve the people. By "uniting with Western medicine", the strategy has been to cull out those elements of ancient Chinese healing which are effective and discard what is not (*8*).

Every Western-style medical school in China (eighty-five of them) contains a department of traditional medicine; similarly, the smaller number of traditional medicine schools each contains a department of Western medicine (*9*).

Practitioners of Chinese medicine are also employed in modern hospitals.

> Western-style and traditional Chinese doctors work together at the (commune health) center according to the policy of integrating the two systems of medicine. Patients may see either type of doctor ... Brigade-based services carried out preventive public health measures, although some curative services provided by traditional doctors were also available (*10*).

The network of barefoot doctors, unique to the Chinese system, cannot be seen as being part of what we understand traditional medicine to mean. Having received intensive short training in both systems for the delivery of primary health care, these intermediaries rather belong to the category of "doctor substitutes" or "physician assistants".

As a recent article (*11*) has warned, the successes of China's health care system are not likely to be repeated in other countries simply by imitating China's methods. The system works in China as it does owing to the Chinese political system, and more particularly to economic policy. Consequently, other countries can scarcely hope to adopt China's system of health care while not adopting its economic policies.

Nepal. The policy of the Government, based on five-year plans, involves a system of integrated health services in which both modern and ayurvedic medicine are applied. Ayurvedic clinics are considered to be part of the basic health services. There is an Ayurvedic Section in the Office of the Director General of Health Services. The programmes for health services included in the fifth Five-Year Plan make provision for four ayurvedic hospitals in each of the four development regions. There is an Ayurvedic Governmental Pharmaceutical Unit, whose objective is to deliver inexpensive medicines. Formal education in Ayurveda is under the direction of the Institute of Medicine of Tribhuwon University.

Democratic People's Republic of Korea. Under sec. 15 of the Public Health Law adopted in April 1980, the State is required, with a view to ensuring the preservation of national therapeutic traditions, to combine traditional therapeutic methods with modern diagnosis in medical establishments. Under sec. 29, health establishments and medical research centres in the country are required to intensify research designed to give traditional medicine a scientific basis, with a view to developing a systematic theory of traditional medicine and further developing traditional medicine and folk remedies. Sec. 36 prescribes that the State is to consolidate centres producing traditional drugs, and is to train establishments, undertakings, organizations, and even individual citizens in the cultivation and collection of medicinal plants. Establishments engaged in the production of traditional drugs and other establishments concerned are required to protect and expand national sources of such drugs and to exploit these sources in a methodical manner.

The above-cited provisions seem to indicate a governmental trend towards integration of modern and traditional medicine. As the terms used are general ("combine methods", "consolidate centres"), some knowledge of the actual implementation of the Public Health Law may be needed to show if the system adopted in the Democratic People's Republic of Korea can be considered "integrated" in the terms of our classification.

Other aspects

A few aspects of traditional medicine merit brief individual attention since they present special features or problems.

Acupuncture

During the past decade, acupuncture has been accepted as a recognized technique in modern medicine, sometimes being subjected to specific regulations, as in the United States of America. There, in at least 15 states non-physicians are permitted to practice acupuncture, at least under some circumstances (*12*). The State of Rhode Island, for example, adopted an Act on 12 May 1978 relating to "the healing art of acupuncture". The legislative declaration preceding the substantive provisions of the Act states that "the practice of the healing art of acupuncture and any branch thereof is declared to be a learned profession, affecting public safety and welfare and charged with the public interest, and therefore subject to protection and regulation by the State". A particularly interesting provision is that no treatment by acupuncture may be performed unless, within a period of 12 months preceding the treatment, the patient has undergone a diagnostic examination by a duly licensed and registered physician with regard to his illness or malady. The doctor of acupuncture (as defined in the Act) or the licensed acupuncture assistant (likewise defined) must have in their possession and be familiar with the results of the said diagnostic examination prior to performing acupuncture. The Act provides for the establishment of a State Board of Acupuncture, and also defines the conditions under which the Board may issue licences for the practice of acupuncture or for the profession of acupuncture assistant.

In Czechoslovakia, acupuncture must be performed by physicians only in specially designated units of the health services.

The attitude of governments towards the practice of acupuncture performed by non-physicians constitutes a different legal issue. In France, like other countries having monopolistic systems, the practice remains illegal. However, in the Federal Republic of Germany it falls within the scope of the *Heilpraktiker* while in the United Kingdom there is no statutory control of acupuncturists. In a few developing countries, there are special provisions regulating the practice of acupuncture. This is, for example, the case in Fiji, where the relevant legal texts are the Acupuncturists, Chiropractors and Chiropodists (Qualification) Regulations, 1976, and the Acupuncturists, Chiropractors and Chiropodists Regulations, 1976. In Algeria, a category of specialized nurses known as "nurse-acupuncturists" was established by an Order dated 10 April 1976.

Traditional birth attendants

TBAs in Africa, Asia and Latin America are reputed to deliver about two-thirds of the children in the world (*13*); it is thus not surprising that this occupation is the frequent subject of special attention on the part of health care administrators and legislators in the countries concerned. Throughout the developing world, the trend is towards providing TBAs with some formal training, as their position and work in the community are based solely on apprenticeship and experience. An excellent report on the worldwide status of traditional birth attendants was recently published by the Population Information Program at Johns Hopkins University (Baltimore, MD, USA), from which the following data are taken (*14*).

As of 1979, TBAs were registered and/or licensed in 33 developing countries (8 in southern and southeastern Asia, 3 in the Middle East, 10 in Africa and 12 in South and Central America). In 1973, a survey undertaken by WHO found that TBAs were legally recognized or registered in some way in 26 countries (*15*). Prohibitive legislation exists in some countries in the Middle East (Egypt, Lebanon and Tunisia), although in practice such legislation is not enforced. In a few countries (such as the Philippines and Belize), TBAs may legally work only in areas where physicians or registered midwives are not available. In several countries, considerable efforts are being made by governments to register and train TBAs and to integrate them into the health care systems, particularly in rural areas (this applies to Afghanistan, Costa Rica, India, Malaysia, Mexico, Panama, and Thailand, among others).

Because of the large numbers of TBAs and the universal respect they enjoy in their communities (except, for cultural and caste reasons, in the Indian subcontinent), and in view of the daily demand from women for their vital assistance, the policy of any health care administration towards these traditional practitioners is particularly important. In addition to their primary tasks in taking care of deliveries, they can be employed as important auxiliaries in propagating hygiene, in family planning, and in efforts to eradicate harmful or dehumanizing customs (such as female circumcision in certain countries).

Chiropractors and osteopaths

Chiropractic and osteopathy are often regulated as distinct professions in some developed countries, notably Australia, Canada, New Zealand and the United States of America. Other countries—such as France in western Europe, Czechoslovakia (by way of special regulations) and other eastern European States—limit such professional practices to physicians. In the United Kingdom, the legal possibilities for a chiropractor to practise the art of healing may not differ from those applicable to any member of the general public.

In many countries, associations of chiropractors have organized attempts to achieve statutory recognition of their profession and some degree of regulation (which would reserve the right to practise chiropractic to those persons who are duly registered or licensed). Some of the developing countries, mainly former British colonies, have regulated chiropractic and osteopathy. This is the case in Fiji (under the Regulations promulgated in 1976), Guyana (under the Medical Service (Amendment) Act of 1979, which provides for the registration of osteopaths and the regulation of the practice of osteopathy in the country), Lesotho (where the practice of both osteopathy and chiropractic is regulated by the Natural Therapeutic Practitioners Act 1976), and Swaziland (where the definition of "natural therapeutic practitioner" contained in the Control of Natural Therapeutic Practitioners Regulations, 1978, includes chiropractors).

The trend to recognize chiropractic as part of a tolerated "parallel medicine" in some developed countries often reflects the idea that a citizen should have a right to decide what kind of treatment he or she will undergo. As both chiropractic and osteopathy are techniques that originated in the second half of the 19th century in the USA, as both need a considerable amount of education and apprenticeship training, and as such occupations show marked features of being performed for profit only and tailored towards practice in developed countries, it may be questionable to what extent they should be treated by legislators as an important part of traditional medicine in developing countries (*16*).

Witchcraft

Various kinds of traditional practitioners—as the definition quoted on page 292 shows—often use as a more or less essential component of their healing procedures "religious background as well as . . . beliefs that are prevalent in the community". Special and difficult problems necessarily arise in considering whether such healing methods should be granted legal recognition or used in the delivery of health care. In some cultures supernatural forces are attributed such importance in the popular concepts of health and disease that religious rites, invocations, magical methods and all forms of witchcraft constitute an integral part of traditional healing, and can be used with beneficial results. On the other hand, the dangers of fraud and of the misuse or harmfulness of some such methods are evident.

Legislative controls of witchcraft are necessary, although it goes without saying that legal intervention in this emotion-loaded field is extremely difficult. Two problems arise: (*a*) what degree of probability that certain forms of witchcraft may cause considerable social danger justifies legal prohibitions and sanctions; and (*b*) what sort of prohibitive legal regulation is, in the particular circumstances, enforceable.

Colonial criminal laws against witchcraft, which are still on the statute book of countries in various parts of the world, follow two broad patterns. Some, such as those of Malawi (1911), the United Republic of Tanzania, (1928), and Uganda (1957), make the practice of witchcraft or the representation of oneself as a person possessing supernatural powers an offence *per se*, whatever the purpose for which the act may be committed. Others, such as the Penal Code of the former Belgian Congo, still in force in Zaire, or the 1925 Witchcraft Ordinance of Kenya, make witchcraft an offence only when it is used or threatened for a harmful purpose—i.e., "with intent to injure", "for the purpose of causing fear", etc.

The excessively broad conception behind the first type of criminal law mentioned above renders such provisions either unenforceable or, possibly, tending to arbitrary if not discriminatory enforcement practice. Laws of the second type may, depending on the dangerous nature of some customs or beliefs, be necessary.

A long series of reported criminal cases from the former British colonies in East Africa show how often and how typically the use of assumed supernatural powers by witch-hunters or witch-doctors led to murders of suspected witches or became a means of extortion. Consequently, the above-mentioned Kenyan Ordinance also provides for the punishment of anyone who "accuses or threatens to accuse any person with being a witch".

Somewhat similar distinctions between harmless and possibly harmful customs, rites and beliefs must necessarily be made by health administrators in considering what methods of healing by supernatural forces can or cannot be used within an intended framework of cooperation with practitioners of traditional medicine.

The strength of the belief in witchcraft and other supernatural forces may be well illustrated by the fact recorded by a law teacher: more than 90% of his undergraduate class of criminal law (average age 20 plus) at a university in Nigeria believed strongly in witchcraft (*17*).

* *
*

There exists a broad consensus in international health circles, as represented in WHO, that traditional medicine should be supported and developed as a means of ensuring that people in the developing world have access to at least some primary health care. Only a few countries, such as India and Sri Lanka, have taken legislative action to promote traditional medicine, while in China there is comprehensive administrative support for the system. In contrast, laws in many of the developing countries are sadly lagging behind the times. Sometimes traditional practitioners are encouraged by flamboyant statements by politicians as to the importance of traditional medicine as a national heritage. At the same time, as the above survey shows, little or nothing has been done by their legislatures to abolish another heritage, that of unrealistic legal barriers, and to create conditions under which all their peoples have access to primary health care.

ACKNOWLEDGEMENTS

The author wishes to express his thanks for the most generous support received from Mr Roland A. Foulkes, of Fort Lauderdale, Florida, USA, whose aid was invaluable during all phases of the preparation of this study. Thanks are also due to Professor Charles Leslie of the University of Delaware, Sir Kenneth Stuart, Medical Adviser to the Commonwealth Secretariat, London, and his colleagues in the Legal Division, Miss A. M. C. Kahn and the late Mr A. R. P. P. K. Cameron of the Department of Health and Social Security, London, who were extremely kind in supplying data and documentation covering the legal situation of traditional medicine in a variety of countries. This survey could not have been undertaken without the comprehensive and detailed texts published in the WHO quarterly journal, the *International Digest of Health Legislation*, in which legislation on traditional medicine has been published regularly in recent years.

REFERENCES

(*1*) *African traditional medicine: report of an expert group*, Brazzaville, WHO Regional Office for Africa, 1976 (AFRO Technical Report Series, No. 1), p. 4.
(*2*) FIELD, M. G. The modern medical system: the Soviet variant. In: Leslie, C., ed. *Asian*

medical systems: a comparative study. Berkeley, CA, University of California Press, 1976, pp. 82–101.

(*3*) *Alternatieve Geneeswijzen in Nederland: rapport van de Commissie Alternatieve Geneeswijzen 1981.* The Hague, Staatsuitgeverij, 1981.

(*4*) KOUMARÉ, M. *La médecine traditionelle au Mali.* Bamako, Institut national de Recherches sur la Pharmacopée et la Médecine traditionelles, 1979, pp. 1 *et seq.*

(*5*) SALL, B. La médecine traditionelle en République de Mali. *Indépendance et Coopération. Revue juridique et politique* (Paris), **35**(1) (1981), p. 117.

(*6*) Data quoted by A. BAGCHI in document SEA/OMC/Trad. Med./Meet. 2/1 (unpublished) presented at the WHO Regional Seminar on the Traditional Medicine Programme, Colombo, 1–5 April 1977.

(*7*) LESLIE, C. Pluralism and integration in the Indian and Chinese medical systems. In: Kleinman, A. et al., ed. *Medicine in Chinese cultures*, Washington, DC, 1976 (DHEW Publication No. NIH 75-653), p. 408.

(*8*) ROEMER, M. I. *Health care systems in world perspective.* Ann Arbor, MI, Health Administration Press, 1976, p. 87.

(*9*) ROEMER, M. I. *Comparative national policies on health care.* New York, Dekker, 1977, p. 73.

(*10*) CHEN, PI-CHAO. *Population and health policy in the People's Republic of China.* Washington, DC, Interdisciplinary Communications Program, Smithsonian Institution, 1976 (Occasional Monograph Series, No. 9), pp. 37–38.

(*11*) BLENDON, R. J. Can China's health care be transplanted without China's economic policies? *New England Journal of Medicine*, **300**:1453 (1979).

(*12*) SCHWARTZ, R. Acupuncture and expertise: a challenge to physician control. *The Hastings Centre report*, **11**(2):5 (1981).

(*13*) OWEN, M. *Legal and policy aspects of the training and utilization of traditional birth attendants.* Unpublished report prepared for the World Health Organization, 1981.

(*14*) *Traditional midwives and family planning*, Baltimore, MD, Johns Hopkins University, Population information program, 1980 (Population Reports, Series J. No. 22).

(*15*) VERDERESE, M. DE L. & TURNBULL, L. M. *The traditional birth attendant in maternal and child health and family planning.* Geneva, World Health Organization, 1975 (WHO Offset Publications No. 18).

(*16*) For a comprehensive publication dealing with many aspects of chiropractic, osteopathy, etc., see the April 1977 report of a Committee of Inquiry set up by the Parliament of the Commonwealth of Australia *Chiropractic, osteopathy, homoeopathy and naturopathy*, Canberra, 1977 (Parliamentary Paper No. 102/1977).

(*17*) AREMU, L. O. Criminal responsibility for homocide in Nigeria and supernatural beliefs. *International and comparative law quarterly*, **29**(1):112–113 (1980).

II. Policy options regulating the practice of traditional medicine
Charles Leslie[1]

The options for improving the role of traditional medicine in health care systems are constrained by the worldwide status of modern or cosmopolitan medicine. The success of modern medicine in preventing or controlling infectious diseases obliges any responsible government to acknowledge its authority in managing public health problems. Compared with traditional medicine, its role in health care planning is enhanced by its nearly perfect adaptation to bureaucratic organization. Furthermore, its technological fecundity and heroic interventions for acute illness are known to peasants in remote villages as well as to city dwellers, and encourage a contemporary faith in medical progress. Anticipating a continuous flow of new cures and improved diagnostic techniques, people throughout the world expect health care in their communities to change. Because the accomplishments of modern science and technology are so much admired, modern medicine commands social priority in most countries.

When traditional medical practitioners organize in African or Asian countries to act as pressure groups for legal changes in health care they challenge the dominance of modern medicine, but the technological advantages, scale of organization, and international character of that system put them at a great disadvantage. Except in revolutionary situations, State policies concerning traditional medicine are largely negotiated and supervised by people trained in modern scientific medicine. The irrational element in this situation derives from the fact that for more than a century the movement to professionalize modern scientific medicine has used the State to eliminate or drastically to curtail and subordinate other forms of practice. This movement has shaped the education of health professionals to an occupational perspective that distorts their comprehension of other systems. Thorsten Veblen called an education of this kind a

[1] Professor of Anthropology and the Humanities, Center for Science and Culture, University of Delaware, Newark, DE, USA.

"trained incapacity". The incapacity among specialists in health care is to observe even-handedly traditional health concepts and practices. Their training, with its regular schedule of examinations, conditions them to hold professionally correct ideas for thinking about health problems. Confronted with different ideas, they must interpret them in the "correct" terms of their own system. In a show of goodwill they may translate indigenous health concepts and practices into those of modern or cosmopolitan medicine, but forced interpretations of this kind are hard to maintain. The more common action is to tolerate traditional medicine by attributing a placebo effect to practices that are otherwise considered harmless. The generosity of this judgement assures the health professional that he has taken a liberal view, justifying his perception of the rest of traditional medicine as a manifestation of ignorance, superstition and quackery. Arthur Kleinman described this trained incapacity in the following way:

> So dominant has the modern medical profession become in the health care systems of most societies (developing and developed) that studies of health care often equate modern medicine with the entire system ... Professional socialization of modern health professionals causes them to regard their own notions as rational and to consider those of patients, the lay public, and other professional and folk practitioners as irrational and "unscientific." ... It is amazing to see how intensely this professional ideology is held by otherwise sensitive and responsible health professionals (1).

Revolutionary actions were used to overcome this myopic view of health professionals toward traditional medicine in China. The integrated system created there commanded the attention of health planners in other countries in the 1970s as they came to realize that monopolistic systems of cosmopolitan medicine were ill suited to developing countries. Even in the industrialized nations where they first evolved, these high technology, hospital oriented systems were being increasingly criticized on utilitarian grounds for failures to be cost-effective and equitable.

The purpose of the fourfold typology of medical systems outlined in the present chapter is to characterize their normative legal structures. This typology is most useful when one remembers that normative institutions are only one aspect of social reality. It has been shown that the exclusive systems which give cosmopolitan medicine a legal monopoly of health care have not abolished other practices, and that many forms of alternative therapy satisfy demands for care that are not met by the regular medical system. In fact, a substantial market exists in Europe and America for traditional health practices imported from Asia. This pluralistic structure of actual practices makes the exclusive systems continuous with the tolerant systems that adopt their legal forms but have even less ability to suppress the so-called irregular or alternative practices.

The integrated systems represented by China select elements from a vast number of traditional practices, and create new settings for them. The selection is made on both political and medical grounds. When acupuncture is used in hospitals for modern surgery it is transformed as a procedure at the same time that it is made a symbol of revolutionary social change. Similarly, barefoot doctors are symbols of a radically new order, and their simple use of herbs and acupuncture attach new cultural values to traditional practices. Meanwhile, laymen, ritual specialists, and folk practitioners may continue the traditional medical use of divination, supernatural curing, and astrology, along with other practices that do not fit the style and ideology of care sponsored by the State. Certainly in Nepal, which has an integrated system, and probably also in China, a great deal of traditional medicine continues to be practised, even though it may be excluded from the normative system organized by the State.

Since the exclusive and tolerant systems either suppress traditional medicine or look the other way to ignore its practice, the models for deliberately using traditional medicine in a State-sponsored system of health care are the integrated systems and the inclusive systems. Our point so far has been that these labels will not be misleading if planners keep in mind the fact that they describe normative institutions which differ from actual practice. Thus, normatively integrated systems only partially integrate practices selected from the repertoire of traditional medicine, leaving a good deal of pluralism in society at large. Similarly, in societies with the inclusive systems actual practices diverge from the normative structure of health care. These systems create separate institutions to segregate traditional and modern medicine, but in fact integration may occur in them, and to an even greater extent in lay society. For example, for many years the Government of India sponsored colleges for traditional medicine with integrated systems of instruction. In the late 1960s a new governmental policy sought to eliminate modern or cosmopolitan medicine from these schools, and to initiate a "pure" curriculum based on ancient medical texts. Despite this change the faculties continue to teach what they know, and their knowledge is entirely grounded in a syncretic tradition of modern and indigenous medicine that began to evolve in South Asia well over a century ago. Registered practitioners of traditional medicine commonly practise this integrated system, and laymen of all social classes combine traditional and modern practices in home care.

The purpose of this conclusion is to clarify our typology for describing the legal role of traditional medicine in different medical systems by showing that: (1) they are all dominated by modern or cosmopolitan medicine, (2) in practice the exclusive systems are pluralistic, and (3) the integrated systems exclude many aspects of traditional medicine. Furthermore, in practice the inclusive and integrated systems form a continuum, just as the exclusive and tolerant systems are continuous with each other. The primary contrast in our typology is therefore between these two sets of normative systems.

One of the paradoxes of life is that we must have rules to have a society, but we cannot have a society without breaking rules. People must be able to do one thing and to say something else, for we must often make a normative system work by pretending that it works, and by adapting rules to circumstances. Moreover, in every society people disagree with each other. Health planners and specialists in modern or cosmopolitan medicine are convinced that they should control health care, but laymen frequently disagree. They resort to irregular and unorthodox therapies, and combine whatever resources are available to them in ways that they hope will be effective. In developing societies laymen are less exposed and committed to professionalized health care than they are in countries with extensive modern medical systems, so that their eclectic and empirical attitudes are even more pronounced. Also, ethnographic studies consistently report that the attitudes of traditional practitioners are similar to those of their clients. They are pragmatic, and curious about new therapies, readily assimilating into their practice any available techniques that seem to them to work. The main task of health planners is to find ways to make appropriate forms of modern scientific knowledge and technology more accessible to traditional practitioners. They will integrate what they learn with their own culture—a task that no outsider can do for them. This syncretism will be disapproved of by the "trained incapacity" of health professionals. Accusations of quackery are inevitable between practitioners from different medical cultures who are also far apart in social status.

Officials do not inspire confidence among humble people anywhere in the world. They are rarely trusted in developing countries when they come from outside the community as inspectors, tax collectors, policemen or health specialists. The customary hierarchy of professional control in contemporary medical institutions is a great barrier to the diffusion of new medical knowledge to traditional practitioners. Yet because they are at home in rural villages, and committed as members of these communities to helping their clients, these practitioners are surely a great potential resource for planning to improve health care in developing countries. Legal actions should legitimize their roles in the normative system of care, and at the same time loosen the professional monopoly of medical resources. These legislative changes will encourage traditional practitioners to improve the efficacy of their practices. Self-help of this kind in local communities is a cornerstone of development.

REFERENCE

(1) KLEINMAN, A. *Patients and healers in the context of culture.* Berkeley, CA, University of California Press, 1980, pp. 56–57.

CHAPTER 28

The role of traditional medicine in primary health care

Robert H. Bannerman[1]

Primary health care is essential health care based on practical, scientifically sound, socially acceptable methods and technology. The principles that are necessary for its effective deployment require a multisectoral approach as determined by various activities and facilities. It is the main vehicle through which an acceptable level of health and near total coverage can be achieved in the foreseeable future.

Primary health care is concerned with the main health problems in the community and the services reflect the political and socioeconomic patterns in the country. In order to make such care readily accessible and acceptable in the community, maximum self-reliance and community participation for health deployment are essential. Such involvement enables communities to deal with their health problems in the most suitable ways, and community leaders are in a better position to make rational decisions concerning primary health care and to ensure appropriate support for health and allied projects. Primary health care workers should, whenever applicable, include the traditional practitioners—healers, birth attendants, etc.

The developed countries are in a more favourable position, as on the whole their facilities and health manpower are both reasonably adequate. What is now required in some developed countries is a redistribution of functions and responsibilities, and more efficient restructuring to reduce costs and at the same time increase efficiency and productivity. In many countries, the soaring costs of health services have become extremely burdensome to the community.

The developing countries, however, pose a picture of want and deprivation with inadequate resources, a dearth of manpower, and no

---

[1] Formerly, Regional Adviser in Maternal and Child Health, WHO Regional Office for Africa, Brazzaville; later, Manager, Traditional Medicine Programme, World Health Organization, Geneva.

definite hope of amelioration in the foreseeable future except through the adoption of unorthodox measures such as the exploitation of useful traditional health practices. This includes a wider use of locally produced herbal medicines and the incorporation of traditional practitioners into the health team. In view of the pressing needs of the developing countries, this chapter will be devoted to those countries.

There is widespread disenchantment with health care in many of these countries for various reasons which are common to nearly all of them. Health resources tend to be concentrated in urban areas, which accommodate only about 20% of the total population. These facilities are so expensive that only the elite and opulent citizens in the city can afford to avail themselves of the specialist services utilizing such costly technology. In the final analysis, only a very small proportion of the total population have ready access to such facilities, which absorb a major part of the total health budget. Meanwhile, the so-called orthodox and conventional health care services devised for Third World populations remain culturally unacceptable and economically unobtainable. The disparity between high costs and low returns in health care has become apparent in both the developed and developing countries, and the economics of health care systems have become a major political issue in many countries. In several developing countries, while about 5% of the national budget is allocated to the health services, some 30% of that amount is absorbed by the drug bill alone and it should be noted that all the drugs for such relatively poor countries are imported against payment in hard currency.

A number of these countries in Africa, Asia and Latin America are therefore exploring the possibility of developing their well known and tested herbal medicines for use in primary health care centres. These medicinal plants are generally locally available and relatively cheap, and there is every virtue in exploiting such local and traditional remedies when they have been tested and proven to be non-toxic, safe, inexpensive and culturally acceptable to the community. The high cost of primary health care has become such a major constraint that what is regarded as basic in health services in the developed countries is considered specialized service in a developing country.

In Ghana, for example, the National Health Planning Unit has stated that at least 70% of the population do not have easy access to the formal health care system and that 75% live in villages that accommodate between 500 and 5000 people. The health budget represents about 3% of the total Government budget and 88% of that amount is used for curative services. Only 1% of the country's total population of 10 million has access to the specialist services on which 40% of the health budget is expended, and another 45% is spent on hospital and clinic services catering for 9% of the population, while the remaining 90%, or 9 million inhabitants, are left with only 15% of the health budget.

Although the national average physician to population ratio was

1:10 000, over 80% of the nearly 1000 Government salaried physicians work in the larger towns and cities which accommodate 15% of the total population. The private practitioners also work almost exclusively in the larger towns. The physician to population ratio for the rural areas is therefore in the region of 1:100 000. It is therefore not surprising that the rural-based indigenous healers should assume so much responsibility for the community's primary health care.

In many of these developing countries primary health care devolves on the healer, herbalist, traditional midwife, and other traditional practitioners. These are the health workers who offer services to the disadvantaged groups that total about 80% of the world's population and have no easy access to any permanent form of health care. Traditional medicine therefore has a major role in primary health care in terms of numbers of people served by that health care system throughout the world and in spite of any defects. The traditional practitioners are the true community health workers in their society. They invariably have the confidence of the people, and whatever their level of skills, it is essential that they should understand the real health needs of their community. There are, however, certain major constraints regarding the use of traditional medicine in primary health care. These are not insurmountable and, with goodwill on all sides, they can be overcome.

The incorporation of traditional health systems into the official health care system requires a major policy decision at very high governmental level.

Categories of traditional practitioners

There are four main categories of traditional practitioners. The first are those who have received a fully integrated training in modern and traditional systems of medicine such as ayurvedic, Unani and Chinese medicine. The second are those trained mainly in traditional medicine but who also have elementary knowledge of modern medicine. Such health workers practise mainly in smaller rural communities, using traditional medicine in general and modern allopathic drugs in emergency situations. The third group are the traditional practitioners without formal training but who have obtained diplomas in some particular traditional system such as Ayurveda after correspondence courses and examinations. They practise only traditional medicine. The fourth group comprises those without either institutional training or qualifications and who practise traditional medicine after several years' apprenticeship with an established traditional practitioner. These include the traditional midwives and some herbalists.

The integration of such a heterogeneous collection of fully-trained, half-trained and untrained practitioners into any official health care system raises many problems. It should be borne in mind, however, that traditional practitioners far outnumber modern health professionals and that over 90% of them work in the rural areas, while the remaining 10% cater mainly for the disadvantaged populations in urban areas. A few have lucrative practices in cities.

In regard to integration, the first group, those with fully integrated training, pose no problem. They are perhaps the ideal practitioners in a traditional society. They seek out and utilize the best practices in both systems, and the well-established and experienced ones often have lucrative consultant practices in big cities or are engaged in research activities. The second category also pose no real problems. They practise almost exclusively in rural areas and some have been engaged in government clinics in India, Burma, Nepal, Sri Lanka, and, of course, China with satisfactory results. Integrated practices have also been introduced into some central hospitals where these traditional practitioners work alongside modern physicians and employ traditional remedies including herbal medicines. Their main function is in the curative aspects of health care, but preventive and community health practices can be inculcated through both basic and in-service training.

The third and fourth categories, those with no institutional or formalized training, however, present several problems. The correspondence courses followed by the third group offer no practical training essential for the acquisition of skills. These are generally part-time practitioners—civil servants, teachers, agricultural officers, etc. Some preliminary orientation courses and in-service training would be required before any form of integration could be considered.

The traditional midwives constitute a special category. In the developing countries, they form the main body of primary health care workers in maternal and child care, and in some countries they are responsible for over 90% of the births. Their role and functions are very well described in Chapter 15 of this volume.

The integration of traditional midwives into health teams has already been initiated by several countries in Africa and Asia during the past two decades. Training programmes have been developed to improve their efficiency and to include family planning activities. Information on TBAs should first be obtained before planning any training programmes with a view to integration. It should include information on their role and functions, numbers and distribution within the community, any training including apprenticeship to established traditional midwives, approximate age, years of practice, etc. By analysing such data, it should be possible to identify the TBAs that would benefit from in-service training and are willing to accept such orientation, and to determine their impact on the health services.

Orientation and training for TBAs require special consideration from the health authorities. TBAs, though illiterate and seldom exposed to any formal educational processes, are experienced, intelligent and respected persons in the community. Their training should therefore be undertaken by health professionals, trainers and supervisors of comparable or preferably greater age and experience, otherwise personality clashes and conflict would occur. The training should be mainly on the job and based on reinforcing useful traditional practices while simultaneously introducing and demonstrating methods that are new but adapted to traditional ones. Leaders of TBAs who have already received orientation and training could later be engaged as teachers and advisers in the training programme.

Development of indigenous healers' training programme

The training and integration of traditional birth attendants is now well accepted in several countries. The situation regarding healers and particularly those without any formal training and education is, however, far less favourable. A major reason is that midwives are primarily concerned with childbirth and mother and child care, while traditional healers perform a wide range of health and allied functions with practices based on supernatural and magic phenomena that are alien to and not readily understood by professional health personnel.

Both national and international training and research projects regarding traditional health practices have focused mainly on traditional birth attendants and very few have concentrated on healers. In view of the urgent need for such training programmes, one such project recently executed in Ghana will be described in some considerable detail.

The Primary Health Training for Indigenous Healers (PRHETIH) Programme, located in Techiman, was designed specifically for the training of healers in that district. The following description is based on a report by the project coordinators, D. M. Warren (Social Anthropologist) and Sr Mary Ann Tregoning (Hospital Matron). The writer's personal knowledge of the project is also incorporated.

The project coordinators undertook extensive consultations with Ministry of Health officials, community leaders, local traditional healers and the staff of the district Catholic Mission Hospital, locally known as The Holy Family Hospital in Techiman. Detailed information was also collected regarding the role and functions of the healers, including healing techniques and beliefs, the needs of individual healers regarding knowledge and skills, and their willingness to participate in the training programme. A total of 45 healers and 7 apprentices were identified, mainly through referral by other healers, and interviewed. A small planning group comprising the project coordinators, Ministry of Health officials and the Secretary of the Healers' Association, analysed the findings on which the training programme was based.

The district hospital had been involved in primary health care since 1972, and in 1975 the hospital staff was invited by the Ministry of Health to participate in an integrated development project in collaboration with the World Health Organization. This involved the training of village health workers and traditional birth attendants, and the extension of nutrition clinics to neighbouring villages. The hospital staff therefore brought to the healers' training programme its valuable field experience of multidisciplinary work with active community involvement. Five years later, the seven TBAs who had been trained in this project were all in active practice within their respective communities, and most of the village health workers trained in the same programme had left the district for various other assignments.

Following these experiences, the hospital staff preferred to cooperate more fully with the indigenous healers who were respected and had well-established practices in the community. Their methods of remuneration, whereby they accepted gifts and not necessarily cash payments for services, were also more convenient and attractive to the community.

By mid-1979, the coordinating committee had completed its work on the objectives and course content and a 60-hour pilot training course was initiated, focusing on environmental health, preventive and promotive measures, family planning, and simple readily available allopathic medicines such as antimalarial tablets. An intensive review was made immediately after this pilot training course and several modifications were introduced. The trainers were given orientation in adult education techniques, and the original 31-week course was reduced to 14 courses of one week each in two seven-week cycles.

The following topics were included:

Cycle I:

1. Hygienic preparation and preservation of medicinal herbs
2. Diarrhoea, dehydration and oral rehydration
3. Houseflies and the spread of disease
4. Vaccination—indigenous and western. Typhoid infection
5. Convulsions
6. Basic nutrition
7. Review—focus on convulsions and basic nutrition

Cycle II:

8. Storage of medicinal herbs in liquid form
9. Weaning foods
10. Basic family planning
11. Basic first-aid (snake bites)
12. Jaundice and leprosy
13. Measles
14. Review

All training was conducted in the local Akan language, and all the trainers could communicate intelligibly in the local language.

Eleven trainers were engaged of which six were from the hospital staff and included the public health nurse, sanitary inspector and medical field unit chief. All the trainers had full-time employment in their respective fields. Classes were held weekly in selected homes of the participating healers and each week the coordinators, trainers and one or two trainees met to preview the subject and make critical remarks. Teaching was mainly by question and answer based on the existing knowledge and practice of healers, demonstration and role-playing. Each healer involved in training was given a personal follow-up visit after each weekly training session. Any difficulties were discussed and solved on an individual basis. This method required a good deal of preliminary preparation, time and patience, but was considered truly worth while. At their request, trained healers now meet periodically to discuss subjects of their choice.

The results of follow-up surveys six months after training have been very encouraging in terms of acquired skills, knowledge and terminal behaviour. All the trainees now store their herbal medicines in clean plastic bags and not mixed in unhygienic containers as was the situation prior to training. The care of sick children had been particularly improved within a remarkably short period. Children with febrile convulsions are now treated with cold-water sponging in preference to herbal enemas (some containing hot peppers, and herbal fumigation.

Oral rehydration for the child with diarrhoea has also been accepted with enthusiasm in preference to the crude cauterization of the child's back and, in contrast to the tabooing of protein, children with kwashiorkor are now given high-protein foods. These salutary changes have been very welcome in regard to child care and several healers in the district who have not yet had the opportunity to join the training courses have already adopted these "new" methods, following information from trained healers regarding the efficacy of such treatment. Although the training programme has been concerned mainly with child care, environmental health has also been given high priority. Ventilated pit latrines have been constructed in several villages and refuse collected in selected locations, covered with leaves and burnt every third day. Plans have been made to shift the focus of the training programme from the Techiman township to the neighbouring villages. Limited financial resources have, however, restricted expansion.

A major factor contributing to the successful implementation of the programme has been the long-standing relationship based on mutual trust and respect between the indigenous healers and the local hospital staff. The constant evaluation of the training courses continues as this has permitted quick response to changing situations and adequate flexibility. Active community participation in overall development has also been generated throughout the district. The approval of the programme by the central Government authorities and especially the Ministry of Health, the cooperation received from the local leaders, healers and health personnel in the district, together with the active community participation encountered, have all contributed to the rapid and satisfactory results recorded above.

Supporting services

When special care or advice on more difficult problems is required, the primary health care worker should have access to more highly trained health personnel with adequate facilities. The types of such personnel will vary according to the resources of each country but they should have full appreciation of the various situations encountered at the primary health care level in order to be able effectively to handle problems referred to them. Their social and educational responsibilities in health education should be emphasized and their main educational function should be to teach the people how to look after themselves. Special attention should be paid to the mothers – "Educate a mother and you educate a family". Health workers could first learn what mothers believe and feel and then, mainly through practical demonstrations, help them to understand how they could improve their own and their family's health.

One major difficulty is to get townsfolk with their culture and education to understand country folk with their non-scholarly belief systems. The effort of understanding must first come from the health authorities and the teachers.

Some serious thought will have to be given to referral arrangements since without such back-up facilities the community would gradually lose confidence in their primary health care systems. Referrals should be carefully explained to both the patient and relatives because in several traditional societies referral to hospital is taken as an indication that the condition is hopeless and the patient is being sent to hospital to die. Patients do not care to be treated far away from their homes and, whenever possible, health interventions should take place at community level.

A clear explanation of these interventions and the technologies employed should always be given in simple language and preferably in the vernacular. Newspapers, films, radio and television could all be employed for mobilizing community interest and support for the development of the primary health care programme.

In communities where health committees are established for the implementation of health programmes it should be ensured that not only government officers and educated persons serve on these committees but that community leaders, literate and illiterate, and senior traditional practitioners and midwives are also included as active participants. Their opinion should be sought on the initial planning, health priorities and overall implementation of the programme. It is mainly through such collaborative efforts involving some devolution of responsibilities coupled with delegation of authority that enthusiasm for community participation can be assured. Traditional practitioners can create a lot of difficulties at primary health care level when they feel, rightly or wrongly, that the administration is discriminating against them. "If you cannot beat them, join them!"

Medicinal plants and herbs

The high cost of drugs and the inability of many developing countries to purchase such drugs have prompted several countries to look for local products in the form of medicinal plants and herbal medicines that have proved to be effective, safe, inexpensive and culturally acceptable. There are many records of traditional therapies employing herbal medicines that are said to be very effective against common ailments and usually without any side-effects. A preliminary task would be to identify the most commonly used formulations for the treatment of common ailments in various localities.

The identification of locally available and commonly used medicinal plants and herbs would have to be effected and a list compiled. In certain Asian and Latin American countries, the cultivation of commonly used medicinal plants is undertaken in home and community gardens to ensure adequate and continuous supplies. This practice can reduce the risk of extinction of endangered plant species.

The cultivation of medicinal plants and herbs can also be conveniently linked with the production of vegetables and fruit with high nutritive value that should be of particular benefit to mothers and children.

In the selection of drugs and herbal medicines for treatment, the health worker is expected to give preference to locally produced and equally effective preparations.

A major constraint in the use of vegetable drugs is the absence of national pharmacopoeias in many countries. A few countries, such as India and China, have developed pharmacopoeias containing recipes of plant and herbal medicines. Others have old manuscripts which describe plants and herbs, including their properties such as taste, odour and changes during digestion, potency and specific therapeutic actions. In most other Third World countries the systematic utilization of these medicinal plants in pharmaceutical industry and for the purpose of health care has not been optimized and remains limited mainly to the production of traditional drugs for local use.

Different drugs are now being combined in one preparation to reduce adverse side-effects, e.g., combining streptomycin with a Chinese traditional drug, or combining active principles of Chinese, Indian, Japanese, and Arab medicines in one mixture so as to obtain an effective but smaller dose.

Primary health care workers should have basic knowledge concerning medicinal plants, their cultivation, identification, collection and preparation for therapeutic applications within the community in which they work. The use of medicinal plants and traditional medicine could make people become more self-reliant.

FURTHER READING

DJUKANOVIC, V. & MACH, E. P., ed. *Alternative approaches to meeting basic health needs in developing countries: a joint UNICEF/WHO study.* Geneva, World Health Organization, 1975.

WORLD HEALTH ORGANIZATION. *Alma-Ata 1978. Primary health care: report of the International Conference on Primary Health Care, Alma-Ata, USSR, 6–12 September 1978,* Geneva, 1978 ("Health for All" series, No. 1).

MAHLER, H. People. *Scientific American,* **243**(3):62–73 (September 1980).

BANNERMAN, R. H. Traditional medicine in modern health care services. *International relations. Journal of the David Davies Memorial Institute of International Studies,* **6**(5):731–747 (May 1980).

WARREN, D. M. & TREGONING, M. A. Indigenous healers and primary health care in Ghana. *Medical anthropology newsletter,* **11**(1):11–13 (November 1979).

WARREN, D. M. ET AL. Ghanaian national policy toward indigenous healers: the case of the primary health training for indigenous healers (PRHETIH) Program. *Social science and medicine,* **16**: 1873–1881 (1982).

NATIONAL HEALTH PLANNING UNIT. *An approach to planning the delivery of health care services.* Accra, Ghana, Ministry of Health, 1979 (Manual No. 1).

Government of Ghana budget estimates book for health. Accra, Ministry of Health, 1979 1980.

Index

Index

Ablution, 35, 126
Abortion, 157
Abrams, Harold, 168
Acorus calamus, 177
Acupressure, 78, 169
Acupuncture, 66, 69–70, 73–74, 76–85, 169, 241, 242, 264–267, 272, 294, 297, 308–309
  ahshi points, 77
  anaesthesia, 81, 267, 269
  analgesia, 81
  attitudes towards, 84
  basic theory, 79–80
  channels, collaterals and acupuncture points, 76–77, 265
  contraindications, 80
  control regulations, 85
  educational programmes, 85
  finger-pressing therapy or acupressure, 78, 169
  future development, 84
  impact on health care, 84
  indications, 80–81
  legislation, 297, 308–309
  national regulations, 85
  needles, 78
  nurse-acupuncturists, 309
  research, 82–85
  technique, 76–78
  technology transfer, 84
  therapeutic methods, 78
  training, 83–84, 242
Aesculapius, 103, 245

Afghanistan, 256, 259, 310
Africa, 19, 25–36, 126, 150, 209–221, 282, 286, 295, 298, 309, 321
  herbal medicines, 319
  intercountry projects, 213
  international cooperation, 214–216
  primary health care, 319
African and Malagasy Committee for Further Education (CAMES), 30, 215
African Region of WHO, 209–221
African traditional medicine, 25–30, 209–211
  activities at regional level, 211
  colonial period, 210
  consultation on, 212
  divination, 125
  education and training, 215
  legislation, 314
  national activities, 213, 218–220
  pharmacopoeia, 29
  postcolonial period, 211
  precolonial situation, 210
  regional activities and developments, 209, 211–213, 216–217
  research, 214, 287
  seminars, symposia and workshops, 221
  traditional birth attendants, 309
  traditional psychiatry, 33–36
  WHO/UNDP collaboration, 215
Agency for Cultural and Technical Cooperation (ACCT), 30

Ahshi points, 77
Algeria, 294, 309
Allopathic medicine, 11, 90–101
  definition, 90
  drugs, 95
  growth of, 91
  influence on health care status, 92
  integrated health care, 99–100
  major disciplines, 92
  medical research, 98–99, 238
  pharmacopoeia, 95–96
  professional organizations, 97
  systems of medical care, 96
Alma-Ata, International Conference on Primary Health Care, 232
Alternative medicine, 243–244
  therapeutic practices and theories, 250
Amehi, see Tibetan system
Americas, 19, 293, 315
  WHO Region, 222–230
Ammi visnaga, 260
Amulets, 42
Angola, 218
Anthroposophical medicine, 163, 248
Arab medicine, *see* Unani medicine
Aretaeus, 90
Asia, 50, 58, 282, 301, 309, 314, 315, 319, 321, 326
Astrology, 59–60, 124, 305
Atharvaveda, 50
Australia, 264, 310
Austria, 81, 240, 241, 242, 244, 245, 246, 248, 293
Autogenic training, 129, 140, 163–164, 167
Autohypnosis, 129
Avicenna, 91, 259
Ayurveda, 17, 19, 20, 22, 50–60, 236, 237, 238, 264, 273, 282, 287, 292, 297, 302, 303–304, 305, 308, 320
  astrology, 59–60
  basic theories, 51
  colour therapy, 165
  diagnosis, 52, 56
  diet, 54
  doctrines of, 50–52
  dosha, 19, 59
  drug action, 55, 303
  drug sources, 54
  efficacy for treatment of rheumatoid arthritis, 235
  examination of patient, 52–53
  materia medica, 180
  meaning of, 50
  nurses, 304
  patient–physician relationship, 55
  pharmacists, 304
  pharmacognosy, 58
  pharmacopoeia, 55
  practitioners, 56, 91, 304
  professional associations, 56
  Rauvolfia serpentina, 178
  research, 57–58, 287
  routines, 52
  specialties, 51
  surgical treatment, 54
  training, 56
  treatment of disease, 53
  way of life, 52

Bach, Edward, 165
Balneotherapy, 120, 241, 245
Bangladesh, 236, 242, 302
  Ayurvedic medicine, 50
  Board of Unani and Ayurvedic Systems of Medicine, 304
  Medical Council Act 1973, 301
  Research Institute, 304
  traditional medicine study, 233
  Unani system, 282
  UNDP intercountry project, 234
Barefoot doctors, 73, 84, 185, 307, 316
Bates' technique of visual education, 164
Belgium, 247, 293, 297
Belize, 310
Benin, 218, 221
Bhutan, 233, 234
Biofeedback, and the autonomic nervous system, 164–165
Birth control, 156–157
Bleeding, as therapy, 241, 246
Bolivia, 42, 46
Bomoh, 273
Bonesetting, 225, 236, 266, 276
Book of Rites, 69
Botanical Institute for Therapeutic Plant Resources, Peru, 228
Brazil, 46, 47, 223

Breast-feeding, association with birth spacing, 156
  relation to kwashiorkor, 105–106
Breathing exercises, 135, 136, 164, 169, 170, 266
Buddhist philosophy, 305
Bulgaria, 245
Burma, 178, 233, 234, 236, 302, 305–306, 321
Burundi, 218

Callawaya, 42, 43, 46
Cameroon, *see* United Republic of Cameroon
CAMES, *see* African and Malagasy Committee for Further Education
Canada, 310
Cancer, 166, 248, 249
Candomble movement, 47
Catharanthus coriaceus, 176
Central African Republic, 218
Central America, 295, 309
Chad, 150
Charismatic healers, 23
Charms, 22, 157
Childbirth, 142, 144, 147
China, 68–75, 76, 103, 282–284, 285, 288, 303, 312
  acupuncture, recognition and use, 85, 267
  acupuncture analgesia, 81
  barefoot doctors, 73, 84, 185, 307
  doctors, types of, 73
  health care system, current trends, 71–74, 307, 312
    integration, 264–266, 315–316
  herbal medicine, 177
    research, 267–268
  hospitals, 72, 307
  medical schools, 86
  midwifery, 155
  policy support of traditional healers, 282
  research institutes, 278
  traditional practitioners, 320, 321
  training in acupuncture, 83
  training courses, 213, 258
  zone therapy, 169
  see also Acupuncture; Chinese medicine
Chinese medicine, 17, 68–75, 86–89, 215, 236, 263, 265–270, 292
  colour therapy, 165
  combined treatments, 74
  dao ying, 69
  development and future prospects, 74
  fracture treatment, 86–89
  herbal drugs, 70, 73, 185, 266, 267–268, 326
  history, 68
  hygiene and preventive measures, 69, 74, 266
  integration with modern medicine, 68, 74, 264–266, 315–316
  Internal Classic, 69–70
  manipulation, 88, 266
  massage, 70, 88, 266
  organization, 72
  pharmacology, 70, 86
  pharmacopoeia, 326
  practitioners, 90, 91
  qi, 265
  research, 72
  scientific elements, 74
  soft-tissue injuries, 88–89
  training, 72, 73, 215, 269
  treatment, 70, 89, 260
  yin-yang, 19, 69, 77, 79, 144, 265, 267
  wuxing, 265
  see also Acupuncture, Moxibustion
Chiropractic, 119, 245, 246, 247, 293, 297, 309, 310–311
Christianity, 104, 126, 241
Christian Science, 292
CITES, *see* Convention of International Trade in Endangered Species of Wild Fauna and Flora
Colombia, 225
Colour therapy, 43, 165
Community development, 288
Community health workers, 285
Concentration of mind, 136
Congo, 218, 221
Contraception, 156–157
Convention of International Trade in Endangered Species of Wild Fauna and Flora (CITES), 178, 179

Costa Rica, 310
Cupping, 241, 246, 266
Curanderos, 20, 225, 226, 229
Curing theories, 250
Cyprus, 257
Czechoslovakia, 294, 309, 310

Darshanas, 50
Dead Sea, 120
Democratic People's Republic of Korea, 294, 307, 308
Dendrobium nobile, 181
Dendrobium pauciflorum, 180
Denmark, 168, 241, 246, 247
Dentistry, legal aspects, 297, 299, 300–301
Developing countries, 24, 67, 196, 197, 198, 204, 206, 216, 318
Diagnosis, 21, 28, 43, 52, 56, 63, 88
Diet, 54, 64, 121, 122, 166
Dioscorea deltoidea, 179, 180
Diplomeris hirsuta, 180
Disease causality, classification, 19
Divination, 28, 34, 42, 43, 124–126, 276
Divine healers, 175, 272
Doctor–patient relationship, 34, 55, 63, 92, 93–95
Do-in, 169
Dominican Republic, 225
Dream analysis, 124
Drugs, allopathic system, 95
  Ayurveda, 54, 55, 303
  convenience, 195
  homoeopathy, 303
  psychotropic, 36
  synthetic, 195
  temperaments of, 62
  Unani, 303
  unorthodox therapies, 249
  see also Herbal medicine and herbal remedies
Dualism concept, 26

East Africa, 311
East European countries, 240, 241, 242, 310
Eastern Mediterranean Region of WHO, 253–262
  research, 259–261
  traditional techniques, 257
  training, 258–259
Ecuador, 225
Egypt, 103, 155, 257, 260, 310
Endangered plants, 175–183
Environment and Development in the Third World (ENDA), 216
Epidemiology of beliefs and customs, 107–109
Epilepsy, 165
Ethiopia, 218
Ethnomedicine, 17–24, 184, 240
  causality concepts, 18–20
  definition, 18
  literature of, 18
Ethnopharmacognostic research, 199, 206
Eurhythmy, 248
Europe, 315
  health care systems, 240
  health laws, 293
  hydrotherapy, 167
  self-care, 249–250
  therapeutic practices and curing theories, 243, 250
  unofficial medicine, 241–249
European Region of WHO, 240–252
Evil eye, 42, 225
Evil spirits, 43, 175
Exorcism, 126–127, 175

Faith healers, 272
Family planning, 158, 286
FAO, *see* Food and Agriculture Organization of the United Nations
Fasting, 122
Fiji, 264, 277–278, 309, 310
Finger pressure, 78, 169
Finland, 241, 242, 246
Fitzgerald, William H., 169
Flower remedies, 165, 244
Folk medicine, 20, 27, 184, 225, 240, 270, 272, 274
Food and Agriculture Organization of the United Nations (FAO), 204, 206
Food cravings, 150
Food roles, 22
  see also Diet
Fracture treatment by integrated methods, China, 86–89

France, acupuncture, 241, 242
  chiropractic, 247
  cupping and bleeding, 246
  homoeopathy, 114, 248
  imported traditional medicine systems, 242
  legislation, 293, 310
  medicinal plants, 244
  medicinal springs, 245
  spiritism, 47
Fright, 41
Fruit, taboos, 145
Fruitarianism, 121

Galenic system, 37, 48, 246, 253
Gambia, 218
Germany, Federal Republic of, acupuncture, 81, 241, 242, 309
  anthroposophical medicine, 163
  autogenic training, 163
  chiropractic, 246-247
  cupping and bleeding, 246
  ethnomedicine, 240
  healing practitioners, 243, 249
  homoeopathy, 248
  iris diagnosis, 119
  legislation, 295-296
  medicinal plants, 244
  medicinal springs, 245
  naturopathy, 119, 121
  negative ion therapy, 168
  teaching of traditional medicine, 240
Gerson treatment, 166
Ghana, 105, 157, 158, 218, 299, 319, 322-324
Ginseng, 175, 176-177
Goitre, 266
Graeco-Arab medicine, *see* Unani medicine
Greece, 103, 242, 245
Greek medicine, 17
Grenada, 227
Guatemala, 144, 147, 150-152, 155, 223, 226-227
Guinea, 218, 221
Guyana, 310

Hahnemann, Samuel, 110-112, 304
Hand healing, 248-249
Healers and healing, 12, 23, 26-30, 32, 33, 63, 166-167, 175, 225, 226, 229, 244, 248-249, 264-265, 268, 271-276, 277-278, 292, 306, 322
Heilpraktiker, 243, 244, 296, 309
Herbal medicine and herbal remedies, 70, 175-182, 194-206, 238, 241, 244, 256, 264, 266, 270, 275, 277, 326
  African pharmacopoeia, 29, 216
  Americas, 228
  amounts as pharmaceutical preparations, 194
  antispasmodics, 180
  appropriate methodology, 200
  brain stimulants, 178
  cancer therapy, 176
  cardiovascular tonics, 178
  carminatives, 180
  contraceptives, 157
  cortisone, 180
  Democratic People's Republic of Korea, 308
  developing countries, 196-197
  dosage forms, 197
  Eastern Mediterranean Region of WHO, 260
  endangered plants, 175-182
  Europe, 244-245
  hypertension control, 179
  industrialized countries, 195-196
  insecticidal action, 177
  intravenous application, 149, 159
  laboratory investigations, 201, 260
  labour, 151
  Papua New Guinea, 274-275
  pharmacology, 185, 278
  Philippines, 270
  pregnancy, 150
  primary health care, 198-206, 319, 326
  production, 73, 194, 195
  reference books, 259
  research, 65-66, 182, 198-206, 267-268, 271
  traditional midwifery and contraception, 157, 159
  see also **NAPRALERT** data base; Phytopharmacology; Phytotherapy
Herbalists, 29, 44, 175, 225, 236
Herbolarios, 271, 272
Hilots, 271
Hinduism, 103, 264, 273

Hippocrates, 61, 90, 253
Hippocratic numeral theory, 37
Hippocratic oath, 23
Homoeopathy, 19, 90, 110–115, 236, 237, 247, 273, 292, 295, 297, 302, 303
  basic assumptions, 110
  basic laws, 111
    chronic diseases, 114
  definition, 90, 304
  drugs, 303
  future possibilities, 115
  individualization, 113–114
  Law of Cure, 114
  Law of Direction of Cure, 112
  Law of Minimum Dose, 113
  Law of Similars, 111
  Law of Single Remedy, 113
  microdosages, 113
  practitioners, 302, 303
  present situation, 114
  preventive medicine, 114
  resurgence of, 110
  training, 115, 247
Honduras, 295
Hong Kong, 299
Hormones, 267
Horoscopes, 59
"Hot" and "cold", 37, 44, 45, 62, 144, 225
  as health regulator, 39
  basic concepts, 38
  in therapy, 40
  research, 45
Humoral pathology, 17, 20, 22
Humoral theory and therapy, 37–46, 61
Humours, temperaments of, 62
Huolitueh huahu, 267
Hydrotherapy, 117, 119–121, 167, 241, 245
Hypnosis, 35, 128–133
  current status, 132
  induction, 131
  limitations and dangers, 132
  selection and preparation of subjects, 131
  termination, 132
  terminology, 129
  therapeutic procedures, 131
  uses, 129

Hypnotherapy, 129

Iatrogenic illness, 122
IMEPLAM, *see* Mexican Institute for the Study of Medicinal Plants
Imhotep, 103
Incantations, 26, 33, 35, 264
India, 233, 242, 302–303
  Acorus calamus, 177
  Ayurvedic medicine, 50
  childbirth, 150
  colour therapy, 165
  herbal medicine, 180–181, 326
  homoeopathic colleges, 115
  iris diagnosis, 119
  legislation, 302–304, 312
  manpower planning, 284
  naturopathy, 121
  policy support, 282, 283
  Rauvolfia serpentina, 178–179
  Siddha system, 58, 303
  traditional birth attendants, 310
  traditional medicine, 236, 237, 242
  traditional practitioners, 237, 321
Indonesia, 145, 158, 233, 234, 238
Infertility, 157
Information systems, 217
  see also NAPRALERT data base
Insanity, 33, 34, 36, 178
  see also Mental health, Psychiatry
Institute of Nutrition of Central America and Panama, Guatemala (INCAP), 227
Integrated systems, 292, 306–308, 315
Internal Classic, 69, 70
International Conference on Asian Medicine, Canberra, 288
International Conference on Primary Health Care, Alma-Ata, 232
International cooperation, 214–216
Ionian medicine, *see* Unani medicine
Iran, 256, 257, 260
Iraq, 257
Iris diagnosis, 119
Israel, 120
Italy, 125, 241, 242, 244, 245
Ivory Coast, 218

Japan, 165, 169, 268, 270, 326
Judaism, 104

Kalia, 26
Kampo medicine, 270
Kenya, 218, 221, 311
Khellin, 260
Kiribati, 276-277, 300
Kleinman, Arthur, 315
Koran, 126-127
Korea, *see* Democratic People's Republic of Korea, Republic of Korea
Kwalwa, 31
Kundalini, 137, 139, 140
Kwashiorkor, 105-106

Lao People's Democratic Republic, 268
Latin America, 37-49, 103, 309, 319, 326
 basic concepts of traditional medicine, 38-39, 146
 herbal medicines, 319
 home deliveries, 223
 "hot" and "cold", 38-42, 44
 humoral theory, 37
 illness due to cold air, 22, 24
 legislation, 295, 298
 medicinal plants, 44-46, 326
 primary health care, 319
 research, 45-46
 spiritism, 46
 traditional birth attendants, 309
  training of, 224
 traditional midwives, 225
 training courses, 224
Lay health practitioner, 296
Lebanon, 310
Leeches, 246
Legislation, 29, 290-317
Leslie, Charles, 303
Lesotho, 300, 310
Liberia, 219
Light baths, 165
Luxembourg, 293

Madagascar, 176, 219, 221
Magic, 20, 241, 275
 in birth control, 157
Magicians, 272
Malawi, 311
Malaysia, 58, 264, 268, 269, 272-274, 299, 310

Maldives, 233, 234, 238
Mali, 26, 212, 219, 298
Manibuog, 277
Manipulation, 88, 264, 266
Manpower planning, 284-285
Massage, 35, 41, 70, 225, 245, 264, 266, 277
Mauritius, 221
Mayas, 145, 155
Medical anthropology, 222, 228
Medical astrology, *see* Astrology
Medical systems, fourfold typology as regards legislation, 315
 history of, 17
 similarities in, 18
 stereotypes, 22
Medicinal plants, *see* Herbal medicine and herbal remedies
Medicine of self, 122
Médicos, 42, 272
Meditation, 136, 138-140, 170
Mental health, 30-36, 125, 126, 136-137, 140, 184, 228, 255, 257, 277, 278, 287
Mexican Institute for the Study of Medicinal Plants, 159, 228
Mexican National Indian Institute, 23
Mexico, births, presence of husbands, 151
 charismatic healers, 23
 family planning programme, 158
 homoeopathic colleges, 115
 "hot" and "cold", 44
 medical anthropology, 222, 227
 sweat baths, 155
 traditional birth attendants, 224, 310
Middle East, 295, 309, 310
Midwifery, *see* Traditional midwifery
Mineral water, 245
Molecular therapy, 201-202
Mongolia, 294
Monodiet, 121
Moxibustion, 69, 70, 74, 76, 78-79
 basic theory, 79-80
 indication for, 79
 methods of application, 79
 procedure, 78
 standardization of technique, 267
 use in therapy, 78
Mozambique, 219
Mud, 245-246

Musicotherapy, 35, 43
Mysticism, 277

NAPRALERT data base, 85, 184–193
  applications in traditional medicine, 189–190
  compound record, 187–188
  current status of access, 191
  data retrieval, 190
  demographic record, 189
  description of, 185
  future plans, 191–193
  major data fields, 186
  organism record, 186
  pharmacology record, 188–189
  sources of information, 186
  work types, 187
National Institute of Natural Medicine, Aymara and Inca Culture, Bolivia, 46
National Institute for Research on the Traditional Pharmacopoeia and Traditional Medicine, Mali, 298
National Institute of Vietnamese Traditional Medicine, 269
Natural therapeutics, 300
Naturopathy, 19, 116–123, 166, 236, 237, 292
Negative-ion therapy, 168
Nepal, 50, 178, 233, 234, 238, 307–308, 316, 321
Netherlands, 297
Newborn, treatment of, 154
New Zealand, 119, 310
Nigella sativa, 260
Niger, 219
Nigeria, 150, 156, 157, 219, 221, 312
Norway, 246, 247

Occult powers, 33
Oceania, 19
Oman, 256
Organizational aspects, 281–289
Organization of African Unity (OAU), 30, 215
Osteopathy, 90, 119, 245, 246, 247, 292, 297, 310–311

Pakistan, 242
  Autonomous Board for Tibb and Homoeopathy, 255
  Ayurvedic medicine, 50
  legislation, 303
  medicinal plants, 260
  recognition of traditional systems, 302
  registration of traditional manpower resources, 258
  research, 256, 260
  traditional birth attendants, 257
  training, 259
  Unani, Ayurvedic and Homoeopathic Practitioners Act 1965, 303
  Unani medicine, 282
Pan American Health Organization (PAHO), 222–223, 226, 227
Pan American Sanitary Conference 1978, technical discussions, 227
Panama, 310
Panax spp., 176–178
Paphiopedilum druryi, 180
Papua New Guinea, 274–276
Paranormal phenomena, 124
Patanjali, 134, 135
Personalistic systems, 19, 20
Peru, 225
Pharmacopoeias, African traditional, 29
  allopathic medicine, 95–96
  Ayurvedic, 55
  Bolivian, 42
  Chinese, 326
  Indian, 326
  medicinal plants, 199, 216, 259
  Unani Tibb, 64
Philippines, 156, 270–272, 310
Physical postures, 135
Phytopharmacology, 194–206
  see also Herbal medicine and herbal remedies
Phytotherapy, 27, 194–206
  new-style, 199, 202
  research, 202
  see also Herbal medicine and herbal remedies
Placenta, 153–154
Plants, classification, 44
  endangered species, 175–183
  see also Herbal medicine and herbal remedies; NAPRALERT data base
Poland, 245–246

Policy options for regulating practice, 314–317
Pregnancy, 142, 144–146, 150, 228
  see also Traditional midwifery
Prenatal care, 149–150
Preventive medicine, 21, 27, 62, 92, 102
  see also Public health
Pribram-Bohm theory, 164
Priest curers, 23
Primary health care, 108–109, 198–206, 213, 281, 283, 285–288, 312, 318–327
Primary Health Training for Indigenous Healers (PRHETIH) Programme, Ghana, 322
Psychiatrist, traditional, 31, 34–35
Psychiatry, traditional, 30–36, 228, 255, 287
  in Africa, traditional, 33–36
Psychosomatic disorders, 11, 136
Psychosomatic medicine, 164
Psychotherapy, 34, 125, 126, 184, 255, 257, 277, 278, 287
Psychotropic drugs, 36, 125
Public health, 92, 102–109
  combined approaches to problems of, 104–107
  development, 102
  history, 102–104
  links with tradition, 104
  scope of, 102–103
  see also Preventive medicine

Qi, 265

Radionics, 168–169
Rauvolfia serpentina, 100, 178–179
Read, Margaret, 106
Reflexology, 169
Relaxation, 164
Remuneration, 29, 35, 64
Republic of Korea, 178, 268, 269–270
Research, acupuncture, 82–85, 287
  Africa, 214, 287
  agrobotanical, 199
  allopathic medicine, 98–99
  Ayurvedic system, 235, 287
  Bandaranaike Ayurvedic Research Institute, Sri Lanka, 238
  birth customs, 157–158
  Chinese system, 72
  coordination, 204, 206
  ethnopharmacognostic, 199
  medicinal plants, 65–66, 159, 260, 267–268, 271
    applied scientific, 202–206
    goal-oriented scientific, 198–202
    molecular therapy, 201–202
  traditional medical practice, 232, 234–235, 259–260, 286–287, 322
  traditional midwifery, 158
  Unani system, 65–66
  WHO's role, 260–261
  Yoga, 287
Rhode Island, 308
Richards, Guyon, 168
Rig Veda, 50
Roga pariksha, 53
Rogi pariksha, 52
Romania, 241, 245, 246
Rwanda, 219

Saussurea lappa, 179, 180
Scandinavia, 297
Schroth's cure, 121
Schulz, J. H., 129, 163
Scientific method, application, 11
Self-care, 62, 93, 164, 165, 167, 169, 170, 249–250
Self-healing, 163, 164, 166
Senegal, 219
Sense organs control, 135
Seychelles, 221
Shamana therapy, 53, 54
Shamans, 23
Shiatsu, 169
Shodana therapy, 53
Siberia, 19
Siddha system, 58, 236, 237, 238, 273, 302, 303
Sierra Leone, 299
Singapore, 58, 268
Smallpox, 104–105
Soft tissue injuries, diagnosis and therapy, China, 88–89
Somalia, 256, 257, 260
Sorcery, 275, 276
Soul substance, 273, 275
South Africa, 300
South America, 295
South Asia, 19, 301, 302

South-East Asia, 155, 231–239, 283, 284
  drug policies, 232
  future efforts, 239
  intercountry consultative meeting, 233
  Region of WHO, 231–239, 283–284
  research, 234–235
  status and functioning of traditional medicine, 236–239
  training and research, 232
South Pacific, 274–278
Spas, 120, 167, 245
Spirits and spiritism, 23, 41, 42, 46–47, 225, 226, 229, 273, 277
Sri Lanka, Ayurvedic medicine, 50, 304
  homoeopathy, 304
  Indigenous Medicine Ordinance, 302
  Rauvolfia serpentina, 178
  recognition of traditional systems, 302
  research, 238
  Siddha system, 58
  traditional medicine studies, 233, 234
  traditional practitioners, 320
  Unani medicine, 238
Steiner, Rudolph, 163, 248
Sudan, 256, 258, 260
Suffism, 140
Supernatural elements, 20–21
Swaziland, 300, 310
Sweat baths, 22
Sweden, 247
Switzerland, 163, 240, 244, 245, 246, 247, 248
  anthroposophical medicine, 163, 248
  chiropractic, 246, 247
  cupping and bleeding, 246
  ethnology, 240
  healing practitioners, 244
  medicinal springs, 245
  plant drug producers, 244
  teaching traditional medicine, 240

T'ai chi, 164, 170
Tanzania, *see* United Republic of Tanzania
Taoism, 104
Tetanus neonatorum, 154

Thaad, 236
Thailand, community-based family planning, 286
  pharmacopoeias, 306
  Rauvolfia serpentina, 179
  traditional birth attendants, 310
  traditional medicine institutions, 233
  traditional medicine studies, 233, 234
  traditional practitioners, 239
  traditional systems, 302, 306
Tibb, *see* Unani medicine
Tibetan system of medicine, 236, 237
Togo, 219, 221
Traditional birth attendant (TBA), Africa, 309
  Asia, 309
  Cuba, 226
  definition, 142–143
  Hilots, 271
  integration, 310
  Latin America, 223, 309
  legislation, 309–310
  manpower resources, 258
  registration, 309
  statistical data, 257
  training, 225, 258–259, 310, 321–322
  training guide, 223
  see also Traditional midwifery
Traditional healers, *see* Healers and healing
Traditional midwifery, 142–162, 228, 321
  coordination with official health system, 159–160
  cross-cultural reviews, 158
  in Ecuador, 225
  in Guatemala, 226
  recruitment and training, 148–149
  research, 157–159
  taboos, 145, 150
  training, 143, 148, 159, 160, 225
Traditional practitioners, 27, 212, 236, 237, 239, 259, 284, 320–322
Traditional psychiatry, *see* Psychiatry
Traditional rites, 22
Training, acupuncture, 83–84
  Africa, 213, 216, 322
  autogenic, 129, 163–164, 167
  Ayurvedic practitioners, 56

barefoot doctors, 84
Callawaya, 42
Chinese medicine, 72, 73, 258, 269
herbalists, 44
homoeopathy, 115
primary health care and public health, 213, 233
Primary Health Training for Indigenous Healers (PRHETIH) Programme, Ghana, 322–324
spiritism, 47
traditional birth attendants, 223, 224, 225, 258–259
traditional medicine, 258–259, 269
traditional midwives, 143, 148, 159–160, 225
traditional practitioners, 233, 259
Unani practitioners, 64, 237
WHO Regional Committee for South-East Asia Resolution, 232
Tunisia, 310

Uganda, 219, 299, 311
Umbanda, 47
Umbilical cord, 153–154
Unani medicine, 20, 61–67, 236, 237, 238, 242, 273, 282, 297, 302, 303, 320, 326
basic concepts and philosophy, 61–63
consultation, 63
control of practice, 303
diagnosis, 63
drug provision, 303
foods, "hot" or "cold", 22
formalized system, 236, 292
healer–patient relationship, 63
history, 17, 253
integration, 66–67
materia medica, 180
pharmacopoeia, 64
practitioners, 63–65
prescriptions, 63
preventive medicine, 62
Rauvolfia serpentina, 178
remuneration, 64
research, 65–66
training, 237, 320
temperament, 62
UNIDO, *see* United Nations Industrial Development Organization

Union of Soviet Socialist Republics (USSR), 168, 241, 242, 245, 248, 243–294
United Arab Emirates, 257
United Kingdom, acupuncture, 241, 242
anthroposophical medicine, 248
flower remedies, 165, 244
chiropractic, 246, 247, 310
healing and healers, 248–249
herbalism, 244
homoeopathy, 247–248
hydrotherapy, 167
legislation, 296, 297
negative ion therapy, 168
osteopathy, 246–247
radionics, 169
reflexology, 169
traditional medicine, 240–241
Unani system, 242
United Nations, 204, 283, 288
United Nations Children's Fund (UNICEF), 160, 204
United Nations Development programme (UNDP), 213, 215, 234, 268, 288
United Nations Educational, Scientific and Cultural Organization (UNESCO), 204
United Nations Industrial Development Organization (UNIDO), 204, 206
United Republic of Cameroon, 220, 221
United Republic of Tanzania, 218, 311
United States of America, acupuncture, 81, 298, 308
allopathic medicine, 95
American Indian cultures, 224
autogenic training, 163
biofeedback, 165
chiropractic, 310
Gerson's treatment, 166
legislation, 293, 298, 308
medical anthropology, 222
negative ion therapy, 168
osteopathy, 310
pharmacopoeia, 95
pregnancy, 144
radionics, 168
reflexology, 169
traditional healers, 224
zone therapy, 169

Upper Volta, 218, 299

Vaccination, 22, 104
Variolation, 104
Veblen, Thorsten, 314
Veda, 50, 90, 134, 178
Vegan diet, 121
Vegetarianism, 121, 122
Viet Nam, 268, 269
Visual education, Bates' technique, 164
Vogt, Oskar, 163

Water treatment, 120, 245
Western Pacific Region of WHO, 263–278
Williams, Cicely, 106
Witchcraft, 22, 157, 273, 305, 311–312
Witch-doctors, 175
Witch-finders, 20
World Health Organization (WHO),
  African Region, 209–221
  Americas, Region of the, 222–230
  areas of action, 283
  cooperation in phytotherapy training, 204
  Eastern Mediterranean Region, 253–262
  European Region, 240–252
  Interregional Consultation on Promotion and Development of Traditional Medicine Programmes, New Delhi, 227
  medical plants inventory, 206
  policy on traditional medicine, 278, 282, 288

primary health care, 108, 213, 312, 322
research, 30, 260, 261, 267
South-East Asia Region, 231–239, 283–284
Special Programme for Research, Development and Research Training in Human Reproduction, 185–186, 190
traditional birth attendants survey, 309–310
traditional medicine programme, 100, 312
Western Pacific Region, 263–278
Wuxing, 265

Yaqona, 277
Yellow Emperor's Internal Classic, 69
Yemen, Democratic, 294
Yin-yang, 19, 69, 71, 77, 79, 144, 265, 267
Yoga, 104, 134–138, 164, 236, 237, 286
  as rehabilitative measure, 138
  integrated, 135
  Kundalini, 137
Yorubas, 46–47, 157
Yugoslavia, 245

Zaire, 220, 221, 311
Zambia, 149, 221
Zar, 257
Zen meditation, 140
Zone therapy, 169

WHO publications may be obtained, direct or through booksellers, from:

ALGERIA: Entreprise nationale du Livre (ENAL), 3 bd Zirout Youcef, ALGIERS

ARGENTINA: Carlos Hirsch, SRL, Florida 165, Galerías Güemes, Escritorio 453/465, BUENOS AIRES

AUSTRALIA: Hunter Publications, 58A Gipps Street, COLLINGWOOD, VIC 3066.

AUSTRIA: Gerold & Co., Graben 31, 1011 VIENNA I

BAHRAIN: United Schools International, Arab Region Office, P.O. Box 726, BAHRAIN

BANGLADESH: The WHO Representative, G.P.O. Box 250, DHAKA 5

BELGIUM: *For books:* Office International de Librairie s.a., avenue Marnix 30, 1050 BRUSSELS. *For periodicals and subscriptions:* Office International des Périodiques, avenue Louise 485, 1050 BRUSSELS.

BHUTAN: *see* India, WHO Regional Office

BOTSWANA: Botsalo Books (Pty) Ltd., P.O. Box 1532, GABORONE

BRAZIL: Centro Latinoamericano de Informação em Ciencias de Saúde (BIREME), Organização Panamericana de Saúde, Sector de Publicações, C.P. 20381 - Rua Botucatu 862, 04023 SÃO PAULO, SP

BURMA: *see* India, WHO Regional Office

CAMEROON: Cameroon Book Centre, P.O. Box 123, South West Province, VICTORIA

CANADA: Canadian Public Health Association, 1335 Carling Avenue, Suite 210, OTTAWA, Ont. K1Z 8N8. (Tel: (613) 725–3769. Telex: 21–053–3841)

CHINA: China National Publications Import & Export Corporation, P.O. Box 88, BEIJING (PEKING)

DEMOCRATIC PEOPLE'S REPUBLIC OF KOREA: *see* India, WHO Regional Office

DENMARK: Munksgaard Export and Subscription Service, Nørre Søgade 35, 1370 COPENHAGEN K (Tel: + 45 1 12 85 70)

FIJI: The WHO Representative, P.O. Box 113, SUVA

FINLAND: Akateeminen Kirjakauppa, Keskuskatu 2, 00101 HELSINKI 10

FRANCE: Arnette, 2 rue Casimir-Delavigne, 75006 PARIS

GERMAN DEMOCRATIC REPUBLIC: Buchhaus Leipzig, Postfach 140, 701 LEIPZIG

GERMANY FEDERAL REPUBLIC OF: Govi-Verlag GmbH, Ginnheimerstrasse 20, Postfach 5360, 6236 ESCHBORN — Buchhandlung Alexander Horn, Kirchgasse 22, Postfach 3340, 6200 WIESBADEN

GREECE: G.C. Eleftheroudakis S.A., Librairie internationale, rue Nikis 4, 105-63 ATHENS

HONG KONG: Hong Kong Government Information Services, Publication (Sales) Office, Information Services Department, No. 1, Battery Path, Central, HONG KONG.

HUNGARY: Kultura, P.O.B. 149, BUDAPEST 62

ICELAND: Snaebjorn Jonsson & Co., Hafnarstraeti 9, P.O. Box 1131, IS-101 REYKJAVIK

INDIA: WHO Regional Office for South-East Asia, World Health House, Indraprastha Estate, Mahatma Gandhi Road, NEW DELHI 110002

IRAN (ISLAMIC REPUBLIC OF): Iran University Press, 85 Park Avenue, P.O. Box 54/551, TEHERAN

IRELAND: TDC Publishers, 12 North Frederick Street, DUBLIN 1 (Tel: 744835–749677)

ISRAEL: Heiliger & Co., 3 Nathan Strauss Street, JERUSALEM 94227

ITALY: Edizioni Minerva Medica, Corso Bramante 83–85, 10126 TURIN; Via Lamarmora 3, 20100 MILAN; Via Spallanzani 9, 00161 ROME

JAPAN: Maruzen Co. Ltd., P.O. Box 5050, TOKYO International, 100–31

JORDAN: Jordan Book Centre Co. Ltd., University Street, P.O. Box 301 (Al-Jubeiha), AMMAN

KENYA: Text Book Centre Ltd, P.O. Box 47540, NAIROBI

KUWAIT: The Kuwait Bookshops Co. Ltd., Thunayan Al-Ghanem Bldg, P.O. Box 2942, KUWAIT

LAO PEOPLE'S DEMOCRATIC REPUBLIC: The WHO Representative, P.O. Box 343, VIENTIANE

LUXEMBOURG: Librairie du Centre, 49 bd Royal, LUXEMBOURG

A/1/88

WHO publications may be obtained, direct or through booksellers, from:

MALAYSIA: The WHO Representative, Room 1004, 10th Floor, Wisma Lim Foo Yong (formerly Fitzpatrick's Building), Jalan Raja Chulan, KUALA LUMPUR 05–10; P.O. Box 2550, KUALA LUMPUR 01–02; Parry's Book Center, 124–1 Jalan Tun Sambanthan, P.O. Box 10960, 50730 KUALA LUMPUR

MALDIVES: *See* India, WHO Regional Office

MEXICO: Librería Interacademica S.A., Av. Sonora 206, 06100-MÉXICO, D.F.

MONGOLIA: *see* India, WHO Regional Office

MOROCCO: Editions La Porte, 281 avenue Mohammed V, RABAT

NEPAL: *see* India, WHO Regional Office

NETHERLANDS: Medical Books Europe BV, Noorderwal 38, 7241 BL LOCHEM

NEW ZEALAND: New Zealand Government Printing Office, Publishing Administration, Private Bag, WELLINGTON; Walter Street, WELLINGTON; World Trade Building, Cubacade, Cuba Street, WELLINGTON, *Government Bookshops at:* Hannaford Burton Building, Rutland Street, Private Bag, AUCKLAND; 159 Hereford Street, Private Bag, CHRISTCHURCH; Alexandra Street, P.O. Box 857, HAMILTON; T & G Building, Princes Street, P.O. Box 1104, DUNEDIN — R. Hill & Son Ltd, Ideal House, Cnr Gillies Avenue & Eden Street, Newmarket, AUCKLAND 1

NORWAY: Tanum — Karl Johan A.S., P.O. Box 1177, Sentrum, N-0107 OSLO 1

PAKISTAN: Mirza Book Agency, 65 Shahrah–E–Quaid–E–Azam, P.O. Box 729, LAHORE 3

PAPUA NEW GUINEA: The WHO Representative, P.O. Box 646, KONEDOBU

PHILIPPINES: World Health Organization, Regional Office for the Western Pacific, P.O. Box 2932, MANILA; National Book Store Inc., 701 Rizal Avenue, P.O. Box 1934, MANILA

PORTUGAL: Livraria Rodrigues, 186 Rua do Ouro, LISBON 2

REPUBLIC OF KOREA: The WHO Representative, Central P.O. Box 540, SEOUL

SAUDI ARABIA: World of Knowledge for Publishing and Distribution, P.O. Box 576, JEDDAH

SINGAPORE: The WHO Representative, 144 Moulmein Road, SINGAPORE 1130; Newton P.O. Box 31, SINGAPORE 9122

SOUTH AFRICA: *Contact major book stores*

SPAIN: Comercial Atheneum S.A., Consejo de Ciento 130–136, 08015 BARCELONA; General Moscardó 29, MADRID 20 — Librería Díaz de Santos, P.O. Box 6050, 28006 MADRID; Balmes 417 y 419, 08022 BARCELONA

SRI LANKA: *see* India, WHO Regional Office

SWEDEN: *For books:* Aktiebolaget C.E. Fritzes Kungl. Hovbokhandel, Regeringsgatan 12, 103 27 STOCKHOLM. *For periodicals:* Wennergren-Williams AB, Box 30004, 104 25 STOCKHOLM

SWITZERLAND: Medizinischer Verlag Hans Huber, Länggassstrasse 76, 3012 BERN 9

THAILAND: *see* India, WHO Regional Office

UNITED KINGDOM: H.M. Stationery Office: 49 High Holborn, LONDON WC1V 6HB; 71 Lothian Road, EDINBURGH EH3 9AZ, 80 Chichester Street, BELFAST BT1 4JY; Brazennose Street, MANCHESTER M60 8AS; 258 Broad Street, BIRMINGHAM B1 2HE; Southey House, Wine Street, BRISTOL BS1 2BQ. *All mail orders should be sent to:* HMSO Publications Centre, 51 Nine Elms Lane, LONDON SW8 5DR

UNITED STATES OF AMERICA: *Copies of individual publications (not subscriptions):* WHO Publications Center USA, 49 Sheridan Avenue, ALBANY, NY 12210. *Subscription orders and correspondence concerning subscriptions should be addressed to the* World Health Organization, Distribution and Sales, 1211 GENEVA 27, Switzerland. *Publications are also available from the* United Nations Bookshop, NEW YORK, NY 10017 (*retail only*)

USSR: *For readers in the USSR requiring Russian editions:* Komsomolskij prospekt 18, Medicinskaja Kniga, MOSCOW — *For readers outside the USSR requiring Russian editions:* Kuzneckij most 18, Meždunarodnaja Kniga, MOSCOW G-200

VENEZUELA: Librería Medica Paris, Apartado 60.681, CARACAS 106

YUGOSLAVIA: Jugoslovenska Knjiga, Terazije 27/II, 11000 BELGRADE

ZIMBABWE: Textbook Sales (PVT) Ltd, 1 Norwich Union Centre, MUTARE

Special terms for developing countries are obtainable on application to the WHO Representatives or WHO Regional Offices listed above or to the World Health Organization, Distribution and Sales Service, 1211 Geneva 27, Switzerland. Orders from countries where sales agents have not yet been appointed may also be sent to the Geneva address, but must be paid for in pounds sterling, US dollars, or Swiss francs. Unesco book coupons may also be used.

Prices are subject to change without notice.